Acute Respiratory Distress Syndrome

Editors

LORRAINE B. WARE
JULIE A. BASTARACHE
CAROLYN S. CALFEE

CLINICS IN CHEST MEDICINE

www.chestmed.theclinics.com

December 2014 • Volume 35 • Number 4

ELSEVIER

1600 John F. Kennedy Boulevard • Suite 1800 • Philadelphia, Pennsylvania, 19103-2899

http://www.theclinics.com

CLINICS IN CHEST MEDICINE Volume 35, Number 4
December 2014 ISSN 0272-5231, ISBN-13: 978-0-323-32642-1

Editor: Patrick Manley
Developmental Editor: Casey Jackson

Clinics in Chest Medicine (ISSN 0272-5231) is published quarterly by Elsevier Inc., 360 Park Avenue South, New York, NY 10010-1710. Months of issue are March, June, September, and December. Periodicals postage paid at New York, NY and additional mailing offices. Subscription prices are $345.00 per year (domestic individuals), $556.00 per year (domestic institutions), $165.00 per year (domestic students/residents), $380.00 per year (Canadian individuals), $690.00 per year (Canadian institutions), $470.00 per year (international individuals), $690.00 per year (international institutions), and $230.00 per year (international and Canadian students/residents). International air speed delivery is included in all Clinics subscription prices. All prices are subject to change without notice. **POSTMASTER:** Send address changes to Clinics in Chest Medicine, Elsevier Health Sciences Division, Subscription Customer Service, 3251 Riverport Lane, Maryland Heights, MO 63043. **Customer Service: Telephone: 1-800-654-2452** (U.S. and Canada); **1-314-447-8871** (outside U.S. and Canada). **Fax: 1-314-447-8029. E-mail: journalscustomerservice-usa@elsevier.com (for print support); journalsonlinesupport-usa@elsevier.com (for online support).**

Reprints. For copies of 100 or more of articles in this publication, please contact the Commercial Reprints Department, Elsevier Inc., 360 Park Avenue South, New York, NY 10010-1710. Tel.: 212-633-3874; Fax: 212-633-3820; E-mail: reprints@elsevier.com.

Clinics in Chest Medicine is covered in *MEDLINE/PubMed (Index Medicus), Current Contents/Clinical Medicine, EMBASE/ Excerpta Medica, Science Citation Index,* and *ISI/BIOMED.*

Contributors

EDITORS

LORRAINE B. WARE, MD
Professor of Medicine; Director, Vanderbilt
Medical Scholars Program, Division of Allergy,
Pulmonary, and Critical Care Medicine,
Department of Medicine, Vanderbilt University
School of Medicine, Nashville, Tennessee

JULIE A. BASTARACHE, MD
Assistant Professor of Medicine, Division of
Allergy, Pulmonary, and Critical Care Medicine,
Department of Medicine, Vanderbilt University
School of Medicine, Nashville, Tennessee

CAROLYN S. CALFEE, MD, MAS
Associate Professor, Departments of Medicine
and Anesthesia, University of California San
Francisco, San Francisco, California

AUTHORS

DARRYL ABRAMS, MD
Assistant Professor of Medicine, Division of
Pulmonary, Allergy and Critical Care, Columbia
University College of Physicians and Surgeons,
New York, New York

RICHARD K. ALBERT, MD
Professor of Medicine, University of Colorado,
Aurora, Colorado; Chief of Medicine,
Department of Medicine, Denver Health,
Denver, Colorado

ALEJANDRO C. ARROLIGA, MD, FCCP
Chairman and Professor of Medicine, Dr. A.
Ford Wolf and Brooksie Nell Boyd Wolf
Centennial Chair of Medicine, Baylor Scott &
White Health, Texas A&M College of Medicine,
Temple, Texas

JULIE A. BASTARACHE, MD
Assistant Professor of Medicine, Division of
Allergy, Pulmonary, and Critical Care
Medicine, Department of Medicine, Vanderbilt
University School of Medicine, Nashville,
Tennessee

JANE BATT, MD, FRCPC, PhD
Department of Medicine, Institute of Medical
Sciences, Keenan Centre for Biomedical
Science, Li Ka Shing Knowledge Institute,
St. Michael's Hospital, University of Toronto,
Toronto, Ontario, Canada

ALEXANDER B. BENSON, MD
Assistant Professor of Medicine, University
of Colorado, Aurora, Colorado; Department
of Medicine, Denver Health, Denver,
Colorado

DANIEL BRODIE, MD
Associate Professor of Medicine, Division of
Pulmonary, Allergy and Critical Care, Columbia
University College of Physicians and Surgeons,
New York, New York

CAROLYN S. CALFEE, MD, MAS
Associate Professor, Departments of
Medicine and Anesthesia, University of
California San Francisco, San Francisco,
California

**GERARD F. CURLEY, MSc, MB, PhD,
FCARCSI**
Assistant Professor, Department of
Anesthesia, Keenan Research Centre for
Biomedical Science, Li Ka Shing Knowledge
Institute, St. Michael's Hospital, University of
Toronto, Toronto, Ontario, Canada

STÉPHANIE DIZIER, MD
Assistance Publique, Hôpitaux de Marseille, Medical Intensive Care Unit APHM, CHU Nord, Marseille, France

CLAUDIA C. DOS SANTOS, MD, FRCPC, MSc
Assistant Professor, Department of Medicine, Institute of Medical Sciences, Keenan Centre for Biomedical Science, Li Ka Shing Knowledge Institute, St. Michael's Hospital, University of Toronto, Toronto, Ontario, Canada

EDDY FAN, MD, PhD
Assistant Professor, Interdepartmental Division of Critical Care Medicine, University of Toronto, Toronto, Ontario, Canada

SHEKHAR A. GHAMANDE, MD, FCCP
Associate Professor of Medicine; Fellowship Director, Pulmonary, Critical Care and Sleep Medicine, Baylor Scott & White Health, Texas A&M College of Medicine, Temple, Texas

JEFFREY E. GOTTS, MD, PhD
Assistant Clinical Professor of Pulmonary & Critical Care Medicine, Departments of Medicine and Anesthesia, Cardiovascular Research Institute, University of California, San Francisco, San Francisco, California

RAY GUO, MD
Fellow, Interdepartmental Division of Critical Care Medicine, University of Toronto, Toronto, Ontario, Canada

MARGARET S. HERRIDGE, MD, FRCPC, MPH
Interdepartmental Division of Critical Care, University of Toronto, Toronto, Ontario, Canada

CATHERINE L. HOUGH, MD, MSc
Associate Professor of Medicine, Division of Pulmonary and Critical Care Medicine, Harborview Medical Center, University of Washington, Seattle, Washington

SAMI HRAIECH, MD
Assistance Publique, Hôpitaux de Marseille, Medical Intensive Care Unit APHM, CHU Nord; Faculté de Médecine, University of Aix-Marseilles, Marseille, France

DAVID R. JANZ, MD, MSc
Section of Pulmonary and Critical Care Medicine, Department of Medicine, LSU School of Medicine, New Orleans, Louisiana

JOSEPH E. LEVITT, MD, MS
Assistant Professor, Division of Pulmonary and Critical Care Medicine, Stanford University, Stanford, California

MICHAEL A. MATTHAY, MD
Professor of Pulmonary & Critical Care Medicine, Departments of Medicine and Anesthesia, Cardiovascular Research Institute, University of California, San Francisco, San Francisco, California

DANIEL F. McAULEY, MB, MD, MRCP
Professor, Intensive Care Medicine, Centre for Infection and Immunity, Queens University Belfast and Royal Victoria Hospital, Belfast, United Kingdom

NUALA J. MEYER, MD, MS
Assistant Professor of Medicine, Pulmonary, Allergy, and Critical Care Medicine, University of Pennsylvania, Perelman School of Medicine, Philadelphia, Pennsylvania

JOHN K. MIDTURI, DO, MPH
Associate Professor of Medicine; Director Infectious Disease Section, Baylor Scott & White Health, Texas A&M College of Medicine, Temple, Texas

FARZAD MOAZED, MD
Division of Pulmonary and Critical Care Medicine, Department of Medicine, University of California San Francisco, San Francisco, California

LAURENT PAPAZIAN, MD, PhD
Assistance Publique, Hôpitaux de Marseille, Medical Intensive Care Unit APHM, CHU Nord; Faculté de Médecine, University of Aix-Marseilles, Marseille, France

JUAN F. SANCHEZ, MD
Assistant Professor of Medicine, Pulmonary and Critical Care; Director Lung Transplantation and Interventional Pulmonology, Baylor Scott & White Health, Texas A&M College of Medicine, Temple, Texas

CIARA M. SHAVER, MD, PhD
Clinical Fellow, Division of Allergy, Pulmonary, and Critical Care Medicine, Department of Medicine, Vanderbilt University Medical Center, Nashville, Tennessee

RENEE D. STAPLETON, MD, PhD
Associate Professor of Medicine, Division of Pulmonary and Critical Care Medicine, Department of Medicine, University of Vermont, Burlington, Vermont

BENJAMIN T. SURATT, MD
Associate Chief, Division of Pulmonary and Critical Care Medicine; Associate Chair of Medicine for Academic Affairs; Associate Professor of Medicine and Cell & Molecular Biology, Department of Medicine, University of Vermont, Burlington, Vermont

ANDREW J. SWEATT, MD
Fellow, Division of Pulmonary and Critical Care Medicine, Stanford University, Stanford, California

CHRISTOPHER J. WALSH, MD, FRCPC
Department of Medicine, Institute of Medical Sciences, Keenan Centre for Biomedical Science, Li Ka Shing Knowledge Institute, St. Michael's Hospital, University of Toronto, Toronto, Ontario, Canada

LORRAINE B. WARE, MD
Professor of Medicine; Director, Vanderbilt Medical Scholars Program, Division of Allergy, Pulmonary, and Critical Care Medicine, Department of Medicine, Vanderbilt University School of Medicine, Nashville, Tennessee

Contents

This article reviews the evolving definitions and epidemiology of the acute respiratory distress syndrome (ARDS) and highlights current efforts to improve identification of high-risk patients, thus to target prevention and early treatment before progression to ARDS. This information will be important for general practitioners and intensivists interested in improving the care of patients at risk for ARDS, and clinical researchers interested in designing clinical trials targeting the prevention and early treatment of acute lung injury.

Acute respiratory distress syndrome (ARDS) remains a major cause of morbidity and mortality in critically ill patients. Over the past several decades, alcohol abuse and cigarette smoke exposure have been identified as risk factors for the development of ARDS. The mechanisms underlying these relationships are complex and remain under investigation but are thought to involve pulmonary immune impairment and alveolar epithelial and endothelial dysfunction. This review summarizes the epidemiologic data supporting links between these exposures and ARDS susceptibility and outcomes and highlights key mechanistic investigations that provide insight into the pathways by which each exposure is linked to ARDS.

The acute respiratory distress syndrome (ARDS) is a heterogeneous group of illnesses affecting the pulmonary parenchyma with acute onset bilateral inflammatory pulmonary infiltrates with associated hypoxemia. ARDS occurs after 2 major types of pulmonary injury: direct lung injury affecting the lung epithelium or indirect lung injury disrupting the vascular endothelium. Greater understanding of the differences between direct and indirect lung injury may refine the classification of patients with ARDS and lead to development of new therapeutics targeted at specific subpopulations of patients with ARDS.

This article discusses obesity, its contribution to clinical outcomes, and the current literature on nutrition. More than one third of Americans are obese. Literature suggests that, among critically ill patients, the relationship between obesity and outcomes is complex. Obese patients may be at greater risk of developing acute respiratory distress syndrome (ARDS) than normal weight patients. Although obesity may confer greater morbidity in intensive care, it seems to decrease mortality. ARDS is a catabolic state; patients demonstrate a profound inflammatory response, multiple organ dysfunction, and hypermetabolism, often with malnutrition. The concept of pharmaconutrition has emerged.

This article summarizes the contributions of high-throughput genomic, proteomic, metabolomic, and gene expression investigations to the understanding of inherited or acquired risk for acute respiratory distress syndrome (ARDS). Although not yet widely applied to a complex trait like ARDS, these techniques are now routinely used to study a variety of disease states. Omic applications hold great promise for identifying novel factors that may contribute to ARDS pathophysiology or may be appropriate for further development as biomarkers or surrogates in clinical studies. Opportunities and challenges of different techniques are discussed, and examples of successful applications in non-ARDS fields are used to illustrate the potential use of each technique.

Given the high incidence and mortality of acute respiratory distress syndrome (ARDS) in critically ill patients, every practitioner needs a bedside approach both for early identification of patients at risk for ARDS and for the appropriate evaluation of patients who meet the diagnostic criteria of ARDS. Recent advances such as the Lung Injury Prediction score, the Early Acute Lung Injury score, and validation of the SpO_2/Fio_2 ratio for assessing the degree of hypoxemia are all practical tools to aid the practitioner in caring for patients at risk of ARDS.

Immunosuppression predisposes the host to development of pulmonary infections, which can lead to respiratory failure and the development of acute respiratory distress syndrome (ARDS). There are multiple mechanisms by which a host can be immunosuppressed and each is associated with specific infectious pathogens. Early invasive diagnostic modalities such as fiber-optic bronchoscopy with bronchoalveolar lavage, transbronchial biopsy, and open lung biopsy are complementary to serologic and noninvasive studies and assist in rapidly establishing an accurate diagnosis, which allows initiation of appropriate therapy and may improve outcomes with relative safety.

Our ability to define appropriate molecular targets for preclinical development and develop better methods needs to be improved, to determine the clinical value of novel acute respiratory distress syndrome (ARDS) agents. Clinical trials must have realistic sample sizes and meaningful end points and use the available observation and meta-analytical data to inform design. Biomarker-driven studies or defined ARDS subsets should be considered to categorize specific at-risk populations most likely to benefit from a new treatment. Innovations in clinical trial design should be pursued to improve the outlook for future interventional trials in ARDS.

a consequence of extracorporeal technology with high risk and unclear benefit. However, advances in component technology, accumulating evidence, and growing experience in recent years have resulted in a resurgence of interest in ECMO. Extracorporeal support, though currently lacking high-level evidence, has the potential to improve outcomes, including survival, in ARDS. In the near future, novel extracorporeal management strategies may, in fact, lead to a new paradigm in the approach to certain patients with ARDS.

The development and severity of acute respiratory distress syndrome (ARDS) are closely related to dysregulated inflammation, and the duration of ARDS and eventual outcomes are related to persistent inflammation and abnormal fibroproliferation. Corticosteroids are potent modulators of inflammation and inhibitors of fibrosis that have been used since the first description of ARDS in attempts to improve outcomes. There is no evidence that corticosteroids prevent the development of ARDS among patients at risk. High-dose and short-course treatment with steroids does not improve the outcomes of patients with ARDS. Additional studies are needed to recommend treatment with steroids for ARDS.

Regenerative medicine has entered a rapid phase of discovery, and much has been learned in recent years about the lung's response to injury. This article first summarizes the cellular and molecular mechanisms that damage the alveolar-capillary barrier, producing acute respiratory distress syndrome (ARDS). The latest understanding of endogenous repair processes is discussed, highlighting the diversity of lung epithelial progenitor cell populations and their regulation in health and disease. Finally, the past, present, and future of exogenous cell-based therapies for ARDS is reviewed.

Survivors of acute respiratory distress syndrome often sustain muscle wasting and functional impairment related to intensive care unit (ICU)–acquired weakness (ICUAW) and this disability may persist for years after ICU discharge. Early diagnosis in cooperative patients by physical examination is recommended to identify patients at risk for weaning failure and to minimize prolongation of risk factors for ICUAW. When possible, early rehabilitation in critically ill patients improves functional outcomes, likely by reducing disuse atrophy. Interventions designed to correct the functional impairment are lacking and further research to delineate the molecular pathways that give rise to ICUAW are needed.

PROGRAM OBJECTIVE

The goal of the *Clinics in Chest Medicine* is to provide practitioners with state-of-the-art information that is clinically useful, concise, well referenced, and comprehensive.

TARGET AUDIENCE

All practicing physicians and healthcare professionals who provide patient care utilizing findings from *Chest Medicine Clinics of North America*.

LEARNING OBJECTIVES

Upon completion of this activity, participants will be able to:
1. Review the epidemiology and definitions of ARDS and early acute lung injury.
2. Discuss environmental risk factors for ARDS.
3. Recognize clinical and biological heterogeneity in ARDS.

ACCREDITATION

The Elsevier Office of Continuing Medical Education (EOCME) is accredited by the Accreditation Council for Continuing Medical Education (ACCME) to provide continuing medical education for physicians.

The EOCME designates this enduring material for a maximum of 15 *AMA PRA Category 1 Credit*(s)™. Physicians should claim only the credit commensurate with the extent of their participation in the activity.

All other health care professionals requesting continuing education credit for this enduring material will be issued a certificate of participation.

DISCLOSURE OF CONFLICTS OF INTEREST

The EOCME assesses conflict of interest with its instructors, faculty, planners, and other individuals who are in a position to control the content of CME activities. All relevant conflicts of interest that are identified are thoroughly vetted by EOCME for fair balance, scientific objectivity, and patient care recommendations. EOCME is committed to providing its learners with CME activities that promote improvements or quality in healthcare and not a specific proprietary business or a commercial interest.

The planning committee, staff, authors and editors listed below have identified no financial relationships or relationships to products or devices they or their spouse/life partner have with commercial interest related to the content of this CME activity:

Darryl Abrams, MD; Richard K. Albert, MD; Alejandro C. Arroliga, MD, FCCP; Julie A. Bastarache, MD; Jane Batt, MD, FRCPC, PhD; Alexander B. Benson, MD; Gerard F. Curley, MB, MCh, MSc, PhD; Stéphanie Dizier, MD; Claudia C. Dos Santos, MD, FRCPC, MSc; Eddy Fan, MD, PhD; Shekhar A. Ghamande, MD, FCCP; Jeffrey E. Gotts, MD, PhD; Ray Guo, MD; Kristen Holm; Margaret S. Herridge, MD, FRCPC, MPH; Catherine L. Hough, MD, MSc; Sami Hraiech, MD; Brynne Hunter; David R. Janz, MD; Sandy Lavery; Joseph E. Levitt, MD, MS; Patrick Manley; Michael A. Matthay, MD; Daniel F. McAuley, MB, MD, MRCP; Jill McNair; Nuala J. Meyer, MD, MS; John K. Midturi, DO, MPH; Farzad Moazed, MD; Palani Murugesan; Laurent Papazian, MD, PhD; Juan F. Sanchez, MD; Ciara M. Shaver, MD, PhD; Renee D. Stapleton, MD, PhD; Benjamin T. Suratt, MD; Andrew J. Sweatt, MD; Christopher J. Walsh, MD, FRCPC; Lorraine B. Ware, MD.

The planning committee, staff, authors and editors listed below have identified financial relationships or relationships to products or devices they or their spouse/life partner have with commercial interest related to the content of this CME activity:

Daniel Brodie, MD is a consultant/advisor for ALung Technologies, Inc.
Carolyn S. Calfee, MD, MAS has research grant from GlaxoSmithKline plc.

UNAPPROVED/OFF-LABEL USE DISCLOSURE

The EOCME requires CME faculty to disclose to the participants:
1. When products or procedures being discussed are off-label, unlabelled, experimental, and/or investigational (not US Food and Drug Administration [FDA] approved); and
2. Any limitations on the information presented, such as data that are preliminary or that represent ongoing research, interim analyses, and/or unsupported opinions. Faculty may discuss information about pharmaceutical agents that is outside of FDA-approved labelling. This information is intended solely for CME and is not intended to promote off-label use of these medications. If you have any questions, contact the medical affairs department of the manufacturer for the most recent prescribing information.

TO ENROLL

To enroll in the *Chest Medicine Clinics* Continuing Medical Education program, call customer service at 1-800-654-2452 or sign up online at http://www.theclinics.com/home/cme. The CME program is available to subscribers for an additional annual fee of USD $225.

METHOD OF PARTICIPATION

In order to claim credit, participants must complete the following:

1. Complete enrolment as indicated above.
2. Read the activity.
3. Complete the CME Test and Evaluation. Participants must achieve a score of 70% on the test. All CME Tests and Evaluations must be completed online.

CME INQUIRIES/SPECIAL NEEDS

For all CME inquiries or special needs, please contact elsevierCME@elsevier.com.

CLINICS IN CHEST MEDICINE

FORTHCOMING ISSUES

March 2015
Non-Tuberculosis Mycobacteria
Gwen A. Huitt and Charles Daley, *Editors*

June 2015
Chest Imaging
David Lynch and Jonathan Chung, *Editors*

September 2015
Critical Care
Shyoko Honiden and Jonathan Siner,
Editors

RECENT ISSUES

September 2014
**Sleep-Disordered Breathing: Beyond
Obstructive Sleep Apnea**
Carolyn M. D'Ambrosio, *Editor*

June 2014
**Pulmonary Rehabilitation: Role and
Advances**
Linda Nici and Richard L. ZuWallack, *Editors*

March 2014
Chronic Obstructive Pulmonary Disease
Peter J. Barnes, *Editor*

RELATED INTEREST

Critical Care Nursing Clinics, Vol. 24, No. 3 (September 2012)
The Lungs in a Mechanical Ventilator Environment
Meredith Mealer and Suzanne C. Lareau, *Editors*

Preface

ARDS: New Mechanistic Insights, New Therapeutic Directions

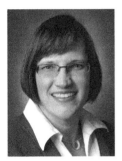

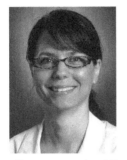

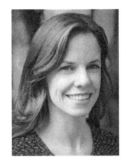

Lorraine B. Ware, MD   Julie A. Bastarache, MD   Carolyn S. Calfee, MD, MAS

Editors

Acute respiratory distress syndrome (ARDS) is a syndrome of acute respiratory failure due to lung inflammation and noncardiogenic pulmonary edema that is familiar to all intensivists regardless of whether they care for adults or children, care for medical or surgical patients, or practice in community or academic medical centers. Despite improvements in outcomes in the last two decades, ARDS remains a major public health problem that generates high health care expenditures and causes major morbidity and mortality. Furthermore, with the aging of the population, and the projected rise in incidence of sepsis, the most common risk factor for ARDS—cases of ARDS are likely to increase.

Since the last issue on ARDS was published in *Clinics in Chest Medicine* in 2006, there have been major advances in our understanding of emerging environmental risk factors for ARDS, such as tobacco smoke exposure; new insights into the clinical heterogeneity of ARDS, particularly with regard to direct versus indirect lung injury and a deeper appreciation for the impact of obesity, nutrition, and immune compromise on the diagnosis

and clinical course of ARDS. Modifications to the original American European Consensus Conference definitions of ARDS by the Berlin Committee have provided some additional clarity on timing of onset and the possibility of coexistent heart failure and ARDS. Although many large, high-profile clinical trials continue to have disappointing outcomes, such as recent trials of statins and high-frequency oscillatory ventilation, there is also encouraging progress on the therapeutic front with new data supporting a potential role for proning and neuromuscular paralysis in severe ARDS. In addition, novel clinical trial designs in ARDS may herald a new era of successful therapies. Finally, the impact of critical illness, including ARDS, on long-term outcomes, including muscle weakness and cognitive dysfunction, is increasingly recognized and studied as a potential modifiable outcome.

In addition to highlighting these advances, this issue provides practical advice for clinicians on the clinical approach to the patient with ARDS, and the unique issues surrounding the diagnostic approach to ARDS in the immunosuppressed. Continuing controversies, such as the role of

Clin Chest Med 35 (2014) xv–xvi
http://dx.doi.org/10.1016/j.ccm.2014.09.001

steroids in treating ARDS, are discussed, as are emerging therapies, such as mesenchymal stromal stem cells. We would like to thank the authors for their outstanding contributions and the editors and publishers for their invaluable assistance in putting together this issue.

Lorraine B. Ware, MD
Director, Vanderbilt Medical Scholars Program
Division of Allergy, Pulmonary, and
Critical Care Medicine
Department of Medicine
Vanderbilt University School of Medicine
T1218 Medical Center North, Nashville
TN 37232-2650, USA

Julie A. Bastarache, MD
Pulmonary and Critical Care Medicine
Vanderbilt University School of Medicine
T-1218 MCN, Nashville
TN 37232-2650, USA

Carolyn S. Calfee, MD, MAS
Departments of Medicine and Anesthesia
University of California, San Francisco
San Francisco, CA 94925, USA

E-mail addresses:
lorraine.ware@vanderbilt.edu (L.B. Ware)
julie.bastarache@Vanderbilt.edu (J.A.
Bastarache)
Carolyn.Calfee@ucsf.edu (C.S. Calfee)

Evolving Epidemiology and Definitions of the Acute Respiratory Distress Syndrome and Early Acute Lung Injury

Andrew J. Sweatt, MD, Joseph E. Levitt, MD, MS*

KEYWORDS

- Acute respiratory distress syndrome • ARDS • Acute lung injury • ALI • Epidemiology • Prevention
- Definition • Criteria

KEY POINTS

- Precise understanding of the epidemiology of the acute respiratory distress syndrome (ARDS) is limited by evolving clinical criteria and lack of an ideal reference standard.
- The recent Berlin Definition of ARDS addressed some limitations of prior definitions and empirically validated current criteria.
- As per the Berlin Definition, acute lung injury (ALI) is no longer a classification and ARDS severity is stratified as mild, moderate, and severe based on the Pao_2/Fio_2 ratio, and predicts mortality better than past definitions.
- The Lung Injury Prediction (LIPS) score and the Early Acute Lung Injury (EALI) score are novel criteria for identifying high-risk patients before progression to ARDS.

INTRODUCTION

Precise understanding of the epidemiology of the acute respiratory distress syndrome (ARDS) has been limited by evolution of the disease criteria over time and lack of an ideal reference standard. Defining ARDS by clinical and physiologic parameters provides feasibility in clinical practice, and has the advantage of conceptualizing the syndrome as a common final pathway of lung injury in response to a variety of inciting causes. However, eschewing pathologic correlation or other reference standards contributes to inclusion of heterogeneous patient populations with differing pathology and potentially very different prognoses. Also, defining a syndrome by criteria that are, in part, dependent on the institution of specific therapies may have significant implications for the epidemiology of the syndrome across countries and time periods because of differences in clinical practice patterns. This review discusses the evolving epidemiology and definition of ARDS, and recent efforts to improve recognition of patients at high risk of developing ARDS and enhance the prevention and early treatment of acute lung injury.

THE EVOLUTION OF ACUTE RESPIRATORY DISTRESS SYNDROME AND LIMITATIONS OF CONSENSUS CRITERIA

ARDS was first described in a series of 12 patients in 1967 by Ashbaugh and colleagues,[1] who recognized a common pattern of severe respiratory

Disclosures: The authors have no funding sources of conflicts of interest to disclose.
Division of Pulmonary and Critical Care Medicine, Stanford University, 300 Pasteur Drive, Stanford, CA 94305, USA
* Corresponding author.
E-mail address: jlevitt@stanford.edu

Clin Chest Med 35 (2014) 609–624
http://dx.doi.org/10.1016/j.ccm.2014.08.002
0272-5231/14/$ – see front matter © 2014 Elsevier Inc. All rights reserved.

distress, refractory cyanosis, loss of lung compliance, and diffuse alveolar infiltrates in a variety of clinical contexts including sepsis, pneumonia, aspiration, and major trauma. Similar syndromes of acute respiratory failure had been previously recognized, but only as distinct conditions named for their specific inciting etiology (eg, Da Nang lung, shock lung, posttraumatic lung, respirator lung). A better understanding of risk factors for ARDS emerged in the early 1980s, but proposed definitions of the syndrome lacked uniformity.[2,3]

In 1994, the American and European Consensus Conference (AECC) established specific clinical criteria for ARDS and acute lung injury (ALI), a novel classification defined by similar criteria but requiring less severe oxygenation impairment.[4] The AECC criteria defined ALI and ARDS as acute respiratory failure with bilateral pulmonary infiltrates on chest radiograph; a partial pressure of arterial oxygen (Pao_2)/fraction of inspired oxygen (Fio_2) ratio less than 300 for ALI and less than 200 for ARDS; and absence of clinical evidence of left atrial hypertension or a pulmonary artery occlusion pressure less than 18 mm Hg. The AECC criteria were subsequently widely adopted, providing uniformity for epidemiologic studies, multicenter clinical trials, and clinical practice guidelines.

Despite offering feasibility and standardization, several limitations of the AECC criteria still exist. First, the meaning of respiratory failure was not clearly defined. Most multicenter clinical trials have limited enrollment to patients receiving mechanical ventilation via an endotracheal tube. However, in the most rigorous epidemiologic study to date, respiratory failure was interpreted to include mechanical ventilation via a noninvasive face mask or endotracheal tube.[5] Other investigators have since expanded interpretation of the consensus criteria to include nonmechanically ventilated patients and those outside of the intensive care unit.[6–9] Whether respiratory failure is interpreted as requiring intubation and/or some level of positive pressure ventilation or purely by Pao_2/Fio_2 ratio and radiographic criteria has major implications for anticipated incidence and outcomes. A pediatric study of patients in the emergency department with acute hypoxic respiratory failure, defined as a Pao_2/Fio_2 less than 300 (using a Pao_2 derived from recorded saturations and charted Fio_2), found that only 5% of patients subsequently required intubation.[8] Another study of adults admitted to respiratory isolation rooms outside the intensive care unit demonstrated that patients with ALI (defined by bilateral infiltrates and hypoxemia) had similar mortality to those without one or both ALI criteria (12% vs 10%).[9]

In 2011, the ARDS Definition Task Force of the European Society of Intensive Care Medicine convened in Berlin to address limitations of the prior AECC definition and provide an empirical review of current and novel ancillary criteria.[10,11] Factors limiting practicality and validity of the definition were identified as: lack of clear delineation of "acute"; confusion over inclusion of ARDS within the definition of ALI; failure to account for positive end-expiratory pressure (PEEP) in assessment of the Pao_2/Fio_2 ratio[12–16]; poor interobserver reliability in interpretation of bilateral infiltrates on chest radiograph[17,18]; inadequate sensitivity of high left atrial pressure for excluding cases of ARDS[19,20]; and absence of requirement of a known risk factor for ARDS. These issues may contribute to misidentification of ARDS, suboptimal stratification of severity of lung injury, and enrollment of a more heterogeneous population into clinical trials.

As proposed solutions, the Berlin Definition (**Table 1**) specifies that "acute" respiratory failure must occur within 1 week of predisposing illness, as supported by observational data revealing that nearly all patients develop ARDS within 7 days of an inciting insult.[21] The prior ALI classification was eliminated, and instead ARDS is categorized by severity: mild (200 < Pao_2/Fio_2 $\leq$300), moderate (100 < Pao_2/Fio_2 $\leq$200), and severe (Pao_2/Fio_2 $\leq$100). This further stratification of severity below a Pao_2/Fio_2 ratio of 200 derives from prior evidence that mortality is highest in the lowest Pao_2/Fio_2 quartile independent of ventilator strategy,[22,23] and prior trials indicating differential success of therapies according to the Pao_2/Fio_2 ratio.[24–26] The Berlin Definition also requires a minimum PEEP of 5 cm H_2O for all severity categories in recognition of the influence of PEEP on the Pao_2/Fio_2 ratio. The panel also clarified radiographic criteria with supporting teaching examples, and recognized the potential for ARDS and hydrostatic edema to coexist in the new definition. Because volume overload is common in patients with ARDS,[20] criteria now exclude clinical evidence of isolated left atrial hypertension but without reference to a specific pulmonary artery occlusion pressure. Finally, the Berlin Definition specifies that use of noninvasive PEEP is allowed but limited to the mild ARDS category. This inclusion is in line with increasing use of noninvasive ventilation worldwide[27] and will likely facilitate further study of noninvasive ventilation for mild ARDS, which continues to be a debated area of research.[28–30]

Importantly the Berlin criteria were empirically derived and validated based on a pooled cohort of patients that comprised separate clinical[5,16,31,32]

Table 1		
The Berlin Definition of the acute respiratory distress syndrome		
	Acute Respiratory Distress Syndrome	
Timing	Within 1 wk of a known clinical insult or new or worsening respiratory symptoms	
Chest imaging[a]	Bilateral opacities not fully explained by effusions, lobar/lung collapse, or nodules	
Origin of edema	Respiratory failure not fully explained by cardiac failure or fluid overload Need objective assessment (eg, echocardiography) to exclude hydrostatic edema if no risk factor present	
Oxygenation		
Mild	$200 < Pao_2/Fio_2 \leq 300$ with PEEP or CPAP ≥ 5 cm H_2O[b]	
Moderate	$100 < Pao_2/Fio_2 \leq 200$ with PEEP or CPAP ≥ 5 cm H_2O	
Severe	$Pao_2/Fio_2 \leq 100$ with PEEP or CPAP ≥ 5 cm H_2O	

Abbreviations: CPAP, continuous positive airway pressure; Fio$_2$, fraction of inspired oxygen; Pao$_2$, partial pressure of arterial oxygen; PEEP, positive end-expiratory pressure.
  [a] Chest radiograph or computed tomography.
  [b] May be delivered noninvasively for mild acute respiratory distress.
  Adapted from Force AD, Ranieri VM, Rubenfeld GD, et al. Acute respiratory distress syndrome: the Berlin Definition. JAMA 2012;307(23):2530. Copyright © (2012) American Medical Association. All rights reserved.

and physiologic[33–35] databases. Of note, 4 proposed ancillary variables (radiographic severity, respiratory system compliance, level of PEEP, and exhaled minute ventilation) were dropped from the empirical definition because they did not enhance the predictive value of the severe ARDS classification. The distribution of ARDS severity in the cohort according to the Berlin Definition was 22% mild, 50% moderate, and 28% severe, with associated mortality rates of 27%, 32%, and 45%, respectively (**Fig. 1**). The Berlin Definition was more predictive of mortality (area under the curve [AUC] 0.58) than the ALI and ARDS classifications by AECC criteria. ARDS severity also correlated with lung weight and shunt fraction in the separate physiologic database.

Whether the Berlin Definition gains the same widespread adoption as the AECC criteria remains to be seen. However, the definition is both pragmatic and empirically derived, addresses many limitations of the prior definition, and will likely improve standardization for clinical care and research. For the purposes of this review, unless otherwise specified, further use of ARDS refers to the Berlin Definition while use of ALI refers to the AECC criteria inclusive or ARDS, with acute lung injury (as opposed to ALI) more generally referring to the pathophysiology leading to ARDS.

EPIDEMIOLOGY OF THE ACUTE RESPIRATORY DISTRESS SYNDROME
Incidence

The current incidence of ARDS, particularly as defined by the Berlin criteria, is not well established.

The most rigorous population-based study to date from Kings County, Washington identified ALI and ARDS in patients receiving mechanical ventilation via an endotracheal tube or noninvasive face mask, similarly to the Berlin Definition.[5] The incidence of ALI and ARDS was estimated at 78.9 and 58.7 cases per 100,000 patient-years, respectively, with an age-adjusted extrapolated incidence of 190,600 cases per year in the United States. Incidence increased with age to a peak of 306 cases per 100,000 patient-years among 75- to 84-year-olds. Pneumonia (46%) and nonpulmonary sepsis (33%) were the most common risk factors. Overall hospital mortality was 38.5%. The incidence of ARDS and ALI in the Kings County study is significantly higher than that reported by other less rigorous epidemiologic studies using AECC criteria before the era of low tidal volume ventilation (**Table 2**). Differences may be explained by underrecognition of the syndrome owing to inadequate screening mechanisms or retrospective study design, extrapolation from less than 1 year of data, and failure to identify all patients at risk within the catchment area in the less rigorous studies. The incidence also appears to be lower in international studies, which may reflect differing demographics and prevalence of risk factors for ARDS in addition to differences regarding availability or use of mechanical ventilation and noninvasive ventilation, particularly in the elderly.

Multiple investigators have also reported the incidence of ALI and ARDS since widespread adoption of lung-protective mechanical ventilation and other improvements in supportive care have occurred (**Table 3**). In the most rigorous of these

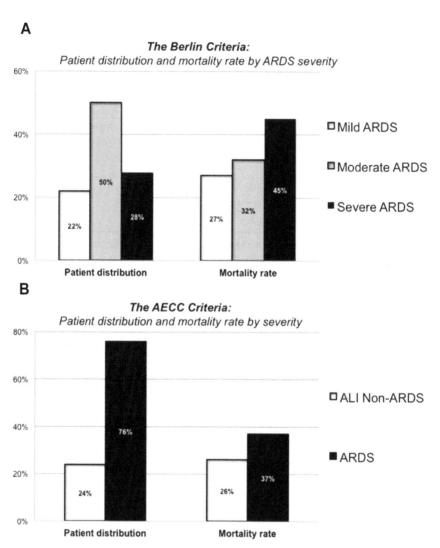

Fig. 1. In the cohort used for Berlin Definition validation and empirical derivation, the distribution of acute respiratory distress syndrome (ARDS) severity and mortality is shown for: (*A*) the Berlin criteria and (*B*) the American and European Consensus Conference (AECC) Consensus criteria. ALI, acute lung injury. (*Data from* Force AD, Ranieri VM, Rubenfeld GD, et al. Acute respiratory distress syndrome: the Berlin definition. JAMA 2012;307(23):2526–33.)

analyses, Li and colleagues[36] demonstrated a temporal decline in ARDS incidence from 2001 to 2008 in a population-based study in Olmstead County, Minnesota. Cases were identified using a well-validated electronic screening tool followed by investigator confirmation. Despite increasing severity of illness and higher rates of risk factors for ARDS at presentation, the incidence of ARDS decreased from 82.4 to 38.9 cases per 100,000 person-years. Of importance, the incidence of patients presenting with ARDS (ie, community-acquired ARDS) did not change and the decline in ARDS was due entirely to what the investigators deemed hospital-acquired ARDS (**Fig. 2**). However, the demographics of Olmstead County

are not representative of the United States, and the Mayo Clinic (in Olmstead County) has been a leader in efforts to standardize health care delivery and limit exposure to potential "second hits" along the pathway to ARDS (see the section Toward Prevention and Early Treatment of Acute Lung Injury). Therefore, these results may not reliably extrapolate to the country as a whole. Moreover, the investigators restricted the definition of ARDS to patients receiving mechanical ventilation via an endotracheal tube. Although this decision is reasonable, some of the observed decline in ARDS incidence may have been attributed to an increasing number of patients treated with non-invasive ventilation that would otherwise have

Table 2
Incidence of ALI and ARDS before the era of lung-protective ventilation

Authors,[Ref.] Year	Location	Study Period	Study Design	ICU Admissions	ALI[a] Incidence	ARDS[a] Incidence
Rubenfeld et al,[5] 2005	Seattle, USA	1999–2000	Prospective, multicenter	Unknown	78.9	58.7
Bersten et al,[31] 2002	Australia	1999 (8 wk)	Prospective, multicenter	1977	34	28
Luhr et al,[88] 1999	Sweden, Denmark	1997 (8 wk)	Prospective, multicenter	13,346	17.9	13.5
Valta et al,[89] 1999	Finland	1993–1995	Retrospective, single center	Unknown	N/A	4.9
Goss et al,[90] 2003	USA (ARDSNet)	1996–1999	Prospective, multicenter	25,392/y	22.4–64.2	N/A
Arroliga et al,[91] 2002	Ohio, USA	1996–1999	Retrospective, single HMO	Unknown	N/A	15.3
Hudson & Steinberg,[92] 1999	Seattle, USA	1997	Retrospective, multicenter	Unknown	18.9	12.6

Abbreviations: ALI, acute lung injury; ARDS, acute respiratory distress syndrome; HMO, health maintenance organization; ICU, intensive care unit; N/A, not applicable.
[a] Incidence per 100,000 patient-years.

Table 3
Incidence of ALI and ARDS in era of lung protective ventilation

Authors,[Ref.] Year	Location	Study Period	Study Design	ICU Admissions	ALI[a] Incidence	ARDS[a] Incidence
Linko et al,[93] 2009	Finland	2007 (8 wk)	Prospective, multicenter	2670	10.6	5.0
Villar et al,[43] 2011	Spain	2008–2009	Prospective, multicenter	11,363	N/A	7.2
Sigurdsson et al,[94] 2013	Iceland	1988–2010	Retrospective, single center	1148/y	N/A	3.63–9.63
Li et al,[36] 2011	Minnesota, USA	2001–2008	Retrospective, 2 centers	~1000/y	N/A	38.9–82.4
Hernu et al,[39] 2013	France	2012 (6 mo)	Prospective, 10 ICUs	3504	N/A	32
Caser et al,[40] 2014	Brazil	2006–2007 (15 mo)	Retrospective, 14 ICUs	7133	N/A	10.1

[a] Incidence per 100,000 patient-years.

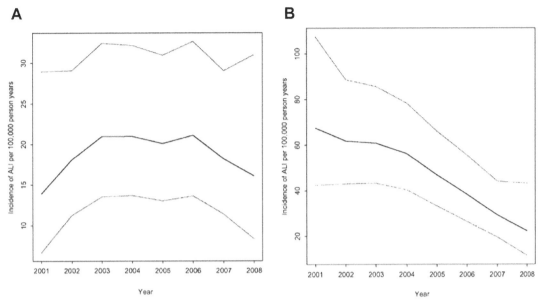

Fig. 2. (*A*) Trends of community-acquired ARDS incidence from 2001 to 2008 in Olmsted County, Minnesota; dotted lines represent 95% confidence intervals. (*B*) Trends of hospital-acquired acute respiratory distress syndrome incidence from 2001 to 2008 in Olmsted County, Minnesota; dotted lines represent 95% confidence intervals. ALI, acute lung injury. (*From* Li G, Malinchoc M, Cartin-Ceba R, et al. Eight-year trend of acute respiratory distress syndrome: a population-based study in Olmsted County, Minnesota. Am J Respir Crit Care Med 2011;183(1):59–66. Reprinted with permission of the American Thoracic Society. Copyright © 2011 American Thoracic Society. Official Journal of the American Thoracic Society.)

been intubated and met criteria for ARDS.[27] Similar dramatic reductions in the incidence of ARDS (from 50% to 90%) have also been demonstrated in smaller cohorts of trauma and nontrauma surgical patients.[37,38] These patient populations are likely less susceptible to temporal changes in the use of noninvasive ventilation, suggesting a real effect on improvements in supportive care. However, these studies lack the rigor of the study by Rubenfeld and colleagues,[5] and a failure to identify all cases of ARDS may explain some of the observed decline in incidence.

Two recent international studies have estimated the incidence of ARDS since the introduction of the Berlin Definition. A 6-month prospective study conducted within 10 adult intensive care units affiliated with the Public University Hospital in Lyon, France screened 3504 critically ill patients and identified 278 who met criteria for ALI and ARDS by AECC criteria.[39] Of these 278 patients, 18 did not meet Berlin criteria because of lack of sufficient PEEP (a similar 12% of patients did not meet ARDS criteria in the original Berlin cohort because PEEP was <5 cm H_2O or missing). An additional 20 patients could not be classified by the Berlin Definition because, despite a Pao_2/Fio_2 of less than 200, they did not meet criteria for moderate or severe ARDS because they were receiving only noninvasive ventilation. Of the remaining 240

patients 18%, 51%, and 31% were classified as mild, moderate, and severe ARDS, respectively. Extrapolated to the population of Lyon, the incidence was estimated at 32 per 100,000 patient-years. However, this estimate does not appear to be adjusted for age or gender, and the observation period from March to September may not have captured potential seasonal variations in the incidence of ARDS.

A retrospective review of a prospective cohort of 14 adult medical and surgical intensive care units collected over 15 months in Southeast Brazil from October 2006 to December 2007 identified 130 cases of ARDS by Berlin criteria among 7133 admissions (1.8%).[40] The cumulative incidence (10.1 cases per 100,000 patient-years) was substantially lower than in Lyon, although the methodology for extrapolating incidence was not described. The distribution of ARDS severity was 38% mild, 52% moderate, and 10% severe, but the study only included patients receiving invasive mechanical ventilation, which likely reduced the number of patients who would have met criteria for mild ARDS.

Predisposing Conditions

The primary etiology of ARDS has remained consistent across studies of established cases of ARDS, with pneumonia (35%–45%) and nonpulmonary sepsis (30%–35%) being the most common followed by aspiration, trauma, pancreatitis, and multiple transfusions.[5,39–43] An in-depth review of risk factors for developing ARDS, including attention to important subgroups, is discussed elsewhere.[44] In contrast to evaluating cases of ARDS or populations of critically ill patients, the Lung Injury Prevention Study (LIPS) prospectively evaluated more than 5000 patients presenting to the emergency department with at least one established risk factor for ARDS.[45] Risk factors were separated into predisposing conditions and risk modifiers. Consistent with other cohorts, sepsis (33%), pneumonia (27%), and shock (19%) were the most common predisposing conditions on presentation among patients who developed ALI. However, cardiac surgery (15%), traumatic brain injury (12%), aspiration (9%), and acute abdominal surgery, lung contusion, and multiple fractures (7% each) were also common. Odds ratios (OR) calculated by multivariable regression for risk factors for developing ALI are shown in **Table 4**.

The presence of multiple comorbidities and chronic pulmonary disease are associated with a

Table 4
Multivariable regression of risk factors for the development of ARDS

	Odds Ratio	95% CI	P value
Predisposing Conditions			
Shock	2.2	1.2–3.7	.008
Aspiration	2.2	1.1–4.3	.02
Sepsis	1.4	0.9–2.4	.14
Pneumonia	0.3	0.02–1.7	.3
High-risk surgery			
Thoracic (noncardiac)	0.9	0.1–3.2	.9
Orthopedic spine	2.1	0.9–4.6	.07
Acute abdomen	2.5	1.1–5.6	.03
Cardiac	3.7	2.0–7.1	<.001
Aortic vascular	5.9	2.5–13.0	<.001
High-risk trauma			
Traumatic brain injury	3.6	2.0–6.8	<.001
Smoke inhalation	2.5	0.8–4.1	.44
Near drowning	5.4	0.06–6.6	.50
Lung contusion	1.5	0.6–3.4	.36
Multiple fractures	1.9	0.8–4.1	.12
Risk Modifiers			
Male gender	1.0	0.7–1.5	.91
Alcohol abuse	1.7	0.9–2.9	.08
Obesity (BMI >30)	1.8	1.2–2.5	.004
Chemotherapy	1.6	0.6–3.6	.32
Diabetes mellitus	0.6	0.2–1.2	.14
Smoking	1.1	0.7–1.5	.4
Emergency surgery	3.1	1.6–5.9	<.01
Tachypnea (RR >30/min)	2.0	1.1–3.5	.02
Spo_2 <95%	1.4	1.0–2.1	.08
Fio_2 >0.35 (>4 L/min)	2.8	1.9–4.1	<.001
Hypoalbuminemia	1.6	1.0–2.4	.03
Acidosis (pH <7.35)	1.7	1.1–2.7	.02

Abbreviations: BMI, body mass index (kg/m^2); CI, confidence interval; Fio_2, fraction of inspired oxygen; RR, respiratory rate; Spo_2, arterial oxygen saturation.

Adapted from Gajic O, Dabbagh O, Park PK, et al. Early identification of patients at risk of acute lung injury: evaluation of lung injury prediction score in a multicenter cohort study. Am J Respir Crit Care Med 2011;183(4):466. Reprinted with permission of the American Thoracic Society. Copyright © 2011 American Thoracic Society. Official Journal of the American Thoracic Society.

higher incidence of acute lung injury.[46] Chronic alcohol abuse and active and passive tobacco exposure also seem to be predisposing factors.[47,48] By contrast, diabetes mellitus may have a protective effect, a relationship that is not well explained but has been found in multiple cohorts.[45,49,50] A recent analysis of the LIPS cohort separately analyzed type 1 and type 2 diabetes and controlled for associated comorbidities such as obesity, acute hyperglycemia, and diabetes-associated medications.[51] Diabetes remained protective (adjusted OR 0.75, 95% confidence interval [CI] 0.59–0.94); moreover, the association was found for both types of diabetes and, in contrast to prior cohorts, in both septic and nonseptic subgroups.[51]

Important gender and racial disparities exist in regard to prevalence of risk factors for ARDS, comorbidities, and severity of illness at presentation in populations of patients at risk. However, race and gender are not clear independent risk factors for developing ARDS. In an observational study of trauma patients, African Americans were more likely to present with shock and penetrating trauma and to receive massive transfusions, but there was no difference in risk-adjusted rates of ALI among whites, African Americans, Hispanics, and Asian/Pacific Islanders.[52] Analysis of a large national database of patients with blunt trauma suggested a protective effect of African American race with respect to ARDS incidence.[53] In the 5000-patient LIPS cohort, African Americans were more likely to present with pneumonia, sepsis, shock, and increased severity of illness, but had lower rates of developing ALI either with or without adjustment for baseline characteristics (adjusted OR 0.66, 95% CI 0.45–0.96).[54] Furthermore, men had higher rates of developing ALI, but not after controlling for baseline imbalances between sexes.

Mortality

Accurate assessment of mortality attributable to ARDS depends on reliable standard diagnostic criteria. A systematic review of more than 3000 patients and 100 studies, between 1967 and 1994 (before AECC criteria), reported a widely ranging but stable mortality rate throughout the study period (55% overall mortality, 95% CI 33%–77%).[55] Although established pharmacologic treatments do not currently exist,[56,57] studies of mortality after adoption of the AECC criteria suggest improved outcomes, likely attributable to improvements in supportive care. A review of 2451 patients enrolled in clinical trials within the ARDS Network from 1995 to 2005 found a decline

in crude mortality from 35% to 26% during the study period.[58] However, clinical trials represent a more highly selected patient population, and results from studies of mortality outside of clinical trials are not consistent. A systematic review of 72 studies and 11,425 patients from 1994 to 2006 found a higher overall mortality rate (44%; 95% CI 40%–46%) than in the ARDS Network trials, but a similar decline in mortality of 1.1% per year over the study period.[59] By contrast, a subsequent systematic review of the same time period found a static mortality rate of 44.0% for observational studies and 36.2% for clinical trials since the introduction of the AECC criteria in 1994.[60] The latter review postulated that disparate findings may be explained by the inclusion of non-English studies, more accurate assignation of study year for high-mortality studies that primarily enrolled patients before 1994 but were completed afterward, better exclusion of studies with overlapping patient populations, and inclusion of 27 additional post-1994 studies.

The Berlin Definition did predict mortality better than AECC criteria in the Task Force's validation cohort; however, prognostic performance was limited when evaluated in recent external cohorts.[39,40,61] Despite the improved empiricism of the Berlin Definition, it remains a purely descriptive clinical phenotype. Significant sources of heterogeneity within the syndrome remain, and these will continue to challenge accurate risk stratification. The prognostic implications of different inciting causes, pathophysiologic phases, mechanisms of lung injury, and responses to mechanical ventilation are unlikely to be adequately accounted for by any pragmatic clinical definition applied to heterogeneous populations.[62]

For example, the predisposing etiology underlying ARDS and patient comorbidities are important independent determinants of outcome. Among ARDS Network study patients enrolled from 1996 through 2005, the rate of in-hospital mortality was highest for sepsis (37%) and pneumonia (30%) while exceptionally low in trauma (11%),[58] although patients with severe trauma were likely underrepresented in these trials. A multicenter clinical trial of activated protein C for treatment of ALI that excluded patients with severe sepsis and an APACHE II score of at least 25 reported an overall mortality rate of only 13%,[63] highlighting the importance of underlying conditions for predicting mortality. Mortality rates with ARDS also increase linearly with age.[5] Body mass index below normal appears be an independent risk factor for mortality, whereas obesity may portend a lower risk of death.[64] Higher acute physiology scores, the presence of shock at admission, immune incompetence, a longer hospital stay before ALI onset, and a shorter stay in the intensive care unit preceding ALI onset are also associated with higher mortatilty.[41,65,66]

In contrast to the risk of developing ARDS, race and ethnicity seem to affect the mortality associated with ARDS. In a case series of greater than 300,000 decedents with ARDS compiled by the National Center for Health Statistics from 1979 to 1996, annual age-adjusted ARDS mortality rates were consistently higher for men than for women, and for African Americans in comparison with other backgrounds.[67] Among patients enrolled in more recent ARDS Network clinical trials, mortality was greater among blacks and Hispanics.[68] After adjustment for demographics, clinical covariates, and severity of illness, mortality among blacks was not significantly higher than in whites (adjusted OR 1.25, 95% CI 0.95–1.66) while the relative mortality among Hispanics actually increased (adjusted OR 2.0, 95% CI 1.37–2.90). The reason for increased mortality among Hispanics is not known, although it deserves further attention given that this finding occurred in patients enrolled in clinical trials where care is presumably more standardized. Similarly, in the aforementioned national database of patients with blunt trauma, Hispanics had higher odds of adjusted ARDS-associated mortality (OR 1.76, 95% CI 1.15–2.62).[53]

Accurate risk stratification of patients with ARDS will be important to the success of future clinical trials. Among ARDS Network study patients, the addition of baseline plasma biomarkers (interlukin-8, soluble tumor necrosis factor receptor 1, and surfactant protein D) to the APACHE III score more accurately predicted mortality.[69] The predictive validity and specificity of future ARDS criteria may be further improved through: identification of novel genetic polymorphisms and biomarkers[70]; more reproducible and practical methods for measuring vascular permeability and extravascular lung water[71,72]; incorporation of Pao_2/Fio_2 responses to standard ventilator settings at 24 hours[13,14]; inclusion of non–plain-film imaging such as fibroproliferation on computed tomography[73] and right ventricular strain on echocardiogram.[74]

TOWARD PREVENTION AND EARLY TREATMENT OF ACUTE LUNG INJURY
Improved Supportive Care

Multiple investigators have identified potentially modifiable risk factors that likely contribute to the incidence of ARDS, including delayed early goal-directed therapy and appropriate antibiotics in patients with sepsis,[49] larger tidal volumes in mechanically ventilated patients,[75–77] and transfusion of blood products.[78–81] With respect to blood products, transfusion of plasma-rich products such as platelets and fresh frozen plasma carries a higher risk than transfusing red blood cells,[79] and recent efforts to remove female donors from the plasma donor pool have reduced the incidence of transfusion-related acute lung injury.[78,80,81] A recent population-based, nested case-control study from the Mayo Clinic in Rochester, Minnesota identified multiple potential hospital exposures related to the development of ARDS.[82] In contrast to other studies, these patients were carefully matched by baseline risk factors for developing ARDS, including their LIPS score. Ascertainment of exposures was blinded, and the screening window for risk-factor exposure was limited to the time from admission to 6 hours before developing ARDS for cases and an equivalent time period (assigned by unblinded statisticians) for controls. In this well-designed study, inadequate empirical antimicrobials, hospital-acquired aspiration, transfusion of blood products, and higher tidal volumes were highly associated with developing ARDS. Over the 10-year study period, the investigators found a significant decline in rates of exposures to these risk factors that correlated with a decline in the rate of hospital-acquired ARDS. Changes implemented to improve standardization of care included: implementation of computerized order entry with decision support for pneumonia, sepsis, and transfusions (with decision support for appropriate antimicrobial delivery and to limit inappropriate transfusions); respiratory therapist driven lung-protective ventilation protocols for mechanically ventilated patients (including use of a validated automated surveillance and notification system with documented reduced time of exposure to larger tidal volumes); and increased staffing of the medical intensive care unit including the addition of a 24-hour on-site intensivist.[36] The relative importance of each of these interventions is unclear; however, there is now abundant evidence that in-hospital exposures to potentially modifiable risk factors contribute to the incidence of ARDS. Efforts to implement commonsense protocols to limit exposures and improve standardization of care are likely low-risk, high-reward strategies for reducing the burden of ARDS.

Identification and Treatment of Early Acute Lung Injury

In the 20 years since publication of the AECC criteria for ALI and ARDS, numerous pharmacologic therapies have been tested and failed to show benefit in large multicenter clinical trials, including several by the National Institutes of Health (NIH)-funded ARDS Network.[83–87] This recognition has led to increased emphasis on earlier identification of high-risk patients, and the restructuring of the ARDS Network into the Network for the Prevention and Early Treatment of Acute Lung Injury (PETAL) forming in 2014. However, established criteria or definitions for early acute lung injury (EALI) to use as inclusion criteria for future trials are lacking.

In a large multicenter prospective study of the more than 5000 patients, the United States Critical Illness and Injury Trials (USCIIT) group developed and validated the LIPS score for the early identification of high-risk patients.[45] The LIPS score targeted patients presenting to the emergency department with at least one established risk factor for ARDS, and was derived from variables present within the first 6 hours of presentation. Risk factors were divided into predisposing conditions (shock, sepsis, aspiration, pneumonia, or high-risk surgery or trauma) and risk modifiers (obesity, alcohol abuse, diabetes, hypoalbuminemia, acidosis, tachypnea, and oxygen supplementation). The overall incidence of ARDS in the cohort was 7%. The LIPS score showed good discrimination (AUC 0.80) and calibration, with rates of ARDS ranging from 1% for a LIPS score of 1 or less to 36% for a LIPS score of 8 or more. A cutoff of a LIPS score greater than 4 had the best overall discrimination with sensitivity of 69% and specificity of 78%; however, it still identified a relatively low-risk population with a positive predictive value of only 18%.

In a prospective single-center study, the authors' research group empirically derived criteria for EALI in patients presenting to the emergency department with bilateral opacities on chest radiograph in the absence of isolated left atrial hypertension. Clinical variables were collected longitudinally for up to 72 hours or 6 hours before meeting criteria for ALI (defined by AECC criteria while receiving positive pressure ventilation via face mask or endotracheal tube). Study investigators performed bedside titration of supplemental oxygen on a daily basis to record the level required to maintain arterial oxygen saturation (SpO_2) greater than 90%. Sixty-two of 256 patients (25%) developed ALI. Oxygen requirement, respiratory rate, and baseline immune suppression were the only independent predictors of progression to ALI. A pragmatic 3-component EALI score (1 point for an oxygen requirement >2–6 L/min or 2 points for >6 L/min; and 1 point each for a respiratory rate >30 per minute and immune suppression) accurately identified patients progressing to ALI and outperformed the LIPS score in this cohort. An EALI score greater than or equal to 2 identified patients who progressed to ALI with 89% sensitivity and 75% specificity. In this cohort (with a 25% prevalence of ALI), this corresponded to positive and negative predictive values of 53% and 95%.

There are substantial differences in design and intent of the EALI and LIPS scores. For some pulmonary specific predisposing conditions and risk factors included in the LIPS (ie, pneumonia, aspiration, SpO_2 <95% or FiO_2 >35%), the distinction between prevention and early identification may be semantic. However, the distinction is real for others (nonpulmonary sepsis, high-risk elective surgery, comorbidities) and may affect not only the incidence but also the time of progression to ALI. The EALI score was derived in patients with at least some evidence of early bilateral opacities on chest radiography. This requirement increased the baseline incidence of developing ALI to 25% compared with 8% in the LIPS cohort, but may also limit sensitivity of identifying patients who progress rapidly without an interval qualifying chest radiograph. Furthermore, the success of the EALI score likely derives from the longitudinal evaluation of physiologic variables for potentially up to 6 hours before the onset of ALI. By contrast, the LIPS score targeted identifying high-risk patients based on variables present within the first 6 hours of admission. It is logical that a scoring system identifying patients at presentation would require consideration of multiple baseline risk factors and risk modifiers, whereas criteria for identifying early but existing lung injury would be more heavily influenced by the acute pulmonary physiology predicting impending respiratory failure.

Selection of criteria to identify appropriate target populations will largely depend on the nature of the intervention. For identifying patients to target for strategies to prevent exposure to modifiable risk factors, sensitive criteria generalizable to multiple patient populations, such as the LIPS score, may be ideal. However, clinical trials testing novel therapies may wish to target higher-risk patients with existing physiologic and radiographic surrogate end points of lung injury. For example, a theoretic clinical trial of an intervention with a predicted 50% reduction in the rate of progression to ARDS would need 400 patients to be appropriately powered if the study population has a baseline 20% risk of developing ARDS (with a 2-tailed α of .05). However, if the baseline risk is 40%, only 160 patients would be needed. As with studies of ARDS, markers of lung injury severity to target as surrogate end points in clinical trials are not well established, which will challenge the design of early exploratory studies and highlights the need for multicenter coordination for appropriately powered clinical trials in this area.

At present, the USCITT Group is conducting 2 multicenter clinical trials for the prevention of ARDS. The Lung Injury Prevention Study with Aspirin (LIPS-A) is a large phase II clinical trial of aspirin versus placebo, targeting 400 patients with a LIPS score of at least 4 and a primary end point of a reduction in the incidence of ALI while receiving invasive mechanical ventilation (NCT01504867). The Lung Injury Prevention Study with Budesonide and Beta Agonists (LIPS-B) is a smaller phase II study of aerosolized budesonide and formoterol versus placebo. This study aims to enroll 40 patients with a LIPS score of at least 4 and a minimal baseline oxygen requirement, with a primary end point of improvement in the Spo_2/Fio_2 ratio (NCT01783821). These trials represent exciting new strategies to reduce the burden of ARDS. This paradigm shift toward prevention and early treatment is now a major focus of the NIH through formation of the PETAL Network. However, with increased emphasis on prevention and early treatment of ARDS, it will be important to continue to refine and standardize criteria to identify the appropriate target populations and inform future clinical trials.

SUMMARY

The AECC criteria for ARDS and ALI have helped to standardize patients for epidemiologic studies, multicenter clinical trials, and clinical practice guidelines. However, lack of consistent interpretation of the AECC criteria has limited precise understanding of the incidence and epidemiology of ARDS. Moreover, ARDS remains underrecognized in clinical practice, and accurate epidemiologic description requires studies with rigorous methodology to reliably identify all cases and relevant patients at risk. Given these limitations, improvements in supportive care apparently have significantly reduced the incidence of ARDS in recent years.

The recently empirically derived and validated Berlin Definition will help codify the inclusion of patients managed with noninvasive positive pressure ventilation and resolve confusion regarding the overlapping criteria of ALI and ARDS. Moreover, establishing mild, moderate, and severe criteria will help risk-stratify patients for research purposes. However, ARDS remains a descriptive clinical phenotype representing heterogeneous inciting causes with likely differing pathology and very different prognoses, which will continue to challenge clinical trials targeting survival benefit.

Developing reliable and clinically available biological markers of lung injury may help identify more homogenous patient populations, and serve as surrogate markers to facilitate future appropriately powered clinical investigations.

The ongoing paradigm shift toward prevention and early treatment may provide further progress toward reducing the significant burden of ARDS. Efforts to implement commonsense protocols to limit exposures to modifiable risk factors and improve standardization of care across institutions are likely to be high-impact strategies to reduce the incidence of ARDS. The LIPS and EALI scores are novel criteria for identifying high-risk patients who may particularly benefit from these strategies. However, it will be important to continue to refine and standardize criteria to further understand the epidemiology of these at-risk populations and to identify the appropriate target patients for future clinical investigations.

REFERENCES

1. Ashbaugh DG, Bigelow DB, Petty TL, et al. Acute respiratory distress in adults. Lancet 1967; 2(7511):319–23.
2. Fowler AA, Hamman RF, Good JT, et al. Adult respiratory distress syndrome: risk with common predispositions. Ann Intern Med 1983;98(5 Pt 1): 593–7.
3. Pepe PE, Potkin RT, Reus DH, et al. Clinical predictors of the adult respiratory distress syndrome. Am J Surg 1982;144(1):124–30.
4. Bernard GR, Artigas A, Brigham KL, et al. The American-European Consensus Conference on ARDS. Definitions, mechanisms, relevant outcomes, and clinical trial coordination. Am J Respir Crit Care Med 1994;149(3 Pt 1):818–24.
5. Rubenfeld GD, Caldwell E, Peabody E, et al. Incidence and outcomes of acute lung injury. N Engl J Med 2005;353(16):1685–93.
6. Ferguson ND, Frutos-Vivar F, Esteban A, et al. Clinical risk conditions for acute lung injury in the intensive care unit and hospital ward: a prospective observational study. Crit Care 2007;11(5):R96.
7. Flori HR, Glidden DV, Rutherford GW, et al. Pediatric acute lung injury: prospective evaluation of risk factors associated with mortality. Am J Respir Crit Care Med 2005;171(9):995–1001.
8. Freishtat RJ, Mojgani B, Mathison DJ, et al. Toward early identification of acute lung injury in the emergency department. J Investig Med 2007;55(8): 423–9.
9. Quartin AA, Campos MA, Maldonado DA, et al. Acute lung injury outside of the ICU: incidence in respiratory isolation on a general ward. Chest 2009;135(2):261–8.

10. Force AD, Ranieri VM, Rubenfeld GD, et al. Acute respiratory distress syndrome: the Berlin Definition. JAMA 2012;307(23):2526–33.

11. Ferguson ND, Fan E, Camporota L, et al. The Berlin definition of ARDS: an expanded rationale, justification, and supplementary material. Intensive Care Med 2012;38(10):1573–82.

12. Villar J, Perez-Mendez L, Kacmarek RM. Current definitions of acute lung injury and the acute respiratory distress syndrome do not reflect their true severity and outcome. Intensive Care Med 1999; 25(9):930–5.

13. Villar J, Perez-Mendez L, Lopez J, et al. An early PEEP/FIO$_2$ trial identifies different degrees of lung injury in patients with acute respiratory distress syndrome. Am J Respir Crit Care Med 2007; 176(8):795–804.

14. Villar J, Perez-Mendez L, Blanco J, et al. A universal definition of ARDS: the PaO$_2$/FiO$_2$ ratio under a standard ventilatory setting–a prospective, multicenter validation study. Intensive Care Med 2013;39(4):583–92.

15. Ferguson ND, Kacmarek RM, Chiche JD, et al. Screening of ARDS patients using standardized ventilator settings: influence on enrollment in a clinical trial. Intensive Care Med 2004;30(6):1111–6.

16. Britos M, Smoot E, Liu KD, et al. The value of positive end-expiratory pressure and Fio(2) criteria in the definition of the acute respiratory distress syndrome. Crit Care Med 2011;39(9):2025–30.

17. Rubenfeld GD, Caldwell E, Granton J, et al. Interobserver variability in applying a radiographic definition for ARDS. Chest 1999;116(5):1347–53.

18. Meade MO, Cook RJ, Guyatt GH, et al. Interobserver variation in interpreting chest radiographs for the diagnosis of acute respiratory distress syndrome. Am J Respir Crit Care Med 2000;161(1):85–90.

19. Ferguson ND, Meade MO, Hallett DC, et al. High values of the pulmonary artery wedge pressure in patients with acute lung injury and acute respiratory distress syndrome. Intensive Care Med 2002; 28(8):1073–7.

20. National Heart, Lung, and Blood Institute Acute Respiratory Distress Syndrome (ARDS) Clinical Trials Network, Wheeler AP, Bernard GR, et al. Pulmonary-artery versus central venous catheter to guide treatment of acute lung injury. N Engl J Med 2006;354(21):2213–24.

21. Hudson LD, Milberg JA, Anardi D, et al. Clinical risks for development of the acute respiratory distress syndrome. Am J Respir Crit Care Med 1995;151(2 Pt 1):293–301.

22. Mercat A, Richard JC, Vielle B, et al. Positive end-expiratory pressure setting in adults with acute lung injury and acute respiratory distress syndrome: a randomized controlled trial. JAMA 2008; 299(6):646–55.

23. Meade MO, Cook DJ, Guyatt GH, et al. Ventilation strategy using low tidal volumes, recruitment maneuvers, and high positive end-expiratory pressure for acute lung injury and acute respiratory distress syndrome: a randomized controlled trial. JAMA 2008;299(6):637–45.

24. Briel M, Meade M, Mercat A, et al. Higher vs lower positive end-expiratory pressure in patients with acute lung injury and acute respiratory distress syndrome: systematic review and meta-analysis. JAMA 2010;303(9):865–73.

25. Cesana BM, Antonelli P, Chiumello D, et al. Positive end-expiratory pressure, prone positioning, and activated protein C: a critical review of meta-analyses. Minerva Anestesiol 2010;76(11):929–36.

26. Papazian L, Forel JM, Gacouin A, et al. Neuromuscular blockers in early acute respiratory distress syndrome. N Engl J Med 2010;363(12):1107–16.

27. Esteban A, Frutos-Vivar F, Muriel A, et al. Evolution of mortality over time in patients receiving mechanical ventilation. Am J Respir Crit Care Med 2013;188(2):220–30.

28. Wang S, Singh B, Tian L, et al. Epidemiology of noninvasive mechanical ventilation in acute respiratory failure–a retrospective population-based study. BMC Emerg Med 2013;13:6.

29. Agarwal R, Aggarwal AN, Gupta D. Role of noninvasive ventilation in acute lung injury/acute respiratory distress syndrome: a proportion meta-analysis. Respir Care 2010;55(12):1653–60.

30. Zhan Q, Sun B, Liang L, et al. Early use of noninvasive positive pressure ventilation for acute lung injury: a multicenter randomized controlled trial. Crit Care Med 2012;40(2):455–60.

31. Bersten AD, Edibam C, Hunt T, et al, Australian and New Zealand Intensive Care Society Clinical Trials Group. Incidence and mortality of acute lung injury and the acute respiratory distress syndrome in three Australian States. Am J Respir Crit Care Med 2002;165(4):443–8.

32. Needham DM, Dennison CR, Dowdy DW, et al. Study protocol: the improving care of acute lung injury patients (ICAP) study. Crit Care 2006; 10(1):R9.

33. Bellani G, Guerra L, Musch G, et al. Lung regional metabolic activity and gas volume changes induced by tidal ventilation in patients with acute lung injury. Am J Respir Crit Care Med 2011; 183(9):1193–9.

34. Terragni PP, Del Sorbo L, Mascia L, et al. Tidal volume lower than 6 ml/kg enhances lung protection: role of extracorporeal carbon dioxide removal. Anesthesiology 2009;111(4):826–35.

35. Terragni PP, Rosboch G, Tealdi A, et al. Tidal hyperinflation during low tidal volume ventilation in acute respiratory distress syndrome. Am J Respir Crit Care Med 2007;175(2):160–6.

36. Li G, Malinchoc M, Cartin-Ceba R, et al. Eight-year trend of acute respiratory distress syndrome: a population-based study in Olmsted County, Minnesota. Am J Respir Crit Care Med 2011;183(1):59–66.

37. Ciesla DJ, Moore EE, Johnson JL, et al. Decreased progression of postinjury lung dysfunction to the acute respiratory distress syndrome and multiple organ failure. Surgery 2006;140(4):640–7 [discussion: 647–8].

38. Martin M, Salim A, Murray J, et al. The decreasing incidence and mortality of acute respiratory distress syndrome after injury: a 5-year observational study. J Trauma 2005;59(5):1107–13.

39. Hernu R, Wallet F, Thiolliere F, et al. An attempt to validate the modification of the American-European consensus definition of acute lung injury/acute respiratory distress syndrome by the Berlin definition in a university hospital. Intensive Care Med 2013;39(12):2161–70.

40. Caser EB, Zandonade E, Pereira E, et al. Impact of distinct definitions of acute lung injury on its incidence and outcomes in Brazilian ICUs: prospective evaluation of 7,133 patients*. Crit Care Med 2014;42(3):574–82.

41. Rubenfeld GD, Herridge MS. Epidemiology and outcomes of acute lung injury. Chest 2007;131(2): 554–62.

42. Thille AW, Esteban A, Fernandez-Segoviano P, et al. Comparison of the Berlin definition for acute respiratory distress syndrome with autopsy. Am J Respir Crit Care Med 2013;187(7):761–7.

43. Villar J, Blanco J, Anon JM, et al. The ALIEN study: incidence and outcome of acute respiratory distress syndrome in the era of lung protective ventilation. Intensive Care Med 2011;37(12):1932–41.

44. Levitt JE, Matthay MA. The utility of clinical predictors of acute lung injury: towards prevention and earlier recognition. Expert Rev Respir Med 2010; 4(6):785–97.

45. Gajic O, Dabbagh O, Park PK, et al. Early identification of patients at risk of acute lung injury: evaluation of lung injury prediction score in a multicenter cohort study. Am J Respir Crit Care Med 2011; 183(4):462–70.

46. Johnson ER, Matthay MA. Acute lung injury: epidemiology, pathogenesis, and treatment. J Aerosol Med Pulm Drug Deliv 2010;23(4):243–52.

47. Moss M, Bucher B, Moore FA, et al. The role of chronic alcohol abuse in the development of acute respiratory distress syndrome in adults. JAMA 1996;275(1):50–4.

48. Calfee CS, Matthay MA, Eisner MD, et al. Active and passive cigarette smoking and acute lung injury after severe blunt trauma. Am J Respir Crit Care Med 2011;183(12):1660–5.

49. Iscimen R, Cartin-Ceba R, Yilmaz M, et al. Risk factors for the development of acute lung injury in patients with septic shock: an observational cohort study. Crit Care Med 2008;36(5):1518–22.

50. Moss M, Guidot DM, Steinberg KP, et al. Diabetic patients have a decreased incidence of acute respiratory distress syndrome. Crit Care Med 2000;28(7):2187–92.

51. Yu S, Christiani DC, Thompson BT, et al. Role of diabetes in the development of acute respiratory distress syndrome. Crit Care Med 2013;41(12): 2720–32.

52. Brown LM, Kallet RH, Matthay MA, et al. The influence of race on the development of acute lung injury in trauma patients. Am J Surg 2011;201(4): 486–91.

53. Ryb GE, Cooper C. Race/ethnicity and acute respiratory distress syndrome: a National Trauma Data Bank study. J Natl Med Assoc 2010;102(10):865–9.

54. Lemos-Filho LB, Mikkelsen ME, Martin GS, et al. Sex, race, and the development of acute lung injury. Chest 2013;143(4):901–9.

55. Krafft P, Fridrich P, Pernerstorfer T, et al. The acute respiratory distress syndrome: definitions, severity and clinical outcome. An analysis of 101 clinical investigations. Intensive Care Med 1996;22(6): 519–29.

56. Calfee CS, Matthay MA. Nonventilatory treatments for acute lung injury and ARDS. Chest 2007; 131(3):913–20.

57. Levitt JE, Matthay MA. Treatment of acute lung injury: historical perspective and potential future therapies. Semin Respir Crit Care Med 2006; 27(4):426–37.

58. Erickson SE, Martin GS, Davis JL, et al, NIH NHLBI ARDS Network. Recent trends in acute lung injury mortality: 1996-2005. Crit Care Med 2009;37(5): 1574–9.

59. Zambon M, Vincent JL. Mortality rates for patients with acute lung injury/ARDS have decreased over time. Chest 2008;133(5):1120–7.

60. Phua J, Badia JR, Adhikari NK, et al. Has mortality from acute respiratory distress syndrome decreased over time? A systematic review. Am J Respir Crit Care Med 2009;179(3):220–7.

61. Costa EL, Amato MB. The new definition for acute lung injury and acute respiratory distress syndrome: is there room for improvement? Curr Opin Crit Care 2013;19(1):16–23.

62. Phua J, Stewart TE, Ferguson ND. Acute respiratory distress syndrome 40 years later: time to revisit its definition. Crit Care Med 2008;36(10): 2912–21.

63. Liu KD, Levitt J, Zhuo H, et al. Randomized clinical trial of activated protein C for the treatment of acute lung injury. Am J Respir Crit Care Med 2008;178(6): 618–23.

64. O'Brien JM Jr, Phillips GS, Ali NA, et al. Body mass index is independently associated with hospital

mortality in mechanically ventilated adults with acute lung injury. Crit Care Med 2006;34(3):738–44.

65. Brun-Buisson C, Minelli C, Bertolini G, et al. Epidemiology and outcome of acute lung injury in European intensive care units. Results from the ALIVE study. Intensive Care Med 2004;30(1):51–61.

66. Luhr OR, Karlsson M, Thorsteinsson A, et al. The impact of respiratory variables on mortality in non-ARDS and ARDS patients requiring mechanical ventilation. Intensive Care Med 2000;26(5):508–17.

67. Moss M, Mannino DM. Race and gender differences in acute respiratory distress syndrome deaths in the United States: an analysis of multiple-cause mortality data (1979-1996). Crit Care Med 2002;30(8):1679–85.

68. Erickson SE, Shlipak MG, Martin GS, et al. Racial and ethnic disparities in mortality from acute lung injury. Crit Care Med 2009;37(1):1–6.

69. Calfee CS, Ware LB, Glidden DV, et al. Use of risk reclassification with multiple biomarkers improves mortality prediction in acute lung injury. Crit Care Med 2011;39(4):711–7.

70. Calfee CS, Eisner MD, Ware LB, et al. Trauma-associated lung injury differs clinically and biologically from acute lung injury due to other clinical disorders. Crit Care Med 2007;35(10):2243–50.

71. Kushimoto S, Endo T, Yamanouchi S, et al. Relationship between extravascular lung water and severity categories of acute respiratory distress syndrome by the Berlin definition. Crit Care 2013;17(4).R132.

72. Jozwiak M, Silva S, Persichini R, et al. Extravascular lung water is an independent prognostic factor in patients with acute respiratory distress syndrome. Crit Care Med 2013;41(2):472–80.

73. Ichikado K. "The Berlin definition" and clinical significance of high-resolution CT (HRCT) imaging in acute respiratory distress syndrome. Masui 2013;62(5):522–31 [in Japanese].

74. Boissier F, Katsahian S, Razazi K, et al. Prevalence and prognosis of cor pulmonale during protective ventilation for acute respiratory distress syndrome. Intensive Care Med 2013;39(10):1725–33.

75. Determann RM, Royakkers A, Wolthuis EK, et al. Ventilation with lower tidal volumes as compared with conventional tidal volumes for patients without acute lung injury: a preventive randomized controlled trial. Crit Care 2010;14(1):R1.

76. Gajic O, Dara SI, Mendez JL, et al. Ventilator-associated lung injury in patients without acute lung injury at the onset of mechanical ventilation. Crit Care Med 2004;32(9):1817–24.

77. Futier E, Constantin JM, Paugam-Burtz C, et al. A trial of intraoperative low-tidal-volume ventilation in abdominal surgery. N Engl J Med 2013;369(5):428–37.

78. Chapman CE, Stainsby D, Jones H, et al. Ten years of hemovigilance reports of transfusion-related acute lung injury in the United Kingdom and the impact of preferential use of male donor plasma. Transfusion 2009;49(3):440–52.

79. Gajic O, Rana R, Winters JL, et al. Transfusion-related acute lung injury in the critically ill: prospective nested case-control study. Am J Respir Crit Care Med 2007;176(9):886–91.

80. Eder AF, Herron RM Jr, Strupp A, et al. Effective reduction of transfusion-related acute lung injury risk with male-predominant plasma strategy in the American Red Cross (2006-2008). Transfusion 2010;50(8):1732–42.

81. Toy P, Gajic O, Bacchetti P, et al. Transfusion-related acute lung injury: incidence and risk factors. Blood 2012;119(7):1757–67.

82. Ahmed AH, Litell JM, Malinchoc M, et al. The role of potentially preventable hospital exposures in the development of acute respiratory distress syndrome: a population-based study. Crit Care Med 2014;42(1):31–9.

83. Ketoconazole for early treatment of acute lung injury and acute respiratory distress syndrome: a randomized controlled trial. The ARDS Network. JAMA 2000;283(15):1995–2002.

84. Randomized, placebo-controlled trial of lisofylline for early treatment of acute lung injury and acute respiratory distress syndrome. Crit Care Med 2002;30(1):1–6.

85. National Heart Lung, Blood Institute Acute Respiratory Distress Syndrome Clinical Trials Network, Matthay MA, Brower RG, et al. Randomized, placebo-controlled clinical trial of an aerosolized beta(2)-agonist for treatment of acute lung injury. Am J Respir Crit Care Med 2011;184(5):561–8.

86. Steinberg KP, Hudson LD, Goodman RB, et al. Efficacy and safety of corticosteroids for persistent acute respiratory distress syndrome. N Engl J Med 2006;354(16):1671–84.

87. Taylor RW, Zimmerman JL, Dellinger RP, et al. Low-dose inhaled nitric oxide in patients with acute lung injury: a randomized controlled trial. JAMA 2004;291(13):1603–9.

88. Luhr OR, Antonsen K, Karlsson M, et al. Incidence and mortality after acute respiratory failure and acute respiratory distress syndrome in Sweden, Denmark, and Iceland. The ARF Study Group. Am J Respir Crit Care Med 1999;159(6):1849–61.

89. Valta P, Uusaro A, Nunes S, et al. Acute respiratory distress syndrome: frequency, clinical course, and costs of care. Crit Care Med 1999;27(11):2367–74.

90. Goss CH, Brower RG, Hudson LD, et al. Incidence of acute lung injury in the United States. Crit Care Med 2003;31(6):1607–11.

91. Arroliga AC, Ghamra ZW, Perez Trepichio A, et al. Incidence of ARDS in an adult population of northeast Ohio. Chest 2002;121(6):1972–6.

92. Hudson LD, Steinberg KP. Epidemiology of acute lung injury and ARDS. Chest 1999;116(1 Suppl):74S–82S.

93. Linko R, Okkonen M, Pettila V, et al. Acute respiratory failure in intensive care units. FINNALI: a prospective cohort study. Intensive Care Med 2009;35(8):1352–61.

94. Sigurdsson MI, Sigvaldason K, Gunnarsson TS, et al. Acute respiratory distress syndrome: nationwide changes in incidence, treatment and mortality over 23 years. Acta Anaesthesiol Scand 2013; 57(1):37–45.

Environmental Risk Factors for Acute Respiratory Distress Syndrome

CrossMark

Farzad Moazed, MD, Carolyn S. Calfee, MD, MAS*

KEYWORDS

- Acute respiratory distress syndrome • Epidemiology • Modifiable risk factors • Alcohol abuse
- Cigarette smoking • Mechanisms • Future interventions

KEY POINTS

- Multiple observational studies have demonstrated that chronic alcohol use is a risk factor for the development of acute respiratory distress syndrome (ARDS).
- Alcohol use may promote the development of ARDS via increased angiotensin II, producing increasing oxidative stress, which creates baseline alveolar epithelial dysfunction and primes the lung for developing noncardiogenic pulmonary edema.
- Although less studied than alcohol use, cigarette smoke exposure also seems likely to be a risk factor for ARDS.
- Cigarette smoke may prime the lung to develop ARDS by creating baseline epithelial and endothelial injury, likely through direct exposure to powerful oxidants contained in cigarettes.

The acute respiratory distress syndrome (ARDS) represents a significant health burden. Despite numerous efforts to identify effective treatments, few have been successful. As a result, considerable attention has now been given to the prevention of ARDS. Although many patients present with risk factors for ARDS, only a certain subset of these patients go on to develop it. Although some of this phenomenon is likely explained by genetic factors, recent research has revealed that modifiable risk factors for ARDS also exist. Alcohol use was the first major modifiable risk factor for ARDS to be identified. Significant details have since emerged over the past 2 decades about the mechanisms that underlie this relationship. These discoveries have spurred the search for additional risk factors. Further investigation has revealed smoking as an additional risk factor for ARDS. Although the data for this second association are newer and less developed, both of

these relationships represent exciting discoveries in the quest to better understand, prevent, and treat ARDS.

ALCOHOL ABUSE

Alcohol is one of the most commonly used and abused drugs worldwide. In the United States, nearly 20 million adults annually meet the criteria for alcohol abuse or dependence.[1,2] Alcohol is known to have numerous systemic health effects, including on the liver and central nervous system.[3] From a respiratory standpoint, alcohol abuse has long been associated with an increased risk of pneumonia.[4,5] More recently, alcohol abuse has been strongly linked in epidemiologic studies to the development of ARDS in at-risk patients.

The first demonstration of an association between chronic alcohol abuse and ARDS was made by Moss and colleagues,[6] who retrospectively

Disclosure: Dr. Calfee has received grant funding from and served on medical advisory boards for Glaxo Smith Kline.

Division of Pulmonary and Critical Care Medicine, Department of Medicine, University of California San Francisco, 505 Parnassus Avenue, M1097 Box 0111, San Francisco, CA 94143-0111, USA

* Corresponding author.

E-mail address: Carolyn.calfee@ucsf.edu

Clin Chest Med 35 (2014) 625–637

http://dx.doi.org/10.1016/j.ccm.2014.08.003

examined 351 patients at risk for ARDS. In this cohort, 43% of patients who chronically abused alcohol developed ARDS compared with only 22% of those who did not abuse alcohol, with the effect most pronounced in patients with sepsis. This study was limited by its retrospective design, particularly because this design required that the history of alcohol use be obtained by chart review and documented history; furthermore, this study did not adjust for concomitant cigarette smoking. Encouraged by these findings, Moss and colleagues conducted a multicenter prospective study of 220 patients with septic shock to further assess this relationship. Methodologically, this study improved on its predecessor by using the Short Michigan Alcohol Screening Test, which has previously been validated as a screening test for chronic alcohol abuse.[7] A multivariate analysis again found that those who chronically abused alcohol developed ARDS more frequently than those who did not, 70% versus 31%, respectively.[8] These two key studies, thus, served as the first major evidence that alcohol use was a risk factor for the development of ARDS.

Several studies have since reinforced the relationship between alcohol use and ARDS. Licker and colleagues[9] examined the incidence of ARDS in 879 patients with non–small cell lung cancer undergoing thoracic surgery. Multivariate logistic regression found that preoperative chronic alcohol consumption was associated with increased odds of developing acute lung injury. In addition, 2 studies examining the risk factors for transfusion-related acute lung injury (TRALI) found that chronic alcohol consumption was associated with the development of TRALI. Gajic and colleagues[10] found that patients who developed TRALI were more likely to be chronic alcohol users when compared with matched controls, 36.5% versus 17.0%, respectively. More recently, Toy and colleagues[11] found that in a multivariate model, chronic alcohol use in patients receiving blood product transfusions significantly increased the odds of developing TRALI. A later study by Gajic and colleagues[12] that evaluated 5584 patients at risk for ARDS to determine a lung injury prediction score found alcohol to be a positive risk factor for the development of ARDS. These studies, thus, supported the prior observations and solidified the association between chronic alcohol use and ARDS (**Table 1**).

Although the relationship between chronic alcohol abuse and ARDS has been demonstrated numerous times, the effect of alcohol on ARDS outcomes has been less clear. Early studies that examined this relationship showed conflicting results. In a retrospective study, Moss and

Table 1 Studies evaluating the relationship between ARDS and alcohol use			
Author, Year	Study Size	Odds Ratio (History of Alcohol Abuse vs No Abuse)	P Value
Moss et al,[6] 1996	351	1.98[a]	<.001
Moss et al,[8] 2003	220	3.70	<.001
Licker et al,[9] 2003	879	1.87	.012
Gajic et al,[10] 2007	148	[b]	.006
Gajic et al,[12] 2011	5584	[c]	.028
Toy et al,[11] 2012	253	5.90	.028

[a] Relative risk.
[b] No odds ratio or relative risk reported. Twenty-seven of 74 patients with acute lung injury had a history of alcohol abuse versus 13 of 74 in matched controls.
[c] No odds ratio or relative risk reported. Forty-four of 377 patients with acute lung injury had a history of alcohol abuse versus 289 of 5207 in patients without acute lung injury.

colleagues[8] found that among patients who developed ARDS, those with a history of chronic alcohol abuse had a significantly higher in-hospital mortality rate compared with those that did not abuse alcohol, 65% versus 36%, respectively.[6] However, a follow-up prospective study that used a more validated measure of alcohol abuse did not demonstrate any difference in mortality in patients with ARDS when stratified by a history of alcohol abuse.

In order to better evaluate the effect of alcohol use on ARDS outcomes, Clark and colleagues[13] performed a secondary analysis of patients enrolled in 3 ARDS Network trials, albuterol to treat acute lung Injury (ALTA), early versus delayed enteral feeding (EDEN), and omega-3 fatty-acid/antioxidant supplementation (OMEGA), which examined the effects of aerosolized albuterol, omega-3 fatty acid supplementation, and early versus delayed parenteral nutrition, respectively, in patients with ARDS. Of note, all 3 studies were stopped early for futility. Participants enrolled in these trials (or their surrogates) completed the Alcohol Use Disorder Identification Test (AUDIT), a previously validated questionnaire[14] developed by the World Health Organization to stratify patients by level of alcohol consumption. In all, 1037 patients, representing 92% of all enrolled patients, had a completed AUDIT and were included in the secondary analysis performed by Clark and colleagues. A multivariate analysis that adjusted for age, sex, severity of illness, history of smoking, acute lung injury risk factor, and baseline comorbidities found that a history of severe alcohol misuse was associated with an increased risk of death or persistent hospitalization at 90 days (odds ratio = 1.78) compared with those with mild alcohol use. The investigators used mild alcohol users rather than nondrinkers as the reference group because nondrinkers had poorer outcomes, thought to be caused by comorbidities that discourage the consumption of alcohol. Thus, it seems likely that chronic alcohol abuse is associated with poor ARDS outcomes, though the data are less extensive for this association than for the association with susceptibility.

Mechanisms

Numerous studies have been performed both in animal models and humans in order to better understand the association between chronic alcohol use and ARDS. These studies have identified a central role for pulmonary immune dysfunction as well as alveolar epithelial dysfunction in the mechanistic link between alcohol and ARDS.

Pulmonary immune dysfunction
Both acute and chronic alcohol use can contribute to a dysfunctional pulmonary immune response. Acute alcohol use impairs neutrophil chemotaxis and function with subsequent decreased phagocytosis and bacterial killing.[15–17] Chronic alcohol use is similarly associated with altered neutrophil function and decreased superoxide production.[18] Chronic alcohol use decreases the levels of granulocyte/macrophage colony-stimulating factor (GM-CSF) receptor and signaling in the lung

epithelium,[19,20] which has been shown to result in defective alveolar macrophage maturation.[21] The net effect of these abnormalities is an increased pulmonary bacterial burden.

In addition to its effects on neutrophils, alcohol use has a variety of effects on cytokine production in the lung. Although acute alcohol use has been shown to impair the production of proinflammatory cytokines, such as tumor necrosis factor (TNF)-α and interleukin (IL)-1β,[22] which may predispose patients to pneumonia, chronic alcohol use has actually been associated with increased levels of proinflammatory cytokines, such as TNF-α, IL-1β, and IL-6, in both human and animal studies.[23–25] Recently, Burnham and colleagues[26] found elevated levels of Chemokine c-c motif ligand-5 (CCL-5) (also known as regulated on activation, normal T-cell expressed and secreted [RANTES]), which is a chemoattractant for a variety of immune cells,[27] in the bronchoalveolar lavage (BAL) fluid of chronic alcoholics. This increase in inflammatory cytokines seems to have a significant effect on downstream inflammation, as IL-6 was recently shown to play a key role in the pulmonary inflammatory response of alcoholic mice in a burn injury model.[26–28] This altered cytokine profile in conjunction with decreased neutrophil and alveolar macrophage function is thought to contribute to the development of ARDS in alcohol abusers.

Alveolar epithelial dysfunction
In addition to its effects on the lung inflammatory response, chronic alcohol use may also predispose to ARDS development by causing increased pulmonary oxidative stress and alveolar epithelial dysfunction. These effects are mediated in part via the renin-angiotensin system (**Fig. 1**). Chronic alcohol use has long been known to increase

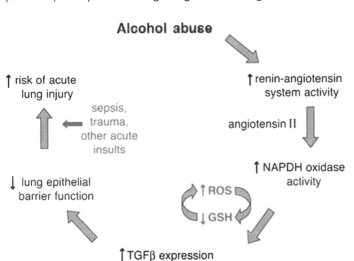

Alcohol abuse

↑ risk of acute lung injury

sepsis, trauma, other acute insults

↓ lung epithelial barrier function

↑ renin-angiotensin system activity

angiotensin II

↑ NAPDH oxidase activity

↑ ROS
↓ GSH

↑ TGFβ expression and activation

Fig. 1. Potential mechanism by which alcohol primes the lung for ARDS. GSH, glutathione; NADPH, nicotinamide adenine dinucleotide phosphate; ROS, reactive oxygen species; TGF-β, transforming growth factor-β. (*From* Kershaw CD, Guidot DM. Alcoholic lung disease. Alcohol Res Health 2008;31(1):71.)

activation of this system, resulting in elevated levels of angiotensin II in humans.[29,30] Angiotensin II may contribute to alveolar epithelial dysfunction through a variety of mechanisms, including via the systemic effects on vascular tone and fluid retention as well as via localized effects, such as promoting apoptosis of alveolar epithelial cells.[31] In addition, angiotensin II activates nicotinamide adenine dinucleotide phosphate (NADPH) oxidase in the lung, resulting in elevated levels of reactive oxygen species.[32,33] This increase in reactive oxygen species (ROS) results in depletion in alveolar levels of the key antioxidant glutathione (GSH) and increases in alveolar oxidized glutathione (GSSG), a phenomenon seen both in animal models[34] and humans who abuse alcohol.[35]

Patients with ARDS have been shown to demonstrate the same derangement with regard to pulmonary glutathione.[36,37] This alteration in glutathione results in decreased antioxidant capacity in the lung and has further been linked to decreased surfactant synthesis[38,39] and increased type II cell apoptosis.[40] Additionally, the depletion of glutathione seems to increase the levels of latent transforming growth factor (TGF)-β, which subsequently contributes to baseline alveolar epithelial dysfunction, manifested by increased permeability and lung edema.[41] The net result of increased activation of this pathway is an alveolar epithelium that is already dysfunctional and, thus, primed for developing ARDS when faced with an acute insult (**Fig. 2**).

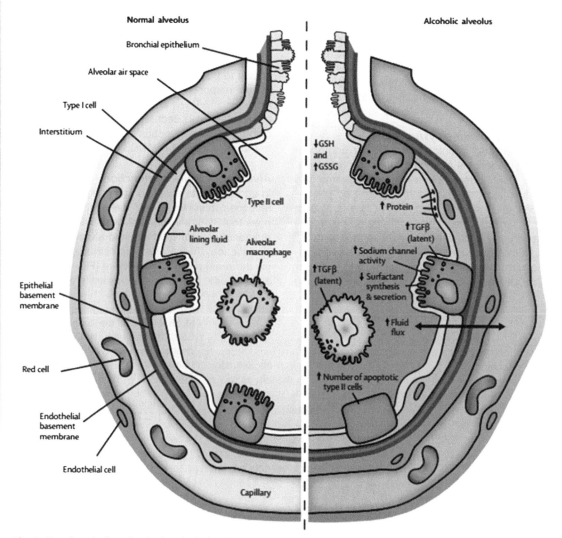

Fig. 2. Baseline dysfunction in the alcoholic alveolus. (*From* Moss M, Burnham EL. Alcohol abuse in the critically ill patient. Lancet 2006;368:2237; with permission.)

Future Interventions

The high prevalence of alcohol abuse worldwide and its association with ARDS present a unique opportunity to improve patient outcomes. Although decreasing the prevalence of alcohol abuse remains an important goal, in addition, the unique mechanistic abnormalities involved in this relationship provide several potentially exciting therapeutic targets for alcoholic patients either at risk for or with ARDS.

One potential therapeutic intervention would be to attempt to increase glutathione levels, which play such a key role in the alveolar epithelial dysfunction observed with alcohol use. The use of N-acetyl-cysteine (NAC), a glutathione precursor, is one potential approach. In both endotoxin and microembolism rat models of ARDS, pretreatment with intravenous (IV) NAC attenuated lung injury.[42,43] Prior small clinical trials have shown that the administration of IV NAC increases glutathione levels in patients with ARDS, although no significant improvement in outcomes was observed (ventilator-free days or mortality).[44–46] However, these studies included small heterogeneous samples of patients with ARDS, rather than focusing on only those with a history of alcohol abuse. It remains unclear whether the administration of glutathione would be a successful therapeutic strategy in alcoholic patients either at risk for or who have already developed ARDS.

Given the role angiotensin II seems to play in altering glutathione levels, the renin-angiotensin system also presents a potential therapeutic target for alcoholic patients with ARDS. Some data suggest that angiotensin-converting enzyme (ACE) polymorphisms that increase angiotensin II levels may affect the risk of developing ARDS and mortality. Marshall and colleagues[47] found that an ACE genotype that causes increased ACE activity was more prevalent in Caucasian patients with ARDS compared with other intensive care unit patients or the general population. Furthermore, among patients with ARDS, this genotype was associated with increased mortality. A later study by Villar and colleagues[48] in Spanish patients did not find a similar relationship. However, a recent meta-analysis by Matsuda and colleagues[49] of nearly 5000 patients with ARDS, including Caucasian and Asian ethnicities, found that ACE genotypes associated with increased activity were associated with an increased risk of mortality from ARDS in Asian populations. These findings, in conjunction with studies in mice that show decreased ACE activity to be protective in animal models of acid aspiration and sepsis-induced ARDS,[50] make the renin-angiotensin system an intriguing therapeutic target. To date, there has been no formal evaluation of the role of ACE inhibitors or angiotensin-receptor blockers (ARB) in patients with ARDS, including alcoholic patients. Although the utility of these agents may be limited because patients with ARDS also often have shock or renal failure, further studies would be required to determine any potential benefits.

The GM-CSF depleted state that is induced by chronic alcohol use also serves as a potential therapeutic target for patients with ARDS. Treatment of alcohol-fed rats with GM-CSF has been shown to improve not only alveolar macrophage function[20] but also decreased alveolar permeability and increased lung edema fluid clearance.[51] Likewise, elevated levels of bronchoalveolar lavage fluid GM-CSF are associated with improved mortality in patients with ARDS.[52] A phase II trial that randomized patients with ARDS to GM-CSF versus placebo showed improved oxygenation with no adverse effects.[53] However, this study as well as a larger phase II randomized clinical trial of GM-CSF versus placebo found no improvement in outcomes, such as ventilator-free days, organ failure–free days, or mortality.[53,54] Whether GM-CSF would improve outcomes in patients with ARDS with a history of chronic alcohol use remains unknown.

SMOKING

Smoking remains a global epidemic. Although antismoking efforts in the United States continue to slowly decrease the rate of smoking among adults (currently 18.1%),[55] tobacco use continues to be the leading cause of preventable death both in the United States and worldwide, killing nearly 6 million people annually.[56] Although many harmful effects of smoking, particularly on the lung, have been known for quite some time, the link between ARDS and smoking has been established only recently.

Early studies investigating the relationship between smoking history and ARDS suggested a possible association, though the findings were inconsistent. Christenson and colleagues[57] studied nearly 4000 patients undergoing cardiac surgery and found in multivariable analysis that a clinical history of being an active smoker was associated with an increased risk of developing ARDS. However, this study did not address or adjust for alcohol use. A later study by Iribarren and colleagues[58] retrospectively studied a large cohort of patients in a single health plan network, 56 of whom went on to develop ARDS. Multivariate analysis showed that a history of active cigarette smoking was associated with increased odds of developing ARDS. Increased amounts of smoking (>20 cigarettes per day) were associated with an even greater odds of developing ARDS. Although this study did adjust for chronic alcohol use among patients, it was limited by its retrospective nature and the use of diagnostic coding, which detects a low prevalence of ARDS. In contrast to these positive studies, a multicenter observational study by Gajic and colleagues[12] of 5584 patients at risk for ARDS did not find cigarette smoking to be a predictive risk factor for developing ARDS. The conflicting findings of these studies may be caused in large part by reliance on smoking history. Recent studies have determined that biomarkers of tobacco use, such as plasma cotinine, are significantly more sensitive for tobacco exposure in critically ill patients compared with self-reported histories.[59]

To further investigate this possible association, Calfee and colleagues[60] prospectively measured plasma cotinine levels in blunt trauma patients at risk for ARDS. Additionally, alcohol exposure was measured by both clinical history and AUDIT surveys. Increasing levels of plasma cotinine were associated with an increased risk of developing ARDS. In a multivariate model, including adjustments for alcohol use, both active smoking as well as moderate to severe passive smoke exposure predicted the development of ARDS. These findings were the first to link smoking to ARDS using biomarkers and also to identify secondhand smoke as a potential risk factor for ARDS development. If confirmed, these findings may have important public health implications, particularly with regard to public smoking bans. Despite the strengths of this study, its findings were limited by its homogenous study population, all of whom were victims of severe blunt trauma enrolled at a single center.

Since then, studies in different patient populations have provided additional evidence in support of an association between smoking and ARDS. Toy and colleagues[11] found that active smoking was associated with an increased risk of TRALI, after adjustment for other predictors. Likewise, Diamond and colleagues[61] conducted a multicenter study of 1255 lung transplant patients to identify risk factors for primary graft dysfunction (PGD), a form of acute lung injury that occurs within 72 hours of lung transplant. In this analysis, donor smoking was associated with increased odds of developing PGD, a finding that persisted after adjustment for other predictors. These studies add to the growing body of literature that supports an association between smoking and ARDS (**Table 2**).

Table 2
Studies examining the relationship between smoking and ARDS

Author, Year	Study Size	Odds Ratio (Active Smokers vs Nonsmokers)	P Value
Christenson et al,[57] 1996	3848	2.01[a]	<.001
Iribarren et al,[58] 2000	121,012	2.85 (<1 pack/d)[a] 4.59 (≥1 pack/d)[a]	<.05 <.05
Gajic et al,[12] 2011	5584	[b]	NS
Calfee et al,[60] 2011	144	2.77	.01
Toy et al,[11] 2012	253	3.40	.02
Diamond et al,[61] 2013	1255	1.80	.002

Abbreviation: NS, not significant.
[a] Relative risk.
[b] No odds ratio or relative risk reported. A total of 107 of 377 patients with acute lung injury had a history of active smoking versus 1239 of 5207 in patients without acute lung injury.

There are limited data on the outcomes of smokers who develop ARDS. One small study examined 47 patients with ARDS and found that nonsurvivors were more likely to be smokers than survivors.[62] A recent study by Hsieh and colleagues[63] sought to better evaluate this question using 381 patients with ARDS from the ALTA and OMEGA ARDS Network randomized controlled trials. Urine 4-(methylnitrosamino)-1-(3-pyridyl)-1-butanol, a well-validated biomarker of tobacco use with a 2-week half-life,[64] was used to stratify patients by smoking exposure status. Although active smokers were found to be younger, with significantly lower severity of illness scores and fewer comorbidities, they had a similar severity of lung injury as measured by either the Berlin Definition or Murray Lung Injury Score, raising the possibility that smokers may be more prone to developing ARDS with a lower severity of illness. Although smoking was associated with lower mortality in unadjusted analysis, a multivariate analysis that controlled for the disparities in age, comorbidities, and severity of illness between smokers and nonsmokers showed no association between smoking status and 60-day mortality.

Mechanism

The mechanisms through which smoking contributes to the development of ARDS remain under investigation (**Fig. 3**). In contrast to alcohol, there are relatively few laboratory-based studies explicitly evaluating the relationship between smoking and ARDS; thus, inferences about the potential mechanisms of association between smoking and ARDS must largely be extrapolated from studies on smoking's effects on the lungs in other experimental settings. With this caveat, the mechanisms linking smoking and ARDS likely involve pulmonary immune dysfunction (as with chronic alcohol use) as well as dysfunction of both the alveolar epithelium and endothelium.

Pulmonary immune dysfunction

Smoking impairs pulmonary immune function through a variety of pathways. Smoking has numerous direct effects on innate and adaptive immunity that increase the risk of infection.[65] These effects include impaired mucociliary function, decreased surfactant production, altered T-cell responses, depressed natural killer cell function, and decreased immunoglobulin levels.[66,67] Additionally, cigarette smoke has been shown to lower the rate of bacterial clearance by alveolar macrophages.[68–70] This decrease in bacterial clearance, in turn, is thought to result in an influx of neutrophils into surrounding tissues, with an associated increase in proinflammatory cytokines and an elevated proteolytic burden.[68] Furthermore, smoking promotes biofilm formation,[71] which plays a role in the increased risk of respiratory infection in smokers.[72,73] This impairment in immunity and predisposition to infection is one potential mechanism by which smoking may increase the risk of ARDS.

Alveolar epithelial dysfunction

Since the 1980s, studies have demonstrated increased alveolar epithelial permeability in smokers compared with nonsmokers,[74] mimicking a key pathophysiologic feature of ARDS. This effect on alveolar permeability may be related to the neutrophil influx observed with smoking, though studies on this mechanistic link have reported conflicting findings. Animal studies by Bhalla and colleagues[75] found that reducing pulmonary neutrophils improved alveolar permeability. However, in similar animal studies, Kleeberger and Hudak[76] found that reducing this neutrophil influx did not attenuate epithelial permeability. A more recent study by Li and colleagues[77] also found that neutrophil depletion did not improve epithelial permeability, suggesting that other mechanisms must also be playing a role.

Since then, several studies have shown that the profound oxidant effect of smoking[78] may be one of the major contributors to the alveolar epithelial dysfunction seen in smokers. Li and colleagues[77] demonstrated that intratracheal inhalation of cigarette smoke in rats resulted in decreased levels of total BAL fluid glutathione with increases in the oxidized form, GSSG. In animal models, this

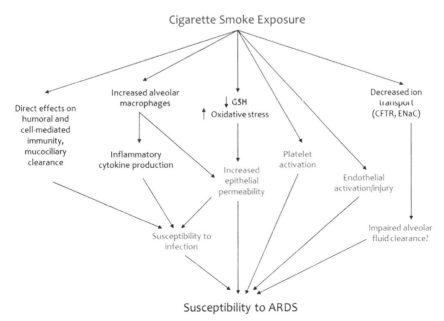

Fig. 3. Mechanisms through which smoking may prime the lung for ARDS. CFTR, cystic fibrosis transmembrane conductance regulator; ENAC, epithelial sodium channel.

phenomenon has been linked to increases in alveolar epithelial permeability, whereas increasing intracellular glutathione has been shown to ameliorate this effect.[79] These findings are remarkably similar to those seen in the setting of alcohol abuse, although the timing of the effects are different: specifically, pulmonary glutathione depletion in alcohol users seems to be more of a chronic phenomenon, whereas in animal models of smoking, the effect is acute, lasting only 6 hours. In an attempt to replicate these findings in humans, Morrison and colleagues[80] performed lung scans to measure alveolar permeability in human subjects. They found that chronic smokers had increased alveolar permeability compared with nonsmokers and that permeability increased even further after chronic smokers acutely smoked a cigarette. However, unlike in animal models, this study did not find any statistically significant difference in BAL fluid glutathione levels between smokers or nonsmokers, suggesting that other mechanisms likely contribute to this phenomenon. Recent evidence shows that cigarette smoke likely disrupts tight junction integrity through an epidermal growth factor receptor pathway,[81,82] which could help explain the increased alveolar permeability seen in smokers. Additionally, cigarette smoke decreases the expression of the primary ion channels responsible for resolving alveolar edema,[83,84] which likely further contributes to baseline epithelial dysfunction.

Endothelial and platelet dysfunction

The damage caused by cigarette smoke on the lungs is not limited to the alveolar epithelium. Smoking also causes vascular endothelial injury and alters endothelial function, a key pathophysiologic change that is also seen in ARDS. Early animal models demonstrated that cigarette smoke increases pulmonary endothelial permeability.[85] Since then, further study has confirmed that cigarette smoke increases lung vascular permeability and worsens lipopolysaccharide-induced lung edema.[86,87] The increased endothelial permeability observed with exposure to cigarette smoke seems to be at least in part mediated by increased levels of ROS in the lung and furthermore is attenuated by NAC.[86,87] This increase in ROS seems to have several downstream targets, including inhibition of Rho A[86] and activation of mitogen-activated protein kinases,[87] that ultimately result in changes to the cytoskeleton resulting in endothelial barrier dysfunction. It is notable that ROS seem to play a key role in both the epithelial and endothelial dysfunction caused by smoking.

Like endothelial dysfunction, to which it is closely linked, platelet dysfunction has long been noted to be a characteristic feature of ARDS.[88,89] Patients with ARDS have been observed to have increased procoagulant and decreased fibrinolytic activity in the alveolar lining layer and microvasculature.[90] These abnormalities promote pulmonary fibrin deposition[91] and can result in microthrombi in small vessels, as pulmonary arterial thrombi and distal filling defects of the microvasculature have been detected in patients with ARDS.[92] These factors likely contribute significantly to gas exchange abnormalities seen in patients with ARDS.[88] Cigarette smoke has been noted to have similar effects on platelets. Both active and passive smoking have been observed to increase platelet activation, predisposing to thrombus.[93] Additionally, platelet activation also results in damage to the endothelium, which can result in vasoconstriction and further prothrombotic and proinflammatory states and cell proliferation in the vessel walls.[93] The effects of secondhand smoke on endothelial and platelet dysfunction are approximately 90% of those of active smoking.[93] Thus, the effects of cigarette smoking on platelets likely plays a key role in contributing to endothelial dysfunction, which may further predispose smokers to ARDS.

Future Directions

Because the mechanistic links between smoking and ARDS are less well defined than those between alcohol and ARDS, the identification of potential targeted therapies is more challenging. One potential area of intervention is the increased oxidative stress caused by cigarettes, which seems to play a key role in both the alveolar epithelial and endothelial abnormalities associated with smoking. Given that chronic alcohol use seems to further affect the antioxidant system and frequently coexists with cigarette smoking in patients, the antioxidant system becomes an even more exciting source for potential intervention. As mentioned previously, studies that examined the use of NAC to replenish the antioxidant system did not show any improvement in outcomes in patients with ARDS. However, this specific population, which may have decreased antioxidant function at baseline, may merit further study. Furthermore, it may be useful to assess the effect of treating this population with NAC while they are at risk for lung injury, as opposed to afterward once the inflammatory response is well established. Further investigation is clearly needed to better understand the relationship between smoking and ARDS in order to identify additional potential therapeutic targets. Meanwhile, continued public health interventions, such as antismoking campaigns and public smoking bans, may help decrease the burden of smoking-associated ARDS.

AIR POLLUTION

Air pollution has been associated with a variety of adverse health outcomes, including all-cause mortality.[94] It is thought that this phenomenon is driven primarily by an increase in cardiorespiratory events. Several epidemiologic studies have shown that air pollution is associated with an increased risk of myocardial infarction and cardiovascular disease mortality.[95–98] The association between air pollution and respiratory mortality is less clear, with some studies showing an increase in respiratory mortality,[94,99,100] whereas other studies have found no such relationship.[101–103] Although the association between air pollution and respiratory mortality is not entirely clear, air pollution has been associated with respiratory morbidities, including increased susceptibility to airway infection[104] and decreased lung function.[105] However, there are no epidemiologic studies that examine the relationship between air pollution and ARDS.

Despite the lack of epidemiologic studies involving a possible association between air pollution and ARDS, there are several reasons to hypothesize that such a relationship may exist. First, cigarette smoke and ambient air pollution share many of the same compounds, such as ozone and particulate matter less than 2.5 μm. Given that cigarette smoke has previously been shown to be a risk factor for ARDS,[11,57,58,60,61] it is plausible that air pollution may pose a similar risk. Second, air pollution and its constituents have been associated with changes in the lung that mimic those of ARDS. Studies in humans demonstrate that air pollution is associated with increased pulmonary inflammation, oxidative stress,[106] and endothelial dysfunction,[107] whereas ozone exposure has been associated with increased epithelial permeability.[108] These findings suggest that, like cigarette smoke, air pollution may prime the lung to develop ARDS by causing increased baseline inflammation as well as epithelial and endothelial dysfunction. However, additional studies are needed to better examine the potential relationship between air pollution and ARDS in humans.

SUMMARY

Significant progress has been made since the search for environmental risk factors for ARDS began nearly 2 decades ago. Chronic alcohol use and smoking have been identified in numerous studies to independently increase the risk of developing ARDS and potentially affect the outcomes of patients who go on to develop the disease. These findings have important implications for public health and for ARDS prevention. Additionally, scientific studies have yielded tremendous insight into many of the mechanisms involved in the relationship between chronic alcohol use and ARDS, and numerous potential viable therapeutic targets have been identified that may enable clinicians to better treat chronic alcohol users with ARDS. Mechanistic studies into the relationship between smoking and ARDS are less developed and represent an important area for future investigation. Future studies are also needed to define the overlap or potential synergy between these two exposures because smoking and alcohol use often coexist in patients. Finally, further epidemiologic study is needed to determine if there are additional environmental factors, such as air pollution, that may also be associated with an increased risk of developing ARDS.

REFERENCES

1. Grant BF, Dawson DA, Stinson FS, et al. The 12-month prevalence and trends in DSM-IV alcohol abuse and dependence: United States, 1991-1992 and 2001-2002. Drug Alcohol Depend 2004;74(3): 223–34.
2. Grant BF. Prevalence and correlates of alcohol use and DSM-IV alcohol dependence in the United States: results of the National Longitudinal Alcohol Epidemiologic Survey. J Stud Alcohol 1997;58(5): 464–73.
3. Moss M, Burnham EL. Alcohol abuse in the critically ill patient. Lancet 2006;368(9554):2231–42.
4. Almirall J, Bolibar I, Serra-Prat M, et al. New evidence of risk factors for community-acquired pneumonia: a population-based study. Eur Respir J 2008;31(6):1274–84.
5. Fernandez-Sola J, Junque A, Estruch R, et al. High alcohol intake as a risk and prognostic factor for community-acquired pneumonia. Arch Intern Med 1995;155(15):1649–54.
6. Moss M, Bucher B, Moore FA, et al. The role of chronic alcohol abuse in the development of acute respiratory distress syndrome in adults. JAMA 1996;275(1):50–4.
7. Selzer ML, Vinokur A, van Rooijen L. A self-administered Short Michigan Alcoholism Screening Test (SMAST). J Stud Alcohol 1975;36(1):117–26.
8. Moss M, Parsons PE, Steinberg KP, et al. Chronic alcohol abuse is associated with an increased incidence of acute respiratory distress syndrome and severity of multiple organ dysfunction in patients with septic shock. Crit Care Med 2003; 31(3):869–77.

9. Licker M, de Perrot M, Spiliopoulos A, et al. Risk factors for acute lung injury after thoracic surgery for lung cancer. Anesth Analg 2003;97(6):1558–65.

10. Gajic O, Rana R, Winters JL, et al. Transfusion-related acute lung injury in the critically ill: prospective nested case-control study. Am J Respir Crit Care Med 2007;176(9):886–91.

11. Toy P, Gajic O, Bacchetti P, et al. Transfusion-related acute lung injury: incidence and risk factors. Blood 2012;119(7):1757–67.

12. Gajic O, Dabbagh O, Park PK, et al. Early identification of patients at risk of acute lung injury: evaluation of lung injury prediction score in a multicenter cohort study. Am J Respir Crit Care Med 2011; 183(4):462–70.

13. Clark BJ, Williams A, Feemster LM, et al. Alcohol screening scores and 90-day outcomes in patients with acute lung injury. Crit Care Med 2013;41(6): 1518–25.

14. Donovan DM, Dunn CW, Rivara FP, et al. Comparison of trauma center patient self-reports and proxy reports on the Alcohol Use Identification Test (AUDIT). J Trauma 2004;56(4):873–82.

15. Boe DM, Nelson S, Zhang P, et al. Acute ethanol intoxication suppresses lung chemokine production following infection with Streptococcus pneumoniae. J Infect Dis 2001;184(9):1134–42.

16. Nilsson E, Lindstrom P, Patarroyo M, et al. Ethanol impairs certain aspects of neutrophil adhesion in vitro: comparisons with inhibition of expression of the CD18 antigen. J Infect Dis 1991;163(3):591–7.

17. MacGregor RR, Spagnuolo PJ, Lentnek AL. Inhibition of granulocyte adherence by ethanol, prednisone, and aspirin, measured with an assay system. N Engl J Med 1974;291(13):642–6.

18. Greenberg SS, Zhao X, Hua L, et al. Ethanol inhibits lung clearance of Pseudomonas aeruginosa by a neutrophil and nitric oxide-dependent mechanism, in vivo. Alcohol Clin Exp Res 1999;23(4):735–44.

19. Joshi PC, Applewhite L, Mitchell PO, et al. GM-CSF receptor expression and signaling is decreased in lungs of ethanol-fed rats. Am J Physiol Lung Cell Mol Physiol 2006;291(6):L1150–8.

20. Joshi PC, Applewhite L, Ritzenthaler JD, et al. Chronic ethanol ingestion in rats decreases granulocyte-macrophage colony-stimulating factor receptor expression and downstream signaling in the alveolar macrophage. J Immunol 2005; 175(10):6837–45.

21. Dranoff G, Crawford AD, Sadelain M, et al. Involvement of granulocyte-macrophage colony-stimulating factor in pulmonary homeostasis. Science 1994;264(5159):713–6.

22. Standiford TJ, Danforth JM. Ethanol feeding inhibits proinflammatory cytokine expression from murine alveolar macrophages ex vivo. Alcohol Clin Exp Res 1997;21(7):1212–7.

23. Deviere J, Content J, Denys C, et al. High interleukin-6 serum levels and increased production by leucocytes in alcoholic liver cirrhosis. Correlation with IgA serum levels and lymphokines production. Clin Exp Immunol 1989;77(2):221–5.

24. Crews FT, Bechara R, Brown LA, et al. Cytokines and alcohol. Alcohol Clin Exp Res 2006;30(4): 720–30.

25. McClain CJ, Cohen DA. Increased tumor necrosis factor production by monocytes in alcoholic hepatitis. Hepatology 1989;9(3):349–51.

26. Burnham EL, Kovacs EJ, Davis CS. Pulmonary cytokine composition differs in the setting of alcohol use disorders and cigarette smoking. Am J Physiol Lung Cell Mol Physiol 2013;304(12): L873–82.

27. Schall TJ, Bacon K, Toy KJ, et al. Selective attraction of monocytes and T lymphocytes of the memory phenotype by cytokine RANTES. Nature 1990; 347(6294):669–71.

28. Chen MM, Bird MD, Zahs A, et al. Pulmonary inflammation after ethanol exposure and burn injury is attenuated in the absence of IL-6. Alcohol 2013; 47(3):223–9.

29. Puddey IB, Beilin LJ, Vandongen R. Regular alcohol use raises blood pressure in treated hypertensive subjects. A randomised controlled trial. Lancet 1987;1(8534):647–51.

30. Linkola J, Fyhrquist F, Ylikahri R. Renin, aldosterone and cortisol during ethanol intoxication and hangover. Acta Physiol Scand 1979;106(1):75–82.

31. Wang R, Ramos C, Joshi I, et al. Human lung myofibroblast-derived inducers of alveolar epithelial apoptosis identified as angiotensin peptides. Am J Physiol 1999;277(6 Pt 1):L1158–64.

32. Bechara RI, Pelaez A, Palacio A, et al. Angiotensin II mediates glutathione depletion, transforming growth factor-beta1 expression, and epithelial barrier dysfunction in the alcoholic rat lung. Am J Physiol Lung Cell Mol Physiol 2005;289(3):L363–70.

33. Polikandriotis JA, Rupnow HL, Elms SC, et al. Chronic ethanol ingestion increases superoxide production and NADPH oxidase expression in the lung. Am J Respir Cell Mol Biol 2006;34(3): 314–9.

34. Guidot DM, Modelska K, Lois M, et al. Ethanol ingestion via glutathione depletion impairs alveolar epithelial barrier function in rats. Am J Physiol Lung Cell Mol Physiol 2000;279(1):L127–35.

35. Moss M, Guidot DM, Wong-Lambertina M, et al. The effects of chronic alcohol abuse on pulmonary glutathione homeostasis. Am J Respir Crit Care Med 2000;161(2 Pt 1):414–9.

36. Pacht ER, Timerman AP, Lykens MG, et al. Deficiency of alveolar fluid glutathione in patients with sepsis and the adult respiratory distress syndrome. Chest 1991;100(5):1397–403.

37. Bunnell E, Pacht ER. Oxidized glutathione is increased in the alveolar fluid of patients with the adult respiratory distress syndrome. Am Rev Respir Dis 1993;148(5):1174–8.

38. Holguin F, Moss I, Brown LA, et al. Chronic ethanol ingestion impairs alveolar type II cell glutathione homeostasis and function and predisposes to endotoxin-mediated acute edematous lung injury in rats. J Clin Invest 1998;101(4):761–8.

39. Velasquez A, Bechara RI, Lewis JF, et al. Glutathione replacement preserves the functional surfactant phospholipid pool size and decreases sepsis-mediated lung dysfunction in ethanol-fed rats. Alcohol Clin Exp Res 2002;26(8):1245–51.

40. Brown LA, Harris FL, Bechara R, et al. Effect of chronic ethanol ingestion on alveolar type II cell: glutathione and inflammatory mediator-induced apoptosis. Alcohol Clin Exp Res 2001;25(7):1078–85.

41. Bechara RI, Brown LA, Roman J, et al. Transforming growth factor beta1 expression and activation is increased in the alcoholic rat lung. Am J Respir Crit Care Med 2004;170(2):188–94.

42. Wegener T, Sandhagen B, Saldeen T. Effect of N-acetylcysteine on pulmonary damage due to microembolism in the rat. Eur J Respir Dis 1987; 70(4):205–12.

43. Davreux CJ, Soric I, Nathens AB, et al. N-acetyl cysteine attenuates acute lung injury in the rat. Shock 1997;8(6):432–8.

44. Suter PM, Domenighetti G, Schaller MD, et al. N-acetylcysteine enhances recovery from acute lung injury in man. A randomized, double-blind, placebo-controlled clinical study. Chest 1994;105(1):190–4.

45. Bernard GR, Wheeler AP, Arons MM, et al. A trial of antioxidants N-acetylcysteine and procysteine in ARDS. The Antioxidant in ARDS Study Group. Chest 1997;112(1):164–72.

46. Domenighetti G, Suter PM, Schaller MD, et al. Treatment with N-acetylcysteine during acute respiratory distress syndrome: a randomized, double-blind, placebo-controlled clinical study. J Crit Care 1997; 12(4):177–82.

47. Marshall RP, Webb S, Bellingan GJ, et al. Angiotensin converting enzyme insertion/deletion polymorphism is associated with susceptibility and outcome in acute respiratory distress syndrome. Am J Respir Crit Care Med 2002;166(5):646–50.

48. Villar J, Flores C, Perez-Mendez L, et al. Angiotensin-converting enzyme insertion/deletion polymorphism is not associated with susceptibility and outcome in sepsis and acute respiratory distress syndrome. Intensive Care Med 2008;34(3):488–95.

49. Matsuda A, Kishi T, Jacob A, et al. Association between insertion/deletion polymorphism in angiotensin-converting enzyme gene and acute lung injury/acute respiratory distress syndrome: a meta-analysis. BMC Med Genet 2012;13:76.

50. Imai Y, Kuba K, Rao S, et al. Angiotensin-converting enzyme 2 protects from severe acute lung failure. Nature 2005;436(7047):112–6.

51. Pelaez A, Bechara RI, Joshi PC, et al. Granulocyte/macrophage colony-stimulating factor treatment improves alveolar epithelial barrier function in alcoholic rat lung. Am J Physiol Lung Cell Mol Physiol 2004;286(1):L106–11.

52. Matute-Bello G, Liles WC, Radella F 2nd, et al. Modulation of neutrophil apoptosis by granulocyte colony-stimulating factor and granulocyte/macrophage colony-stimulating factor during the course of acute respiratory distress syndrome. Crit Care Med 2000;28(1):1–7.

53. Presneill JJ, Harris T, Stewart AG, et al. A randomized phase II trial of granulocyte-macrophage colony-stimulating factor therapy in severe sepsis with respiratory dysfunction. Am J Respir Crit Care Med 2002; 166(2):138–43.

54. Paine R 3rd, Standiford TJ, Dechert RE, et al. A randomized trial of recombinant human granulocyte-macrophage colony stimulating factor for patients with acute lung injury. Crit Care Med 2012;40(1):90–7.

55. Centers for Disease Control and Prevention (CDC). Vital signs: current cigarette smoking among adults aged >/=18 years–United States, 2005–2010. MMWR Morb Mortal Wkly Rep 2011; 60(35):1207–12.

56. World Health Organization. WHO report on the global tobacco epidemic. Geneva (Switzerland): World Health Organization; 2013.

57. Christenson JT, Aeberhard JM, Badel P, et al. Adult respiratory distress syndrome after cardiac surgery. Cardiovasc Surg 1996;4(1):15–21.

58. Iribarren C, Jacobs DR Jr, Sidney S, et al. Cigarette smoking, alcohol consumption, and risk of ARDS: a 15-year cohort study in a managed care setting. Chest 2000;117(1):163–8.

59. Hsieh SJ, Ware LB, Eisner MD, et al. Biomarkers increase detection of active smoking and secondhand smoke exposure in critically ill patients. Crit Care Med 2011;39(1):40–5.

60. Calfee CS, Matthay MA, Eisner MD, et al. Active and passive cigarette smoking and acute lung injury after severe blunt trauma. Am J Respir Crit Care Med 2011;183(12):1660–5.

61. Diamond JM, Lee JC, Kawut SM, et al. Clinical risk factors for primary graft dysfunction after lung transplantation. Am J Respir Crit Care Med 2013; 187(5):527–34.

62. Ando K, Doi T, Moody SY, et al. The effect of comorbidity on the prognosis of acute lung injury and acute respiratory distress syndrome. Intern Med 2012;51(14):1835–40.

63. Hsieh SJ, Zhuo H, Benowitz NL, et al. Prevalence and impact of active and passive cigarette smoking

in acute respiratory distress syndrome. Crit Care Med 2014;42(9):2058–68.

64. Goniewicz ML, Eisner MD, Lazcano-Ponce E, et al. Comparison of urine cotinine and the tobacco-specific nitrosamine metabolite 4-(methylnitrosamino)-1-(3-pyridyl)-1-butanol (NNAL) and their ratio to discriminate active from passive smoking. Nicotine Tob Res 2011;13(3):202–8.

65. Edwards D. Immunological effects of tobacco smoking in "healthy" smokers. COPD 2009;6(1): 48–58.

66. Sopori M. Effects of cigarette smoke on the immune system. Nat Rev Immunol 2002;2(5):372–7.

67. Mehta H, Nazzal K, Sadikot RT. Cigarette smoking and innate immunity. Inflamm Res 2008;57(11): 497–503.

68. Drannik AG, Pouladi MA, Robbins CS, et al. Impact of cigarette smoke on clearance and inflammation after Pseudomonas aeruginosa infection. Am J Respir Crit Care Med 2004;170(11):1164–71.

69. Phipps JC, Aronoff DM, Curtis JL, et al. Cigarette smoke exposure impairs pulmonary bacterial clearance and alveolar macrophage complement-mediated phagocytosis of Streptococcus pneumoniae. Infect Immun 2010;78(3):1214–20.

70. Marti-Lliteras P, Regueiro V, Morey P, et al. Nontypeable Haemophilus influenzae clearance by alveolar macrophages is impaired by exposure to cigarette smoke. Infect Immun 2009;77(10):4232–42.

71. Mutepe ND, Cockeran R, Steel HC, et al. Effects of cigarette smoke condensate on pneumococcal biofilm formation and pneumolysin. Eur Respir J 2013;41(2):392–5.

72. Sanz Herrero F, Blanquer Olivas J. Microbiology and risk factors for community-acquired pneumonia. Semin Respir Crit Care Med 2012;33(3): 220–31.

73. Fung HB, Monteagudo-Chu MO. Community-acquired pneumonia in the elderly. Am J Geriatr Pharmacother 2010;8(1):47–62.

74. Jones JG, Minty BD, Lawler P, et al. Increased alveolar epithelial permeability in cigarette smokers. Lancet 1980;1(8159):66–8.

75. Bhalla DK, Daniels DS, Luu NT. Attenuation of ozone-induced airway permeability in rats by pretreatment with cyclophosphamide, FPL 55712, and indomethacin. Am J Respir Cell Mol Biol 1992;7(1):73–80.

76. Kleeberger SR, Hudak BB. Acute ozone-induced change in airway permeability: role of infiltrating leukocytes. J Appl Physiol (1985) 1992;72(2):670–6.

77. Li XY, Rahman I, Donaldson K, et al. Mechanisms of cigarette smoke induced increased airspace permeability. Thorax 1996;51(5):465–71.

78. Church DF, Pryor WA. Free-radical chemistry of cigarette smoke and its toxicological implications. Environ Health Perspect 1985;64:111–26.

79. Li XY, Donaldson K, Rahman I, et al. An investigation of the role of glutathione in increased epithelial permeability induced by cigarette smoke in vivo and in vitro. Am J Respir Crit Care Med 1994; 149(6):1518–25.

80. Morrison D, Rahman I, Lannan S, et al. Epithelial permeability, inflammation, and oxidant stress in the air spaces of smokers. Am J Respir Crit Care Med 1999;159(2):473–9.

81. Petecchia L, Sabatini F, Varesio L, et al. Bronchial airway epithelial cell damage following exposure to cigarette smoke includes disassembly of tight junction components mediated by the extracellular signal-regulated kinase 1/2 pathway. Chest 2009; 135(6):1502–12.

82. Heijink IH, Brandenburg SM, Postma DS, et al. Cigarette smoke impairs airway epithelial barrier function and cell-cell contact recovery. Eur Respir J 2012; 39(2):419–28.

83. Xu H, Ferro TJ, Chu S. Cigarette smoke condensate inhibits ENaC alpha-subunit expression in lung epithelial cells. Eur Respir J 2007;30(4): 633–42.

84. Cantin AM, Hanrahan JW, Bilodeau G, et al. Cystic fibrosis transmembrane conductance regulator function is suppressed in cigarette smokers. Am J Respir Crit Care Med 2006;173(10):1139–44.

85. Holden WE, Maier JM, Malinow MR. Cigarette smoke extract increases albumin flux across pulmonary endothelium in vitro. J Appl Physiol (1985) 1989;66(1):443–9.

86. Lu Q, Sakhatskyy P, Grinnell K, et al. Cigarette smoke causes lung vascular barrier dysfunction via oxidative stress-mediated inhibition of RhoA and focal adhesion kinase. Am J Physiol Lung Cell Mol Physiol 2011;301(6):L847–57.

87. Schweitzer KS, Hatoum H, Brown MB, et al. Mechanisms of lung endothelial barrier disruption induced by cigarette smoke: role of oxidative stress and ceramides. Am J Physiol Lung Cell Mol Physiol 2011; 301(6):L836–46.

88. Ware LB, Matthay MA. The acute respiratory distress syndrome. N Engl J Med 2000;342(18): 1334–49.

89. Looney MR, Nguyen JX, Hu Y, et al. Platelet depletion and aspirin treatment protect mice in a two-event model of transfusion-related acute lung injury. J Clin Invest 2009;119(11):3450–61.

90. Gunther A, Mosavi P, Heinemann S, et al. Alveolar fibrin formation caused by enhanced procoagulant and depressed fibrinolytic capacities in severe pneumonia. Comparison with the acute respiratory distress syndrome. Am J Respir Crit Care Med 2000;161(2 Pt 1):454–62.

91. Idell S. Coagulation, fibrinolysis, and fibrin deposition in acute lung injury. Crit Care Med 2003;31(4 Suppl):S213–20.

92. Greene R. Pulmonary vascular obstruction in the adult respiratory distress syndrome. J Thorac Imaging 1986;1(3):31–8.

93. Barnoya J, Glantz SA. Cardiovascular effects of secondhand smoke: nearly as large as smoking. Circulation 2005;111(20):2684–98.

94. Atkinson RW, Kang S, Anderson HR, et al. Epidemiological time series studies of PM2.5 and daily mortality and hospital admissions: a systematic review and meta-analysis. Thorax 2014;69(7):660–5.

95. Mustafic H, Jabre P, Caussin C, et al. Main air pollutants and myocardial infarction: a systematic review and meta-analysis. JAMA 2012;307(7): 713–21.

96. Pope CA 3rd, Burnett RT, Krewski D, et al. Cardiovascular mortality and exposure to airborne fine particulate matter and cigarette smoke: shape of the exposure-response relationship. Circulation 2009;120(11):941–8.

97. Brunekreef B, Holgate ST. Air pollution and health. Lancet 2002;360(9341):1233–42.

98. Brunekreef B, Beelen R, Hoek G, et al. Effects of long-term exposure to traffic-related air pollution on respiratory and cardiovascular mortality in the Netherlands: the NLCS-AIR study. Res Rep Health Eff Inst 2009;(139):5–71 [discussion: 73–89].

99. Beelen R, Hoek G, van den Brandt PA, et al. Long-term effects of traffic-related air pollution on mortality in a Dutch cohort (NLCS-AIR study). Environ Health Perspect 2008;116(2):196–202.

100. Dong GH, Zhang P, Sun B, et al. Long-term exposure to ambient air pollution and respiratory disease mortality in Shenyang, China: a 12-year population-based retrospective cohort study. Respiration 2012;84(5):360–8.

101. Dockery DW, Pope CA 3rd, Xu X, et al. An association between air pollution and mortality in six U.S. cities. N Engl J Med 1993;329(24):1753–9.

102. Pope CA 3rd, Thun MJ, Namboodiri MM, et al. Particulate air pollution as a predictor of mortality in a prospective study of U.S. adults. Am J Respir Crit Care Med 1995;151(3 Pt 1):669–74.

103. Dimakopoulou K, Samoli E, Beelen R, et al. Air pollution and nonmalignant respiratory mortality in 16 cohorts within the ESCAPE Project. Am J Respir Crit Care Med 2014;189(6):684–96.

104. Noah TL, Zhou H, Zhang H, et al. Diesel exhaust exposure and nasal response to attenuated influenza in normal and allergic volunteers. Am J Respir Crit Care Med 2012;185(2):179–85.

105. Schultz ES, Gruzieva O, Bellander T, et al. Traffic-related air pollution and lung function in children at 8 years of age: a birth cohort study. Am J Respir Crit Care Med 2012;186(12):1286–91.

106. Huang W, Wang G, Lu SE, et al. Inflammatory and oxidative stress responses of healthy young adults to changes in air quality during the Beijing Olympics. Am J Respir Crit Care Med 2012;186(11): 1150–9.

107. Bind MA, Baccarelli A, Zanobetti A, et al. Air pollution and markers of coagulation, inflammation, and endothelial function: associations and epigene-environment interactions in an elderly cohort. Epidemiology 2012;23(2):332–40.

108. Que LG, Stiles JV, Sundy JS, et al. Pulmonary function, bronchial reactivity, and epithelial permeability are response phenotypes to ozone and develop differentially in healthy humans. J Appl Physiol (1985) 2011;111(3):679–87.

Clinical and Biological Heterogeneity in Acute Respiratory Distress Syndrome
Direct Versus Indirect Lung Injury

Ciara M. Shaver, MD, PhD*, Julie A. Bastarache, MD

KEYWORDS

- Direct lung injury • Indirect lung injury • Acute respiratory distress syndrome • Acute lung injury

KEY POINTS

- Acute respiratory distress syndrome (ARDS) is caused by both direct (pulmonary, primary) and indirect (extrapulmonary, secondary) causes.
- Direct ARDS causes epithelial injury and indirect ARDS causes endothelial injury.
- There are important clinical differences between direct ARDS and indirect ARDS in pathologic abnormality, radiography, respiratory mechanics, response to treatment, and outcomes.
- Animal models of direct and indirect lung injury highlight different mechanisms of injury, particularly early in disease.
- Greater understanding of the mechanisms of direct and indirect ARDS in humans and in animal models is needed for development and testing of new therapeutics.

INTRODUCTION

Twenty years ago, the American-European Consensus Conference on ARDS emphasized the complexity of the pathogenesis of acute respiratory distress syndrome (ARDS) and suggested that separation of ARDS patients into more homogeneous subgroups could be a useful strategy to facilitate understanding of this syndrome. The consensus panel authors proposed 2 broad groups of patients with ARDS: those with direct injury to the lung parenchyma and those with indirect lung injury in the setting of systemic inflammation.[1] These 2 categories are appealing because they are based solely on clinical information readily available at the patient's bedside, and it is reasonable to

hypothesize that direct lung insults may be distinct from bystander lung damage. However, it is important to note that there are many alternative ways to separate patients into groups. For example, patient groups could be defined using panels of recently identified biomarkers, by severity of disease (mild, moderate, or severe by Berlin definition[2]), or by more specific inciting cause, such as trauma or sepsis. As emphasized by the consensus panel authors, distinct mechanisms underlying lung injury may affect clinical response to therapeutics and impact clinical trial design. For the purposes of this review, comparisons between direct and indirect causes of ARDS have been chosen to be the focus.

Funding Sources: National Institutes of Health, grant HL087738 (C.M. Shaver); National Institutes of Health, grant HL090785, American Heart Association, grant 11CRP7820021 (J.A. Bastarache).
Conflicts of Interest: None.
Division of Allergy, Pulmonary, and Critical Care Medicine, Department of Medicine, Vanderbilt University School of Medicine, Medical Center North, T-1218, Nashville, TN 37232-2650, USA
* Corresponding author.
E-mail address: ciara.shaver@vanderbilt.edu

Clin Chest Med 35 (2014) 639–653
http://dx.doi.org/10.1016/j.ccm.2014.08.004
0272-5231/14/$ – see front matter

The underlying causes of ARDS are summarized in **Table 1**. Direct (pulmonary or primary) lung injury results in local damage to the lung epithelium, whereas indirect (extrapulmonary or secondary) lung injury occurs in the setting of systemic disorders that diffusely damage the vascular endothelium. Pneumonia and aspiration of gastric contents account for most direct lung injury, while sepsis is the major cause of indirect injury.[3,4] Although there is substantial overlap, studies estimate that approximately 55% of ARDS is caused by direct lung injury.[5] Although a direct cause of ARDS from pneumonia may be the initiating factor, almost 80% of patients with ARDS have sepsis, with 46% resulting from a direct pulmonary infection and the remainder resulting from extrapulmonary sources.[4]

Many patients have multiple potential contributors to ARDS. In one study, up to 21% of ARDS patients had mixed causes of lung injury.[5] Furthermore, even with illness restricted to the thoracic cavity, there may be elements of both direct and indirect injury. For example, a direct injury from lobar pneumonia may have indirect inflammatory effects in the contralateral lung. This type of clinical heterogeneity makes it difficult to focus clinical trials on defined nonoverlapping subgroups and presents challenges to interpretation of data from experimental animal models of ARDS. Nonetheless, separation of underlying causes of ARDS into direct and indirect causes provides a useful framework for understanding the pathogenesis of lung injury and for explaining some of the clinical

heterogeneity seen in patients. In addition, the distinction between direct and indirect lung injury allows for improved study design in animal models and more specific therapeutic trials in subsets of patients with ARDS.

This review focuses on the distinctions between ARDS from direct or indirect causes in both human patients and experimental lung injury models. Because of variability in study design and outcome measures, the authors have chosen to limit their discussion to studies that separated patients according to the underlying cause of ARDS (direct vs indirect) and to those mechanisms that have been studied specifically in both direct and indirect injury models, with an emphasis on studies that tested both types of models in a single study.

CLINICAL DIFFERENCES BETWEEN DIRECT AND INDIRECT ACUTE RESPIRATORY DISTRESS SYNDROME

The Berlin definition of ARDS defines this syndrome as acute onset respiratory failure associated with bilateral pulmonary infiltrates and hypoxemia that is not fully explained by cardiac disease or fluid overload.[2] In this section, the existing clinical evidence that outlines important differences between direct and indirect ARDS in humans is summarized. **Table 2** is designed to highlight distinctions between these 2 groups of ARDS patients, recognizing that there may be significant overlap between direct and indirect ARDS with more subtle differences between these groups.

Pathologic Findings

Table 1 Causes of acute respiratory distress syndrome	
Direct Lung Injury	**Indirect Lung Injury**
Pneumonia (bacterial, viral, fungal)	Sepsis syndrome
Aspiration	Nonthoracic trauma
Mechanical ventilation (barotrauma, volutrauma)	Transfusion
Lung contusion	Cardiopulmonary bypass
Inhalation injury	Pancreatitis
Near-drowning	Drug overdose
Fat emboli	Burn injury
Reperfusion injury	

Adapted from Bernard GR, Artigas A, Brigham KL, et al. The American-European consensus conference on ARDS. Definitions, mechanisms, relevant outcomes, and clinical trial coordination. Am J Respir Crit Care Med 1994;149(3 Pt 1):821; and Ware LB, Matthay MA. The acute respiratory distress syndrome. N Engl J Med 2000;342(18):1338.

When examined pathologically, lung biopsies from patients with ARDS from direct and indirect causes show different properties.[6] One retrospective study showed that direct ARDS had significantly more alveolar collapse, fibrin deposition, and alveolar wall edema than ARDS from indirect causes.[7] Increased amounts of collagen, but not elastin, were present in early ARDS from direct injury but not in ARDS from indirect injury.[8] Lamy and colleagues[9] demonstrated that patients with limited response to positive end-expiratory pressure (PEEP) had more severe tissue injury with greater alveolar hemorrhage and exudate on lung biopsy. An elegant study of patients by Peres and colleagues[2] described the hyaline membranes seen in direct and indirect ARDS in great detail (**Fig. 1**). In direct ARDS, hyaline membranes were discontinuous and thickly deposited, whereas the hyaline membranes in indirect ARDS were thin and more evenly distributed. Indirect ARDS had reduced expression of factor VIII, consistent with endothelial injury, and increased expression of

Table 2
Clinical features that may differ between direct and indirect acute respiratory distress syndrome

	Direct Causes	Indirect Causes
Pathology	Epithelial injury may be more prominent	Endothelial injury may be more prominent
	Hyaline membranes tend to be more discontinuous and thick	Hyaline membranes tend to be more evenly distributed and thin
	Increased fibrin and collagen tend to be more prominent	Increased factor VIII tends to be more prominent
	May have more edema	May have less edema
Radiographic	Consolidation tends to be equivalent to GGO	GGO tends to be more prominent than consolidation
	GGO tends to be more diffuse	GGO tends to be more centrally located
	Consolidation tends to be more asymmetric and patchy	Consolidation tends to be less prominent
	Opacities tend to be in the nondependent lung regions	Opacities tend to be in the dependent lung regions
Respiratory mechanics	Lung elastance tends to be increased	Lung and chest wall elastance tends to be increased
	Tends to be less responsive to PEEP	Tends to be more responsive to PEEP
Therapeutic response	Tends to be more responsive to prone positioning	Tends to be more responsive to alveolar recruitment maneuvers
	Better with surfactant	Worse with surfactant
Genetic risk	Tends to have an increased RAGE level	Tends to have increased Ang-2 and vWF levels
	POPDC3 (reduced risk)	FAAH (increased risk)
	-308A allele of TNF (reduced risk)	TNFB22 allele of TNF (reduced risk)
		Tends to have a reduced expression of apoA-IV, C-II, B-100
Outcomes	Tends to have an increased mortality	
	Tends to be associated with more mild QOL impairments	Tends to be associated with more severe QOL deficits

Abbreviation: QOL, quality of life.

cytokeratin AE1/AE3, consistent with an intact epithelium.[2] This study illustrates the concept that direct ARDS is a more localized injury to the epithelium as compared with the more diffuse endothelial injury seen during indirect ARDS.

Radiographic Appearance

Consistent with different underlying pathophysiologic processes, ARDS from direct and indirect causes have distinct characteristics on computed tomography (CT) scans.[10–14] Goodman and colleagues[11] performed a prospective study analyzing imaging patterns on CT of 33 patients with ARDS. Direct ARDS had equivalent areas of consolidation and ground glass opacification (GGO) and tended to have asymmetry of the consolidated areas. In contrast, indirect ARDS was predominantly GGO that was more centrally distributed than in direct ARDS. These findings are supported by a second study in which Pelosi and colleagues[12] demonstrated that direct ARDS had more patchy

densities compared with indirect ARDS. Rouby and colleagues[14] prospectively studied CT scans and pulmonary mechanics in 71 patients with ARDS and showed that patients with direct ARDS had bilateral hypoattenuation that was either diffuse or patchy and was more prominent than in indirect ARDS. Finally, opacities in nondependent areas of the lung were more common in direct ARDS.[10,13]

Respiratory Mechanics

Several studies over the last 20 years have demonstrated that the underlying cause of ARDS affects respiratory mechanics differently depending on mechanism of injury.[15–20] Gattinoni and colleagues[15] were the first to compare characteristics of patients with direct and indirect ARDS when they measured pulmonary mechanics of 21 patients with ARDS. Patients with direct lung injury had increased lung elastance at baseline that did not improve with increased PEEP. In contrast,

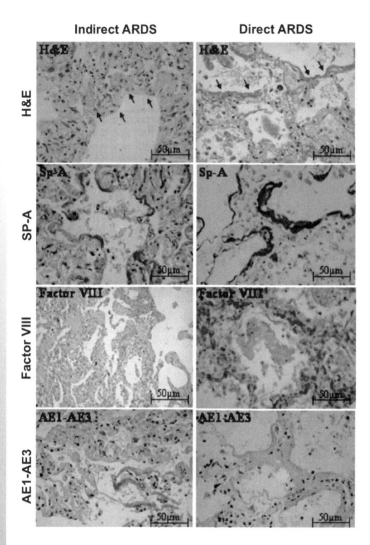

Fig. 1. Histopathology and immunohistochemistry of direct and indirect ARDS. Hematoxylin and eosin (H&E) staining shows that SP-A-positive hyaline membranes (*arrows*) are thick layers in direct ARDS, but thin and discontinuous layers in indirect ARDS. Direct ARDS shows lack of AE1-AE3 staining, consistent with epithelial injury. In contrast, indirect ARDS shows increased anti-factor VIII staining, consistent with endothelial damage. (*From* Peres e Serra A, Parra ER, Eher E, et al. Nonhomogeneous immunostaining of hyaline membranes in different manifestations of diffuse alveolar damage. Clinics (Sao Paulo) 2006;61(6):499.)

patients with indirect injury had increased elastance of both the lung and the chest wall that was reduced with increased PEEP, reflecting increased alveolar recruitment in response to PEEP therapy. These results are consistent with the differences in the underlying pathophysiology with direct injury primarily exhibiting lung consolidation and indirect injury having interstitial edema and vascular congestion. The authors speculated that PEEP in the setting of direct lung injury may lead to alveolar stretch in relatively normal areas of lung, causing secondary lung injury, whereas PEEP in the setting of indirect lung injury, applied more evenly across a more homogenously affected lung, results in increased alveolar recruitment. These data are further supported by additional data showing that patients with direct ARDS have reduced lung compliance and increased chest wall compliance relative to those with indirect ARDS.[20]

Another study demonstrated that use of sigh breaths given with high PEEP was more effective in patients with indirect ARDS compared with direct ARDS.[19] Patients treated with sigh breaths and lung protective ventilation had increased oxygenation and reduced elastance compared with those treated only with lung protective ventilation. Subsequently, Lim and colleagues[17] performed a prospective clinical trial that demonstrated that an alveolar recruitment maneuver followed by increased PEEP improved oxygenation in 47 patients with ARDS. Patients with indirect causes of ARDS had significantly greater improvement in oxygenation parameters and radiographic appearance compared with those with direct causes of ARDS. These findings were confirmed in another prospective study of 24 ARDS patients in which increased PEEP as a recruitment strategy showed greater improvement in oxygenation and increased lung compliance in patients with indirect lung injury.[18]

Risk Factors for Acute Respiratory Distress Syndrome

Genetic risk

Several studies have used genomic or proteomic techniques to assess for risk of developing ARDS after direct or indirect lung injury.[21–23] One study of 417 patients with ARDS assessed for single nucleotide polymorphisms (SNP) associated with the risk of developing ARDS.[21] A SNP in POPDC3 was associated with a reduced risk for direct ARDS (odds ratio [OR] 0.65). This gene is 1 of 3 genes in the Popeye-domain-containing family involved in skeletal muscle regeneration, but how it impacts lung injury is unclear. Additional SNPs in PDE4B, ABCC1, and TNFRSF11A were associated with increased risk of direct ARDS in this meta-analysis. Similarly, a SNP in FAAH (fatty acid amine hydrolase) conveyed an OR of 1.70 for indirect ARDS. The authors speculated that this gene may increase risk for ARDS through alterations in HDL metabolism. Interestingly, no polymorphisms associated with both direct and indirect ARDS were identified. Another study investigated whether polymorphisms in the TNF gene were associated with the risk of ARDS[22] and found that the -308A allele was associated with reduced risk for direct ARDS (OR 0.53) and increased 60-day mortality (OR 2.1). In contrast, the TNFB22 allele was associated with a reduced risk of indirect ARDS (OR 0.48), but was not associated with mortality. The mechanisms through which these polymorphisms affect risk of ARDS are unknown.

Protein biomarkers

A great deal of research has identified measurable biomarkers that are elevated in patients with ARDS (reviewed by Janz and Ware[24]) and can serve as useful tools to separate patients into meaningful subgroups for further study. However, biomarkers are inherently variable and the optimal cutoff values to separate between direct and indirect injury are not straightforward. A few studies have analyzed markers of epithelial or endothelial damage in human patients with ARDS. For example, the receptor for advanced glycation end-products (RAGE), a marker of type I epithelial cell damage, and KL-6/MUC1, a marker of type II epithelial cell injury, are more elevated in pulmonary edema fluid from patients with direct ARDS compared with those with hydrostatic pulmonary edema.[25–27] Conversely, angiopoietin-2 (Ang-2) and von Willebrand factor (vWF), markers of endothelial damage, are more elevated in plasma of patients with indirect ARDS in the setting of sepsis than those with direct injury from pneumonia and are associated with increased mortality.[28–33] Importantly, many of these studies include mixed populations of patients and the distinctions between direct and indirect ARDS are imperfect. Chen and colleagues[23] recently used a proteomic approach to identify proteins that were differentially expressed in plasma of patients with ARDS from direct or indirect causes. This proteomic approach revealed that expression of apolipoproteins A-IV, C-II, and B-100 were decreased in patients with indirect lung injury compared with those with direct lung injury. Eleven proteins were associated with both direct and indirect injury, underscoring possible overlap between biomarker levels among ARDS patients. These common pathways involved acute phase responses, clathrin-mediated endocytosis, nitric oxide, and reactive oxygen species production in macrophages, and complement system activation (among others). Another study identified distinct circulating glycosaminoglycan signatures in direct and indirect ARDS.[34] This group collected plasma samples from 17 patients with ARDS and used mass spectrometry to show that patients with direct ARDS have increased hyaluronic acid levels, whereas patients with indirect ARDS have increased heparan sulfate levels. Indirect ARDS was also associated with increased sulfation of heparan disaccharides.

Response to Treatment

Patients with direct and indirect lung injury have demonstrated different responses to several clinical therapeutics. As described above, patients with indirect ARDS have greater improvements in oxygenation and pulmonary mechanics in response to increased PEEP or recruitment maneuvers.[15,17–20] Several authors have investigated the response of patients with ARDS to prone positioning according on the type of underlying lung injury.[12,17,35,36] Lim and colleagues[35] demonstrated that patients with direct ARDS had slower and less marked improvement of oxygenation and radiographic appearances after 2 hours of prone positioning than those with indirect injury. More recently, Pelosi and colleagues[16] prospectively assessed 73 patients ARDS and found that improvement in oxygenation with 6 hours of prone positioning was greater in patients with indirect ARDS. In contrast, other smaller studies did not demonstrate any differences in the clinical benefit between direct and indirect ARDS despite prone positioning improving oxygenation.[17,36]

There are also limited data suggesting that adults with indirect ARDS may have greater response to exogenous surfactant administration.

In 2 randomized controlled trials of 448 patients with ARDS, Spragg and colleagues[37] demonstrated improved oxygenation in patients who received intratracheal (IT) surfactant therapy compared with the control group. A post-hoc analysis of the effects of surfactant therapy on direct or indirect ARDS showed that patients with direct ARDS tended toward reduced mortality ($P<.002$ for interaction between direct ARDS and mortality), particularly in patients with pneumonia as the cause of ARDS. In contrast, patients with indirect ARDS tended to have higher mortality (41% vs 28%) with surfactant therapy. A subsequent study of the association of direct lung injury with mortality did not confirm this difference. In addition, several other studies of surfactant therapy in adults with ARDS have been performed and failed to show any clinical benefit[38,39] and, therefore, the ultimate utility of surfactant in ARDS remains uncertain.[40]

Finally, a subgroup analysis from the randomized controlled trial assessing low tidal volume ventilation[41] demonstrated that the benefit of low tidal volumes occurred regardless of underlying cause of ARDS, despite there being significant differences in overall mortality between the 2 etiologic groups.[42]

Patient Outcomes

Monchi and colleagues[43] retrospectively demonstrated that patients with direct ARDS had increased mortality compared with those with indirect ARDS, even when adjusted for overall severity of illness and comorbidities (OR 2.6, 95% confidence interval 1.1–6.9, $P<.05$). In another study, patients with direct ARDS and diffuse radiographic abnormalities with low lung compliance had increased mortality compared with those with lobar infiltrates (75% vs 41%).[14] A small prospective study of outcomes in 177 patients with ARDS showed a trend toward increased mortality (42% vs 23%, $P = .1$) in direct ARDS with no differences in measures of pulmonary function.[44] This conclusion is supported by a more recent study of 180 ARDS patients that showed a trend toward increased mortality in direct ARDS (57% vs 24%) with the cause of ARDS being a significant predictor of outcome in a univariate analysis.[45]

In an attempt to definitively show whether direct lung injury had increased mortality compared with indirect lung injury, Agarwal and colleagues[46] performed a meta-analysis comparing the overall mortality in ARDS from direct or indirect causes. This analysis included 34 studies with 4311 patients that separately reported mortality of patients with direct and indirect ARDS. The odds ratio of death with direct lung injury was 1.04 or 1.11 (depending on the statistical model used) compared with indirect injury, suggesting that the underlying cause of ARDS may not affect overall mortality. Importantly, this meta-analysis had significant heterogeneity among studies and many important studies of ARDS were excluded.

Aside from mortality, there have now been several studies that have measured indicators of quality of life after critical illness.[47–51] Patients with ARDS have worse quality-of-life (QOL) scores than patients without ARDS during critical illness, and these impairments persisted over several years.[48,49,51] A meta-analysis by Dowdy and colleagues,[52] which included 557 ARDS survivors, showed impaired physical and mental quality-of-life scores in patients compared with controls, independent of the underlying cause of ARDS. One prospective study by Parker and colleagues[47] followed 73 patients with ARDS for 1 year after critical illness to specifically assess whether the underlying cause of ARDS affected QOL scores. In fact, this group showed that patients with indirect ARDS had worse QOL on most domains tested, even when adjusted for duration of illness and comorbidities.

PATHOGENETIC MECHANISMS OF EXPERIMENTAL ACUTE RESPIRATORY DISTRESS SYNDROME

Clinically, patients with ARDS are all treated similarly with a focus on use of low tidal volume ventilation. However, as described above, there are numerous studies that suggest that clinical and biological heterogeneity in ARDS may influence response to treatment. Use of experimental models of acute lung injury are critical for defining the specific mechanisms involved in development of ARDS, with the ultimate goal being identification of novel therapeutic targets that may impact specific subgroups of patients with ARDS.

Experimental Models of Direct and Indirect Acute Respiratory Distress Syndrome

The American Thoracic Society has recommended that animal models of ARDS have at least 3 of 4 key features similar to ARDS in humans: (1) histologic evidence of tissue injury, (2) alteration of the alveolar capillary barrier, (3) presence of an acute inflammatory response, and (4) evidence of physiologic dysfunction.[53] Studies have shown differences between direct and indirect injury in all 4 of these pathophysiologic features.

The most common models of direct lung injury are IT lipopolysaccharide (LPS) administration, mechanical ventilation, and acid aspiration

(**Table 3**).[53] In general, these direct lung injury models cause epithelial dysfunction. The most common models of indirect lung injury include systemic LPS administration (intravenous or intraperitoneal [IP]), cecal ligation and puncture (CLP), or hemorrhage. These indirect models of lung injury primarily cause diffuse damage to the vascular endothelium. Which model is most appropriate to use depends on the specific research question being addressed. In addition, because some experimental models cause less severe lung injury in general, many studies combine 2 injury models, such as IT LPS with mechanical ventilation or hemorrhage followed by CLP, to better mimic human illness and to induce more severe injury to facilitate mechanistic investigations. Another approach frequently used in comparative studies of experimental lung injury is titration of different injurious stimuli to cause equivalent severity of ARDS. This strategy allows distinction between direct and indirect lung injury instead of only measuring differences in disease severity.

In this section, the similarities and differences in experimental lung injury caused by both direct and indirect insults (**Table 4**) are reviewed, and studies highlighting differences in the pathophysiology of ARDS from different causes are focused on. As with the human data shown in **Table 2**, **Table 4** is designed to emphasize the distinctions between experimental direct and indirect lung injury, knowing that there is likely some significant overlap between these groups.

Table 3
Experimental models of direct and indirect lung injury

Direct Lung Injury	Indirect Lung Injury
Intratracheal LPS	Intravenous LPS
Acid aspiration	Intraperitoneal lipopolysaccharide
Mechanical ventilation	Cecal ligation and puncture
Infectious organisms	Hemorrhage
Bleomycin	Ischemia-reperfusion injury
Hyperoxia	Oleic acid injection
Surfactant depletion	Infectious organisms
	Thiourea injection
	MHC-I antibody injection
	Femur fracture with hemorrhage
	Ischemic renal injury

Abbreviation: MHC-I, major histocompatibility complex-I.

Markers of Epithelial or Endothelial Injury

Data from both human and animal studies support the concept that direct lung injury first causes epithelial damage, whereas indirect lung injury initially causes endothelial dysfunction. Su and colleagues[54] demonstrated that RAGE, a marker of epithelial damage, was increased in 3 models of direct lung injury (IT LPS, acid aspiration, and *Escherichia coli* pneumonia), but not in 2 models of indirect lung injury (major histocompatibility complex-I monoclonal antibody injection to simulate transfusion-related lung injury and thiourea injection). Similar to human ARDS,[55] higher levels of RAGE in the airspaces were associated with more severe lung injury in direct experimental lung injury.[54] In mice, indirect lung injury caused by hemorrhage followed by CLP showed that Ang-2 levels were increased systemically in affected mice, consistent with endothelial injury.[56] Furthermore, IP injection of Ang-2 alone was sufficient to cause increased pulmonary capillary leak,[31] supporting the concept that endothelial dysfunction contributes to lung injury. These data support the existing data from human patients suggesting differences in biomarkers of epithelial and endothelial damage during direct and indirect ARDS.

Histologic Injury

The histologic appearance of injured lungs varies depending on the inciting stimulus.[6] In general, injury caused by direct stimuli damages the alveolar epithelium, whereas injury caused by indirect stimuli damages the vascular endothelium. Menezes and colleagues[57] compared the effects of direct and indirect lung injury caused by LPS. The doses of LPS given IT or IP were selected to cause similar degrees of pulmonary mechanical dysfunction and cellular inflammation within the lung parenchyma 24 hours after injury. Direct injury from IT LPS caused destruction of the alveolar epithelium with hyaline deposition and significant neutrophil apoptosis. In contrast, indirect injury from systemic LPS caused pulmonary interstitial edema with intact epithelial and endothelial layers by electron microscopy (**Fig. 2**). Another distinction between direct and indirect lung injury is the amount of collagen and elastin deposition. Twenty-four hours after injury from either IT or IP LPS, there is increased deposition of collagen, but not elastin, in all animals regardless of the cause of lung injury.[57] However, in direct lung injury, the increases in collagen deposition persisted for up to 8 weeks and were associated with prolonged impairment in pulmonary mechanics. In contrast, after indirect injury, early collagen deposition was quickly reversed.[58] These data suggest that direct stimuli

Table 4
Features that may differ between direct and indirect lung injury in animal models

	Direct Causes	Indirect Causes
Histology	Tends to have more prominent epithelial injury Tends to have more alveolar destruction Tends to have more prominent hyaline deposition Tends to have more neutrophil apoptosis	Tends to have more prominent endothelial injury Tends to have more interstitial edema Tends to have a normal barrier by microscopy
Alveolar capillary barrier	Defective Tends to have more severely impaired alveolar fluid clearance	Defective Tends to have less severely impaired alveolar fluid clearance
Inflammation	Tends to be more neutrophilic Tends to be persistent Regulatory T cells tend to have a more prominent role in the later stages IL-6 tends to be more anti-inflammatory	Tends to be more monocytic Tends to resolve more quickly Regulatory T cells tend to have a more prominent role in the earlier stages IL-6 tends to be more pro-inflammatory
Physiology	Abnormalities tend to persist Tends to be more resistant to recruitment maneuvers Tends to be associated with an increased risk for ventilator-induced injury and barotrauma	Abnormalities tend to resolve more rapidly Tends to be more responsive to recruitment with PEEP

may impair lung repair mechanisms, in contrast to the more transient damage from indirect causes of lung injury, which remodels quickly.

Disruption of the Alveolar-Capillary Barrier

Integrity of the alveolar-capillary barrier and continued clearance of fluid from the alveolar space are critical elements for maintaining adequate lung function. Ultimately, pulmonary edema develops when both epithelial and endothelial barrier integrity are lost.

There are human studies that show that the kinetics of pulmonary edema development differ according to the cause of ARDS. In trauma patients, those with direct lung injury develop pulmonary edema more quickly than patients with indirect injury.[59] Initially, edema is localized to the injured region, but becomes more widespread over several days. In contrast, indirect injury caused diffuse pulmonary edema later after injury. Another study of alveolar fluid clearance in ARDS patients showed that patients with direct lung injury had impaired resolution of pulmonary edema compared with those with indirect lung injury.[60] Furthermore, patients with maximal alveolar fluid clearance were less likely to have sepsis as the underlying cause of ARDS.

There have been few studies that have specifically assessed differences in alveolar permeability and alveolar fluid clearance in both direct and indirect experimental lung injury models, partially because increased alveolar capillary permeability is a key feature for lung injury models. Those studies that have compared different models of injury show that TRPC6 and αENaC ion channels are each similarly involved in both direct and indirect lung injury.[61,62] In the latter study, mice with direct lung injury from hyperoxia had greater increases in pulmonary edema with loss of αENaC than those with indirect lung injury from thiourea injection.[62]

Inflammation

The impact of different elements of the innate and adaptive immune systems on development of lung injury is the most studied feature of experimental ARDS. There have been several excellent detailed reviews of the role of individual cell types, cytokines, and pathways.[63–66] Here, the elements of inflammation that are different between direct and indirect ARDS are focused on.

Inflammatory cell influx

Several studies have demonstrated that direct lung injury causes greater alveolar inflammation

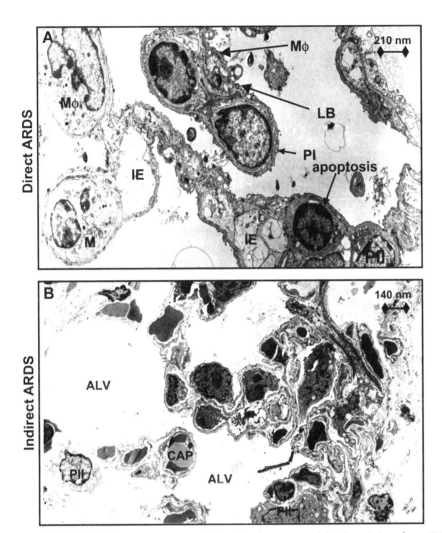

Fig. 2. Electron microscopy of experimental direct (*A*) and indirect ARDS (*B*). Direct injury from IT LPS caused destruction of the alveolar epithelium with hyaline deposition and significant neutrophil apoptosis. In contrast, indirect injury from IP LPS caused pulmonary interstitial edema with intact epithelial and endothelial layers. ALV, alveolar space; CAP, capillary; IE, interstitial edema; LB, lamellar bodies; Mφ, macrophage; PI and PII, types I and II pneumocytes. (*From* Menezes SL, Bozza PT, Neto HC, et al. Pulmonary and extrapulmonary acute lung injury: inflammatory and ultrastructural analyses. J Appl Physiol (1985) 2005;98(5):1780; with permission.)

than indirect lung injury, even when overall pulmonary inflammation and mechanical dysfunction have been equalized.[57,58,67,68] Menezes and colleagues[57] showed that mice with direct lung injury from LPS had 4-fold increased inflammatory cell recruitment into the airspace compared with mice with indirect lung injury from systemic LPS. Most cells in bronchoalveolar lavage (BAL) fluids were neutrophils in direct injury, but monocyte/macrophages in indirect injury. In addition, the BAL fluid of mice with direct lung injury had 2-fold to 3-fold increased levels of keratinocyte chemoattractant (KC, CXCL-1), interleukin (IL)-10, and IL-6 compared with those with indirect injury.[57] As with collagen deposition, the airspace inflammation in mice with direct lung injury persisted for

up to 3 weeks, whereas the inflammation in those with indirect injury resolved within a few days.[58] Bhargava and colleagues[67] showed that IT LPS, IP LPS, or ischemic acute kidney injury each caused similar degrees of inflammation in the lung interstitium. However, intra-alveolar neutrophil accumulation only occurred in direct lung injury. Another study demonstrated that direct lung injury from IT LPS induced greater alveolar inflammation and less fibrosis than indirect injury from IP LPS.[68]

Role of T cells and dendritic cells

Although inflammation in lung injury is typically thought to be mediated by neutrophils and macrophage populations, there is increasing evidence that other cells types are important.[69–72] Venet and colleagues[70] recently demonstrated that dendritic cells are recruited to the lung and exert anti-inflammatory effects on monocytes and that $CD4^+CD25^+Foxp3^+$ regulatory T cells limit inflammation[69] during indirect lung injury caused by hemorrhage followed by CLP. Reduction of the regulatory T-cell population exacerbated indirect lung injury through effects on IL-10 expression. Similar studies using a direct model of lung injury show a key role for regulatory T cells in epithelial repair after LPS-mediated direct lung injury through reduction in fibrocyte recruitment and fibroblast proliferation.[71,72] However, in contrast with the early effects of regulatory T cells after indirect lung injury in the previous study, the importance of regulatory T cells in repair of direct lung injury is not apparent until several days after lung injury begins.

Cytokine expression

Several studies have investigated the role of IL-6 in lung injury.[67,73–75] IL-6 had been previously associated with increased mortality in ARDS[76,77] and in acute kidney injury in critically ill patients.[78] In animal studies, IL-6 has distinct roles in direct versus indirect lung injury and has different effects in the airspace compared with the circulation. During indirect lung injury, IL-6 is critical for the development of inflammation in the airspace.[74,79] For example, Mommsen and colleagues[74] showed that $IL-6^{-/-}$ mice had impaired cytokine production by alveolar macrophages after hemorrhagic shock and femur fracture, an indirect cause of lung injury. Meng and colleagues[79] showed that IL-6 was required for post-hemorrhage neutrophil accumulation in the lung. Although these models of indirect injury showed a pro-inflammatory role for IL-6 in the airspace, loss of IL-6 resulted in increased cytokine expression in the serum of mice with indirect lung injury.[73] During direct lung injury caused by IT LPS, $IL-6^{-/-}$ mice had *increased* BAL inflammation.[73] Bhargava and colleagues[67] showed that IL-6 levels were markedly increased in direct lung injury from LPS, but not after indirect lung injury from either IP LPS or acute kidney injury. Surprisingly, administration of additional IL-6 into the airspace reduced inflammation after direct injury, but had no role in lung injury from indirect causes. This study is interesting because of its suggestion that intra-alveolar therapies may be beneficial in the setting of direct epithelial cell injury and less useful in systemic causes of lung damage.

Physiologic Dysfunction

Although modeling of histology, permeability, and inflammation is critical to understand ARDS, it is equally important to understand the physiologic consequences of experimental lung injury.

Several studies have demonstrated that direct lung injury results in more persistent inflammation and prolonged collagen deposition after LPS treatment,[57,58,68] which could lead to decreased lung compliance. Santos and colleagues[58] measured pulmonary mechanics in mice with direct or indirect lung injury caused by LPS to determine whether persistent inflammation was detrimental to respiratory mechanics. Interestingly, despite similar pulmonary dysfunction after 24 hours, mice with direct lung injury had increased resistive pressures and viscoelastic pressures for at least 8 weeks. In contrast, these parameters normalized in less than 1 week in indirect injury. The authors hypothesized that the indirect injury resolved more quickly because of the lack of type II pneumocyte damage and intact repair mechanisms.

Consistent with the data described in human patients with ARDS, Riva and colleagues[80] determined whether the response to recruitment maneuvers differed depending on the type of lung injury. Rats were treated with IT or IP LPS and then placed on low tidal volume mechanical ventilation with 3 sequential 40-second recruitment maneuvers at high PEEP. Similar to humans, alveolar recruitment was more effective in rats with indirect lung injury. Lung resistance and static elastance were more significantly reduced and atelectasis more limited in indirect lung injury. Another study by Kuiper and colleagues[81] showed that direct lung injury from acid aspiration reduced oxygenation and lung compliance, effects that were not seen in indirect lung injury from CLP.

Another set of studies demonstrated that direct lung injury increased susceptibility to additional lung injury related to mechanical ventilation. In one study, rats were mechanically ventilated with either low or high tidal volumes after direct injury from acid aspiration or indirect injury from CLP.[81] Rats with direct lung injury were more susceptible to secondary injury from ventilation. Another study comparing dogs with direct lung injury from surfactant depletion to dogs with indirect lung injury from oleic acid infusion showed that direct lung injury cause more focal lung injury and was more susceptible to hyperinflation from PEEP.[82]

Therapeutic Responses

Because of the proposed differences in the underlying pathogenesis of direct and indirect ARDS, several investigators have hypothesized that the cause of ARDS might affect responses to therapy. Different responses to ventilator parameters are discussed above. One study by Leite-Junior and colleagues[68] studied whether early treatment with corticosteroids had differential effects on lung injury from direct or indirect causes. Mice were treated with IT or IP LPS followed by intravenous methylprednisolone or saline 6 hours later. Steroid treatment reduced lung mechanical dysfunction and cytokine production (transforming growth factor-β, IL-6, and KC) in the setting of direct, but not indirect, lung injury. In contrast, steroids in indirect injury stimulated increased endothelial repair. These data suggest that steroids have different effects based on the underlying injury mechanism.

Cellular therapies
Several studies have investigated whether administration of mesenchymal stem cells (MSC) or bone marrow–derived mononuclear cells (BMDMC) could mitigate lung injury.[83,84] Araujo and colleagues[84] treated mice with intravenous BMDMC after IT or IP LPS and found that BMDMC therapy had a greater impact on pulmonary mechanics after indirect lung injury, with no differences in inflammation or fibrosis after 7 days. More recently, Maron-Gutierrez and colleagues[83] treated mice with IT or IP LPS followed by intravenous MSC 24 hours later. MSC reduced cellular inflammation in both BAL fluid and peripheral blood and reduced cytokine expression in response to both types of injury, although the effect of cellular therapy was greater in direct lung injury.[83] In addition, in direct injury, but not in indirect injury, stem cells impaired the transition of macrophage subpopulations to the M2 phenotype that typically facilitates tissue repair.[83] Arginase-1 expression was reduced and IL-12 and GM-CSF expression increased in animals with direct lung injury also treated with stem cell therapy. As a result, mice with direct lung injury treated with MSC had reduced collagen deposition.[83]

Epithelial versus systemic therapy administration
There is increasing evidence that the airspace is a separate biological compartment from the circulation, even during severe ARDS when the alveolar capillary barrier is compromised. For example, in a model of indirect lung injury from hemorrhage followed by CLP, inhibition of the Fas and Fas ligand pathway locally in the airspace limited alveolar inflammation, cytokine expression, and epithelial destruction during indirect lung injury.[85,86] In contrast, systemic delivery of the same inhibitors had no effect on lung injury. In a similar way, Bhargava and colleagues[67] showed that administration of additional IL-6 into the airspace reduced inflammation after direct injury, but had no role in lung injury from indirect causes.

These data suggest that delivery of therapy may need to be focused on the major cell of injury, using inhaled or IT administration for epithelial injury and systemic administration for endothelial injury.

SUMMARY

ARDS remains a significant clinical problem with limited effective therapies outside use of low tidal volume ventilation. It is becoming increasingly clear that the underlying process that leads to ARDS plays a critical role in patient outcomes. ARDS from direct causes, including pneumonia, aspiration, and mechanical ventilation, leads predominantly to epithelial injury, whereas ARDS from indirect causes, such as sepsis, results mainly in endothelial damage. Early in the course of disease, the different sources of cellular injury activate distinct inflammatory pathways, leading to differences in wound healing and survival. These differences seen in human populations have been recapitulated in animal models of direct and indirect lung injury. As reviewed here, direct and indirect lung injury have distinct patterns of epithelial and endothelial injury, respectively, which occurs in part because of differences in the degree and characteristics of the alveolar inflammatory infiltrate, repair of abnormal pulmonary mechanics, resolution of pulmonary edema resulting from destruction of the alveolar-capillary barrier, and responses to therapies.

The separation of ARDS into direct and indirect lung injury is appealing in the sense that it may allow more focused and rigorous investigation in more homogeneous patient and animal populations. However, it is equally important to acknowledge that most patients with ARDS have complicated critical illnesses with multiorgan failure and likely have features of both direct and indirect lung injury. Even a clear case of direct lung injury from community-acquired pneumonia likely has some "indirect" inflammatory effects in the contralateral lung. Although the clinical complexity is certainly real, to make advances in the mechanistic understanding of the development and resolution of ARDS using animal models, it is necessary to simplify experimental models and compare several different insults that result in lung injury. This comparison will allow further definition of pathways distinct to either direct or indirect injury and will also allow refinement of pathways common to any cause of ARDS. Use of cell-specific biomarkers of epithelial or endothelial damage, like RAGE and Ang-2, may facilitate separation of patients into appropriate groups for clinical trials or may help direct appropriate therapies to the airspace or circulation. In addition, there are several alternative strategies to separate patients into clinically meaningful subgroups for ongoing investigation.

Overall, ARDS from direct causes is distinct from ARDS due to indirect causes, in both human populations and experimental animal models. Future studies could harness these differences to identify more homogenous patient populations to identify subgroups that may benefit from specific therapeutic interventions and will allow more rigorous scientific investigation into critical steps underlying the pathogenesis of this devastating disease. It is hoped that comparison of direct and indirect ARDS can lead to novel successful therapies for this devastating disease.

REFERENCES

1. Bernard GR, Artigas A, Brigham KL, et al. The American-European consensus conference on ARDS. Definitions, mechanisms, relevant outcomes, and clinical trial coordination. Am J Respir Crit Care Med 1994;149(3 Pt 1):818–24.

2. Peres e Serra A, Parra ER, Eher E, et al. Nonhomogeneous immunostaining of hyaline membranes in different manifestations of diffuse alveolar damage. Clinics (Sao Paulo) 2006;61(6):497–502.

3. Ware LB, Matthay MA. The acute respiratory distress syndrome. N Engl J Med 2000;342(18):1334–49.

4. Rubenfeld GD, Caldwell E, Peabody E, et al. Incidence and outcomes of acute lung injury. N Engl J Med 2005;353(16):1685–93.

5. Brun-Buisson C, Minelli C, Bertolini G, et al. Epidemiology and outcome of acute lung injury in European intensive care units. Results from the ALIVE study. Intensive Care Med 2004;30(1):51–61.

6. Capelozzi VL. What have anatomic and pathologic studies taught us about acute lung injury and acute respiratory distress syndrome? Curr Opin Crit Care 2008;14(1):56–63.

7. Hoelz C, Negri EM, Lichtenfels AJ, et al. Morphometric differences in pulmonary lesions in primary and secondary ARDS. A preliminary study in autopsies. Pathol Res Pract 2001;197(8):521–30.

8. Negri EM, Hoelz C, Barbas CS, et al. Acute remodeling of parenchyma in pulmonary and extrapulmonary ARDS. An autopsy study of collagen-elastic system fibers. Pathol Res Pract 2002;198(5):355–61.

9. Lamy M, Fallat RJ, Koeniger E, et al. Pathologic features and mechanisms of hypoxemia in adult respiratory distress syndrome. Am Rev Respir Dis 1976;114(2):267–84.

10. Desai SR, Wells AU, Suntharalingam G, et al. Acute respiratory distress syndrome caused by pulmonary and extrapulmonary injury: a comparative CT study. Radiology 2001;218(3):689–93.

11. Goodman LR, Fumagalli R, Tagliabue P, et al. Adult respiratory distress syndrome due to pulmonary and extrapulmonary causes: CT, clinical, and functional correlations. Radiology 1999;213(2):545–52.

12. Pelosi P, D'Onofrio D, Chiumello D, et al. Pulmonary and extrapulmonary acute respiratory distress syndrome are different. Eur Respir J Suppl 2003;42:48s–56s.

13. Winer-Muram HT, Steiner RM, Gurney JW, et al. Ventilator-associated pneumonia in patients with adult respiratory distress syndrome: CT evaluation. Radiology 1998;208(1):193–9.

14. Rouby JJ, Puybasset L, Cluzel P, et al. Regional distribution of gas and tissue in acute respiratory distress syndrome. II. Physiological correlations and definition of an ARDS severity score. CT Scan ARDS Study Group. Intensive Care Med 2000;26(8):1046–56.

15. Gattinoni L, Pelosi P, Suter PM, et al. Acute respiratory distress syndrome caused by pulmonary and extrapulmonary disease. Different syndromes? Am J Respir Crit Care Med 1998;158(1):3–11.

16. Pelosi P, Brazzi L, Gattinoni L. Prone position in acute respiratory distress syndrome. Eur Respir J 2002;20(4):1017–28.

17. Lim CM, Jung H, Koh Y, et al. Effect of alveolar recruitment maneuver in early acute respiratory distress syndrome according to antiderecruitment strategy, etiological category of diffuse lung injury, and body position of the patient. Crit Care Med 2003;31(2):411–8.

18. Tugrul S, Akinci O, Ozcan PE, et al. Effects of sustained inflation and postinflation positive end-expiratory pressure in acute respiratory distress syndrome: focusing on pulmonary and extrapulmonary forms. Crit Care Med 2003;31(3):738–44.

19. Pelosi P, Cadringher P, Bottino N, et al. Sigh in acute respiratory distress syndrome. Am J Respir Crit Care Med 1999;159(3):872–80.

20. Albaiceta GM, Taboada F, Parra D, et al. Differences in the deflation limb of the pressure-volume curves in acute respiratory distress syndrome from pulmonary and extrapulmonary origin. Intensive Care Med 2003;29(11):1943–9.

21. Tejera P, Meyer NJ, Chen F, et al. Distinct and replicable genetic risk factors for acute respiratory distress syndrome of pulmonary or extrapulmonary origin. J Med Genet 2012;49(11):671–80.

22. Gong MN, Zhou W, Williams PL, et al. -308GA and TNFB polymorphisms in acute respiratory distress syndrome. Eur Respir J 2005;26(3):382–9.

23. Chen X, Shan Q, Jiang L, et al. Quantitative proteomic analysis by iTRAQ for identification of candidate biomarkers in plasma from acute respiratory distress syndrome patients. Biochem Biophys Res Commun 2013;441(1):1–6.

24. Janz DR, Ware LB. Biomarkers of ALI/ARDS: pathogenesis, discovery, and relevance to clinical trials. Semin Respir Crit Care Med 2013;34(4):537–48.

25. Uchida T, Shirasawa M, Ware LB, et al. Receptor for advanced glycation end-products is a marker of type I cell injury in acute lung injury. Am J Respir Crit Care Med 2006;173(9):1008–15.

26. Ishizaka A, Matsuda T, Albertine KH, et al. Elevation of KL-6, a lung epithelial cell marker, in plasma and epithelial lining fluid in acute respiratory distress syndrome. Am J Physiol Lung Cell Mol Physiol 2004;286(6):L1088–94.

27. Kondo T, Hattori N, Ishikawa N, et al. KL-6 concentration in pulmonary epithelial lining fluid is a useful prognostic indicator in patients with acute respiratory distress syndrome. Respir Res 2011;12:32.

28. van der Heijden M, Pickkers P, van Nieuw Amerongen GP, et al. Circulating angiopoietin-2 levels in the course of septic shock: relation with fluid balance, pulmonary dysfunction and mortality. Intensive Care Med 2009;35(9):1567–74.

29. Calfee CS, Gallagher D, Abbott J, et al. Plasma angiopoietin-2 in clinical acute lung injury: prognostic and pathogenetic significance. Crit Care Med 2012;40(6):1731–7.

30. van der Heijden M, van Nieuw Amerongen GP, Koolwijk P, et al. Angiopoietin-2, permeability oedema, occurrence and severity of ALI/ARDS in septic and non-septic critically ill patients. Thorax 2008;63(10):903–9.

31. Parikh SM, Mammoto T, Schultz A, et al. Excess circulating angiopoietin-2 may contribute to pulmonary vascular leak in sepsis in humans. PLoS Med 2006;3(3):e46.

32. Rubin DB, Wiener-Kronish JP, Murray JF, et al. Elevated von Willebrand factor antigen is an early plasma predictor of acute lung injury in nonpulmonary sepsis syndrome. J Clin Invest 1990;86(2):474–80.

33. Ong T, McClintock DE, Kallet RH, et al. Ratio of angiopoietin-2 to angiopoietin-1 as a predictor of mortality in acute lung injury patients. Crit Care Med 2010;38(9):1845–51.

34. Schmidt EP, Li G, Li L, et al. The circulating glycosaminoglycan signature of respiratory failure in critically ill adults. J Biol Chem 2014;289(12):8194–202.

35. Lim CM, Kim EK, Lee JS, et al. Comparison of the response to the prone position between pulmonary and extrapulmonary acute respiratory distress syndrome. Intensive Care Med 2001;27(3):477–85.

36. Rialp G, Betbese AJ, Perez-Marquez M, et al. Short-term effects of inhaled nitric oxide and prone position in pulmonary and extrapulmonary acute respiratory distress syndrome. Am J Respir Crit Care Med 2001;164(2):243–9.

37. Spragg RG, Lewis JF, Walmrath HD, et al. Effect of recombinant surfactant protein C-based surfactant on the acute respiratory distress syndrome. N Engl J Med 2004;351(9):884–92.

38. Anzueto A, Baughman RP, Guntupalli KK, et al. Aerosolized surfactant in adults with sepsis-induced acute respiratory distress syndrome. Exosurf Acute Respiratory Distress Syndrome Sepsis Study Group. N Engl J Med 1996;334(22):1417–21.

39. Kesecioglu J, Beale R, Stewart TE, et al. Exogenous natural surfactant for treatment of acute lung injury and the acute respiratory distress syndrome. Am J Respir Crit Care Med 2009;180(10):989–94.

40. Willson DF, Notter RH. The future of exogenous surfactant therapy. Respir Care 2011;56(9):1369–86 [discussion: 1386–8].

41. The Acute Respiratory Distress Syndrome Network. Ventilation with lower tidal volumes as compared with traditional tidal volumes for acute lung injury and the acute respiratory distress syndrome. N Engl J Med 2000;342(18):1301–8.

42. Eisner MD, Thompson T, Hudson LD, et al. Efficacy of low tidal volume ventilation in patients with different clinical risk factors for acute lung injury and the acute respiratory distress syndrome. Am J Respir Crit Care Med 2001;164(2):231–6.

43. Monchi M, Bellenfant F, Cariou A, et al. Early predictive factors of survival in the acute respiratory distress syndrome. A multivariate analysis. Am J Respir Crit Care Med 1998;158(4):1076–81.

44. Suntharalingam G, Regan K, Keogh BF, et al. Influence of direct and indirect etiology on acute outcome and 6-month functional recovery in acute respiratory distress syndrome. Crit Care Med 2001;29(3):562–6.

45. Agarwal R, Aggarwal AN, Gupta D, et al. Etiology and outcomes of pulmonary and extrapulmonary acute lung injury/ARDS in a respiratory ICU in North India. Chest 2006;130(3):724–9.

46. Agarwal R, Srinivas R, Nath A, et al. Is the mortality higher in the pulmonary vs the extrapulmonary ARDS? A meta analysis. Chest 2008;133(6):1463–73.

47. Parker CM, Heyland DK, Groll D, et al. Mechanism of injury influences quality of life in survivors of acute respiratory distress syndrome. Intensive Care Med 2006;32(11):1895–900.

48. Schelling G, Stoll C, Vogelmeier C, et al. Pulmonary function and health-related quality of life in a sample of long-term survivors of the acute respiratory distress syndrome. Intensive Care Med 2000;26(9):1304–11.

49. Orme J Jr, Romney JS, Hopkins RO, et al. Pulmonary function and health-related quality of life in survivors of acute respiratory distress syndrome. Am J Respir Crit Care Med 2003;167(5):690–4.

50. Herridge MS. Recovery and long-term outcome in acute respiratory distress syndrome. Crit Care Clin 2011;27(3):685–704.

51. Herridge MS, Tansey CM, Matte A, et al. Functional disability 5 years after acute respiratory distress syndrome. N Engl J Med 2011;364(14):1293–304.

52. Dowdy DW, Eid MP, Dennison CR, et al. Quality of life after acute respiratory distress syndrome: a meta-analysis. Intensive Care Med 2006;32(8): 1115–24.

53. Matute-Bello G, Downey G, Moore BB, et al. An official American Thoracic Society workshop report: features and measurements of experimental acute lung injury in animals. Am J Respir Cell Mol Biol 2011;44(5):725–38.

54. Su X, Looney MR, Gupta N, et al. Receptor for advanced glycation end-products (RAGE) is an indicator of direct lung injury in models of experimental lung injury. Am J Physiol Lung Cell Mol Physiol 2009;297(1):L1–5.

55. Calfee CS, Ware LB, Eisner MD, et al. Plasma receptor for advanced glycation end products and clinical outcomes in acute lung injury. Thorax 2008;63(12):1083–9.

56. Lomas-Neira J, Venet F, Chung CS, et al. Neutrophil-endothelial interactions mediate angiopoietin-2-associated pulmonary endothelial cell dysfunction in indirect acute lung injury in mice. Am J Respir Cell Mol Biol 2014;50(1):193–200.

57. Menezes SL, Bozza PT, Neto HC, et al. Pulmonary and extrapulmonary acute lung injury: inflammatory and ultrastructural analyses. J Appl Physiol (1985) 2005;98(5):1777–83.

58. Santos FB, Nagato LK, Boechem NM, et al. Time course of lung parenchyma remodeling in pulmonary and extrapulmonary acute lung injury. J Appl Physiol (1985) 2006;100(1):98–106.

59. Putensen C, Waibel U, Koller W, et al. Assessment of changes in lung microvascular permeability in posttraumatic acute lung failure after direct and indirect injuries to lungs. Anesth Analg 1992; 74(6):793–9.

60. Ware LB, Matthay MA. Alveolar fluid clearance is impaired in the majority of patients with acute lung injury and the acute respiratory distress syndrome. Am J Respir Crit Care Med 2001;163(6): 1376–83.

61. Tauseef M, Knezevic N, Chava KR, et al. TLR4 activation of TRPC6-dependent calcium signaling mediates endotoxin-induced lung vascular permeability and inflammation. J Exp Med 2012;209(11): 1953–68.

62. Egli M, Duplain H, Lepori M, et al. Defective respiratory amiloride-sensitive sodium transport predisposes to pulmonary oedema and delays its resolution in mice. J Physiol 2004;560(Pt 3): 857–65.

63. Perl M, Lomas-Neira J, Venet F, et al. Pathogenesis of indirect (secondary) acute lung injury. Expert Rev Respir Med 2011;5(1):115–26.

64. Galani V, Tatsaki E, Bai M, et al. The role of apoptosis in the pathophysiology of acute respiratory distress syndrome (ARDS): an up-to-date cell-specific review. Pathol Res Pract 2010;206(3):145–50.

65. Reiss LK, Uhlig U, Uhlig S. Models and mechanisms of acute lung injury caused by direct insults. Eur J Cell Biol 2012;91(6–7):590–601.

66. Puneet P, Moochhala S, Bhatia M. Chemokines in acute respiratory distress syndrome. Am J Physiol Lung Cell Mol Physiol 2005;288(1):L3–15.

67. Bhargava R, Janssen W, Altmann C, et al. Intratracheal IL-6 protects against lung inflammation in direct, but not indirect, causes of acute lung injury in mice. PLoS One 2013;8(5):e61405.

68. Leite-Junior JH, Garcia CS, Souza-Fernandes AB, et al. Methylprednisolone improves lung mechanics and reduces the inflammatory response in pulmonary but not in extrapulmonary mild acute lung injury in mice. Crit Care Med 2008;36(9):2621–8.

69. Venet F, Chung CS, Huang X, et al. Lymphocytes in the development of lung inflammation: a role for regulatory CD4+ T cells in indirect pulmonary lung injury. J Immunol 2009;183(5):3472–80.

70. Venet F, Huang X, Chung CS, et al. Plasmacytoid dendritic cells control lung inflammation and monocyte recruitment in indirect acute lung injury in mice. Am J Pathol 2010;176(2):764–73.

71. D'Alessio FR, Tsushima K, Aggarwal NR, et al. CD4+CD25+Foxp3+ Tregs resolve experimental lung injury in mice and are present in humans with acute lung injury. J Clin Invest 2009;119(10): 2898–913.

72. Garibaldi BT, D'Alessio FR, Mock JR, et al. Regulatory T cells reduce acute lung injury fibroproliferation by decreasing fibrocyte recruitment. Am J Respir Cell Mol Biol 2013;48(1):35–43.

73. Xing Z, Gauldie J, Cox G, et al. IL-6 is an antiinflammatory cytokine required for controlling local or systemic acute inflammatory responses. J Clin Invest 1998;101(2):311–20.

74. Mommsen P, Barkhausen T, Frink M, et al. Productive capacity of alveolar macrophages and pulmonary organ damage after femoral fracture and hemorrhage in IL-6 knockout mice. Cytokine 2011;53(1):60–5.

75. Gurkan OU, He C, Zielinski R, et al. Interleukin-6 mediates pulmonary vascular permeability in a two-hit model of ventilator-associated lung injury. Exp Lung Res 2011;37(10):575–84.

76. Meduri GU, Headley S, Kohler G, et al. Persistent elevation of inflammatory cytokines predicts a poor outcome in ARDS. Plasma IL-1 beta and IL-6 levels are consistent and efficient predictors of outcome over time. Chest 1995;107(4):1062–73.

77. Parsons PE, Eisner MD, Thompson BT, et al. Lower tidal volume ventilation and plasma cytokine markers of inflammation in patients with acute lung injury. Crit Care Med 2005;33(1):1–6 [discussion: 230–2].

78. Simmons EM, Himmelfarb J, Sezer MT, et al. Plasma cytokine levels predict mortality in patients with acute renal failure. Kidney Int 2004;65(4):1357–65.

79. Meng ZH, Dyer K, Billiar TR, et al. Essential role for IL-6 in postresuscitation inflammation in hemorrhagic shock. Am J Physiol Cell Physiol 2001; 280(2):C343–51.

80. Riva DR, Oliveira MBG, Rzezinski AF, et al. Recruitment maneuver in pulmonary and exptrapulmonary experimental acute lung injury. Crit Care Med 2008; 36(6):1900–8.

81. Kuiper JW, Plotz FB, Groeneveld AJ, et al. High tidal volume mechanical ventilation-induced lung injury in rats is greater after acid instillation than after sepsis-induced acute lung injury, but does not increase systemic inflammation: an experimental study. BMC Anesthesiol 2011;11:26.

82. Yang Y, Chen Q, Liu S, et al. Effects of recruitment maneuvers with PEEP on lung volume distribution in canine models of direct and indirect lung injury. Mol Biol Rep 2014;41(3):1325–33.

83. Maron-Gutierrez T, Silva JD, Asensi KD, et al. Effects of mesenchymal stem cell therapy on the time course of pulmonary remodeling depend on the etiology of lung injury in mice. Crit Care Med 2013;41(11):e319–33.

84. Araujo IM, Abreu SC, Maron-Gutierrez T, et al. Bone marrow-derived mononuclear cell therapy in experimental pulmonary and extrapulmonary acute lung injury. Crit Care Med 2010;38(8):1733–41.

85. Perl M, Chung CS, Lomas-Neira J, et al. Silencing of Fas, but not caspase-8, in lung epithelial cells ameliorates pulmonary apoptosis, inflammation, and neutrophil influx after hemorrhagic shock and sepsis. Am J Pathol 2005;167(6):1545–59.

86. Thakkar RK, Chung CS, Chen Y, et al. Local tissue expression of the cell death ligand, fas ligand, plays a central role in the development of extrapulmonary acute lung injury. Shock 2011;36(2):138–43.

Obesity and Nutrition in Acute Respiratory Distress Syndrome

Renee D. Stapleton, MD, PhD*, Benjamin T. Suratt, MD

KEYWORDS

- ARDS • Acute lung injury • Obesity • Nutrition • Enteral nutrition • Parenteral nutrition

KEY POINTS

- Among critically ill patients, obesity may be associated with a greater risk of development of acute respiratory distress syndrome (ARDS), but is also associated with better survival.
- Rising body mass index is associated with increased length of mechanical ventilation, intensive care stay, and hospital stay.
- Many elements of the metabolic syndrome have been implicated in the effects of obesity on ARDS risk and outcomes.
- Enteral nutrition should be used in the vast majority of ARDS patients, and the role for parenteral nutrition is extremely limited.
- Enteral nutrition should be started within 24 to 48 hours of ICU admission, and either full or trophic feedings for the first few days are reasonable.
- Consideration should be given to not monitor gastric residual volumes in most critically ill patients; new evidence suggests this is safe and does not lead to worse outcomes.

OBESITY AND ACUTE RESPIRATORY DISTRESS SYNDROME

The prevalence of obesity, especially extreme obesity (body mass index [BMI] $\geq$40 kg/m^2), has been rapidly increasing for the past 2 decades in the United States and other developed countries.[1] More than one third of the American population is obese, and more than 5% is extremely obese.[2] The public health consequences of this rise in obesity are considerable, because obesity is associated with significant morbidities and increased all-cause mortality in both men and women.[1] However, in critically ill patients including those with acute respiratory distress syndrome (ARDS), the relationship between obesity and morbidity and mortality seems to be more complex and at times counterintuitive. A decade of observational evidence suggests that obese patients may be at greater risk of developing ARDS and other organ failures in the intensive care unit (ICU), and of having protracted ICU and hospital lengths of stay (LOS) compared with normal weight patients. Yet, obese patients seem to have greater survival rates compared with similarly ill lean patients. Therefore, in contrast with what might be assumed by clinicians, although obesity may confer greater ICU morbidity, it seems to simultaneously decrease mortality. The mechanisms for these findings are not yet clear, but recent biologic data may begin to provide an explanation.

Disclosure Statement: Neither of the authors has any conflicts of interest.
Division of Pulmonary and Critical Care Medicine, Department of Medicine, University of Vermont, 149 Beaumont Avenue, Burlington, VT 05405, USA
* Corresponding author. 149 Beaumont Avenue, HSRF 222, Burlington, VT 05405.
E-mail address: renee.stapleton@uvm.edu

Clin Chest Med 35 (2014) 655–671
http://dx.doi.org/10.1016/j.ccm.2014.08.005
0272-5231/14/$ – see front matter © 2014 Elsevier Inc. All rights reserved.

Clinical Course and Outcomes of Acute Respiratory Distress Syndrome in Obese Patients

Studies in acute respiratory distress syndrome and general critical illness: risk

Although the protective effects of diabetes against the development of ARDS were first demonstrated 15 years ago,[3] little has been reported on the effects of obesity and other components of the metabolic syndrome on the development of ARDS. Obesity-associated comorbid illnesses, such as cardiovascular disease, undoubtedly increase the overall risk of developing critical illness, and recent studies have suggested that the obese are at increased risk for critical illness from infectious etiologies, such as the H1N1 influenza virus.[4] However, obesity's effects on the relative risk of developing ARDS, independent of comorbid conditions and other confounding factors, have only recently been examined. Work by Gong and colleagues,[5] examining a cohort of critically ill patients at risk for ARDS, suggests that the risk of developing ARDS rises with BMI, independent of severity illness, gender, diabetic status, or identified risk factor for ARDS. Obese BMI categories were associated with the development of ARDS compared with normal weight, with adjusted odds ratio of 1.66 (95% CI, 1.21–2.28) for obese and 1.78 (95% CI, 1.12–2.92) for severely obese. Additional work by this group has shown a similar association between BMI and the risk for acute kidney injury (AKI) in patients with ARDS.[6] Interestingly, this latter study also demonstrated an association between elevated BMI and decreased 60-day mortality in patients with ARDS and acute kidney injury.

Studies in acute respiratory distress syndrome and general critical illness: outcomes

Over the last decade, a growing number of observational studies have shown that, despite having elevated risks for the development of ARDS and other organ failures, obese critically ill patients paradoxically have similar to significantly improved survival compared with normal weight critically ill patients.[7–24] Although the majority of these reports have included general medical, surgical, and trauma ICU patients, several prior studies have specifically focused on ARDS (**Table 1**).[5,6,10,17,18,25]

Of these reports, most were performed as secondary analyses of other studies of ARDS, including the Molecular Epidemiology of ARDS study,[5,6] ARDS Network ARMA and ALVEOLI trials,[17,25] and King County Lung Injury Project (KCLIP) in Seattle,[18] and one was an observational study utilizing the Project Impact database.[10] All

but one[17] of these reports showed a significant association between BMI and ARDS mortality at their respective endpoints (ICU, hospital, or 28–90 days) in unadjusted analyses, in which mortality fell with rising BMI. The association between BMI and mortality was maintained after multivariate analyses in 2 of these studies,[6,17] in which the overweight and obese subjects were found to have reduced mortality compared with normal weight subjects, except possibly for those with a BMI of greater than 50 kg/m^2,[10] suggesting a 'J-curve' relationship between BMI and mortality. Three studies[5,10,18] also examined LOS and discharge disposition in their cohorts. Of these, 2 showed significant associations between rising BMI and the duration of mechanical ventilation, ICU, and hospital LOS, and the likelihood of subsequent discharge to a rehabilitation or skilled nursing facility.[5,18] Although in aggregate these studies do not yield a clear picture of BMI's effects on mortality, it is worth noting that the studies finding either no association between BMI and mortality or a loss of such association after multivariate analyses examined cohorts with relatively lower mean BMIs compared with the studies that showed significant associations. Thus, what can be surmised to date is that obesity has consistently been shown not to increase the risk of death from ARDS, and may even be protective in this disease.

In addition to these studies and many others that have examined general ICU patients, 3 meta-analyses[26–28] and a large observational study of outcomes in obese critically ill patients[23] have recently been published. The metaanalyses included 62,000 to 88,000 subjects from up to 22 published studies and found that critically ill overweight and obese subjects had significantly lower hospital mortality compared with normal weight subjects. The Dutch National Intensive Care Evaluation (NICE) observational study examined more than 154,000 critically ill patients from 1999 to 2010 and found a significant association between BMI and mortality, with an adjusted odds ratio that ranged from 0.86 to 0.96 in the overweight, obese, and severely obese BMI categories using a reference BMI of 25, whereas the adjusted OR for subjects in the normal BMI range was 1.07. As seen in several other studies, a slight upslope in mortality ('J curve') was noted as BMI rose above 40 kg/m^2 in this study, but it remained below that seen in the normal BMI range.

In summary, current evidence suggests that overweight, obese, and extremely obese critically ill patients may be at greater risk for the development of ARDS and may experience greater associated morbidity including ICU LOS and duration of mechanical ventilation with ARDS, yet these

Table 1
Summary of published studies of clinical outcomes in obese critically ill patients with ARDS

	O'Brien et al,[17] 2004	O'Brien et al,[10] 2006	Morris et al,[18] 2007	Stapleton et al,[25] 2010	Gong et al,[5] 2010	Soto et al,[6] 2012
Participants	807	1488	825	1409	1795	751
Design	Secondary analysis of data from 1 ARDS Network RCT	Cohort study using Project Impact database	Secondary analysis of prospectively collected data from King County Lung Injury Project	Secondary analysis of data from 2 ARDS Network RCTs	Retrospective cohort study of patients at risk for ARDS from 2 Boston hospitals	Retrospective cohort study of ARDS patients from 2 Boston hospitals
ARDS definition	AECC	Diagnosis codes from database	AECC	AECC	AECC	AECC
Primary Outcome (adjusted analyses)	No difference in 28-d mortality between obese and normal weight patients.	Significantly decreased hospital mortality in obese compared with normal weight patients.	No difference in hospital mortality between obese and normal weight patients.	No difference in 90-d mortality between obese and normal weight patients.	Increasing BMI (either as linear or categorical variable) significantly associated with development of ARDS.	Increasing BMI significantly associated with AKI.
Secondary Outcomes (adjusted analyses)	No differences in VFDs, achieving unassisted ventilation, or 180-day mortality between obese and normal weight patients.	No difference in ICU LOS, hospital LOS, or discharge location between obese and normal weight patients.	Significantly longer DMV, ICU LOS, and hospital LOS in severely obese survivors compared with normal weight patients. Severely obese patients also more likely to be discharged to a rehabilitation or skilled nursing facility than to home.	No differences in VFDs or OFFDs between obese and normal weight patients.	Increasing BMI associated with longer time from ICU admission to development of ARDS. Among 547 patients who developed ARDS, BMI not associated with 60-day mortality.[a]	Increasing BMI associated with significantly decreased 60-d mortality.[a]

Abbreviations: AECC, American–European Consensus Conference; AKI, acute kidney injury; ARDS, acute respiratory distress syndrome; BMI, body mass index; ICU, intensive care unit; LOS, length of stay; OFFDs, organ failure–free days; RCT, randomized controlled trial; VFDs, ventilator–free days.

[a] Although these 2 studies presumably included many of the same patients, one found no significant association between BMI and death although the other found that increasing BMI was associated with a significant decrease in death. One explanation may be that the multivariable models used in each study adjusted for different variables.

same patients seem to have equal to lower mortality from ARDS compared with normal weight patients (**Box 1**).

Limitations of prior investigations

There are several limitations to prior studies in outcomes in critically ill patients with and without ARDS. First, BMI has been used in all studies as the measure of obesity, but it may not accurately reflect obesity syndromes compared with other measurements, such as waist circumference.[29] Furthermore, measurement of BMI may be altered by intravenous fluid administration in ICU patients before weight is obtained or erroneous assessment of height in supine critically ill patients.[30] Third, a tool for assessing severity of illness specifically in obese patients does not exist and current assessment tools, including Acute Physiologic and Chronic Health Evaluation (APACHE) and Simplified Acute Physiology Score (SAPS),[31,32] may not accurately reflect mortality risk in obese patients owing to unknown factors that may be specific to the obese population. Fourth, processes of care for obese and extremely obese patients in different hospitals and ICUs are likely to be highly variable and may bias results, either toward improved or worse outcomes for obese patients.[33] Finally, diagnosing ARDS and assessing the degree of critical illness in extremely obese patients can be very difficult (eg, measuring noninvasive blood pressure measurements[34] or interpreting chest radiographs), thus leading to misclassification and incorrect case ascertainment, although many studies report an improvement in outcomes in the overweight and obese groups where such misclassification is less likely.[25] However, the study of critically ill patients at risk for ARDS by Gong and colleagues[5] found that increasing BMI was significantly associated with the subsequent development of ARDS owing to a greater incidence of hypoxemic respiratory failure (PaO_2/FiO_2 ratio <200) and not a greater incidence of bilateral pulmonary infiltrates on chest radiograph. Thus, misinterpretation of chest radiographs in obese patients is unlikely to be responsible for incorrect ascertainment.[5]

Possible explanation of findings

Results of these clinical studies have now prompted interest in investigating mechanisms by which obesity may influence ICU course and outcomes. Reasons for increased duration of mechanical ventilation and ICU LOS in obese patients with ARDS observed in some studies may be owing to physiologic factors that lead to longer duration of care, but do not increase mortality. For example, lung derecruitment owing to the weight of the abdomen and chest wall and provider reluctance to extubate an extremely obese patient may contribute to longer duration of ventilation.[35]

However, explanations of why the incidence of ARDS may be higher, yet survival better in obese patients compared with normal weight patients, are less clear. It is possible that the obese may be 'primed' for the development of ARDS through baseline low-grade inflammation and vascular activation and injury,[36,37] yet the subsequent sustained inflammation of ARDS is curtailed by as of yet unknown factors. In support of this, a recent study found that obese patients with established ARDS have higher levels of circulating von Willebrand factor, thought to be a marker of vascular injury, yet lower levels of proinflammatory cytokines (interleukin [IL]-6, IL-8) and surfactant protein D (a marker of alveolar epithelial injury) that are known to be increased in ARDS and to be associated with increased mortality,[25] thus suggesting that innate immunity and the inflammatory response may be altered in obesity.

Biologic Relationship of Obesity and Acute Respiratory Distress Syndrome

Obesity and the pathogenesis of acute respiratory distress syndrome

Despite decades of research, the pathogenesis of ARDS remains incompletely understood. It is increasingly recognized, however, that the pathogenesis and outcome of ARDS may be influenced by host factors, including genetic polymorphisms and comorbid conditions.[38,39] In this light, the clinical evidence that obesity may both promote and ameliorate ARDS suggests that obesity may be one such factor. In the case of ARDS promotion, such an interaction would not be surprising, because obesity is itself believed to be an inflammatory state with baseline increased circulating neutrophil levels,[40,41] elevations in blood tumor necrosis factor-α, IL-1β, IL-6, and IL-8,[42,43] and innate immune cell activation[44–46] with endothelial injury,[47–49] perhaps predictive of inflammatory

---

Box 1
Clinical effects of obesity on acute respiratory distress syndrome (ARDS)

- Risk of developing ARDS ↑
- Mortality from ARDS ↔/↓
- Duration of mechanical ventilation ↑
- Length of hospital stay ↑

Abbreviations: ↓, decreased; ↑, increased; ↔, no effect.

synergy between the obese state and inciters of ARDS. However, evidence that plasma IL-6 and IL-8 decrease with increasing BMI in ARDS patients[25] suggests that, although obesity may increase the risk of developing ARDS,[5] it may paradoxically have an attenuating effect on ARDS-associated inflammation and hence the progression of the disease.

Although human studies examining the effects of obesity on ARDS pathophysiology are scarce, recent reports in animal models suggest that such models may recapitulate the clinical effects of obesity, allowing further dissection of the underlying mechanisms. Most animal studies examining obesity-associated effects on pulmonary immunity and inflammation have focused on models of asthma and pneumonia, and although some forms of airway inflammation seem to be amplified by obesity,[50] the response to pneumonia is blunted,[51–53] suggesting that the inflammatory response in the alveoli (the site of ARDS) is impaired. In published reports examining obesity's effects on ARDS models, obese mice and rats demonstrate reduced inflammation, lung injury, and mortality from lipopolysaccharide-, hyperoxia-, and ozone-induced ARDS,[54–58] although in the case of ozone exposure, findings are mixed and seem to vary with the acuity of exposure.[57,59,60]

Obesity and its effects on the inflammatory response in acute respiratory distress syndrome

Given the systemic abnormalities associated with obesity and the accompanying metabolic syndrome, obesity's effects on the pathogenesis of ARDS almost certainly reflect interaction between multiple facets of the obese state. Although few reports focus on obesity itself, a growing literature examines the effects of the metabolic syndrome on ARDS pathogenesis and outcome. The most extensively investigated element of the metabolic syndrome in this regard is diabetes.

Diabetes has been convincingly shown to be associated with a reduced risk of developing ARDS in 4 large clinical studies of high-risk patients, including those with sepsis, aspiration, trauma, and massive transfusion, with an adjusted odds ratios ranging from 0.33 to 0.76.[3,61–63] Although this protective effect is reproducible in animal models of diabetes,[54,64–66] the underlying mechanisms remain unclear. Diabetes is associated with an impaired innate immune response[67,68] that, although believed to drive the increased risk of infection in diabetics through impairment of neutrophil function among other effects,[69] might conversely attenuate inappropriate inflammatory states such as ARDS. Evidence supporting roles for either hyperglycemia or insulin resistance in the attenuation of ARDS is conflicting, but a recent study has suggested that the protective effects of occur in both types 1 and 2 diabetes and are independent of diabetic therapy.[63] Interestingly, diabetic status was not associated with change in mortality in any of the 4 studies.

Comparable studies investigating dyslipidemia and its effects on ARDS risk and pathogenesis have not yet been published. However, as with obesity in general, dyslipidemia is associated with baseline elevations in circulating neutrophil levels in both humans and mouse models, often in the absence of accompanying obesity.[70–73] Persistent activation of both monocytes and neutrophils are described in dyslipidemic states, accompanied by endothelial injury,[74] and may be driven by direct effects of lipid species on leukocytes.[75–77] Yet, in this setting there seem to be defects in neutrophil and monocyte function,[78,79] and recently animal models of hypercholesterolemia without obesity have suggested that the development of lipopolysaccharide-induced ARDS is blunted[80] and that neutrophil chemotaxis and pulmonary macrophage activation are impaired in this model.[58] Whether such defects might reflect tonic activation of the innate immune system with "desensitization" to acute stimuli or other effects of the dyslipidemic state is not yet known.

Another significant feature of the metabolic syndrome and obesity in general is the dysregulation of adipokine release and response. Although initially described as hormonelike signaling molecules released by adipose tissue and involved in metabolic homeostasis, adipokines such as leptin, adiponectin, and visfatin have recently been shown to have protean effects, including modulation of both innate and adaptive immune systems.[81,82] The best studied of these molecules is leptin, which was originally described as a regulator of appetite. Leptin has been shown to be important in the marrow development of the myelomonocytic lineages,[83,84] and to serve as an activation and survival signal for neutrophils in the periphery.[85–87] Interestingly, leptin also seems to act as a neutrophil chemoattractant[88–91] and may be released by the injured lung,[91–93] whereas serum levels of leptin are increased in critical illness.[94–96] These findings, together with recent animal and human studies,[91,97] suggest a possible role for leptin in the development and progression of ARDS, and thus leptin resistance, as occurs in obesity, might yield a protective effect.

How leptin's effects on innate immune function may be altered in obesity is poorly understood.

Obesity is typically accompanied by a state of hyperleptinemic leptin resistance in which leptin response is blunted despite high circulating levels of this cytokine, presumably owing to receptor desensitization. Elevated leptin levels in patients with end-stage renal disease have been implicated in the neutrophil dysfunction that accompanies that state,[90] although animal models of aleptinemia and leptin resistance suggest that the development of hyperoxic and lipopolysaccharide-induced ARDS is blunted in this setting.[55,56,91] Whether hyperleptinemia with leptin resistance may affect the development of human ARDS has not yet been addressed.

Obesity and its effects on pulmonary mechanics in acute respiratory distress syndrome

A further possibility that must be considered when examining the potential interaction between obesity and ARDS focuses on the biomechanical effects of obesity. Obese individuals manifest altered pulmonary mechanics compared with lean individuals, at baseline and when mechanically ventilated (**Fig. 1**). Obese patients with ARDS demonstrate similar changes, with a combination of reduced chest wall and lung compliance leading to a lower functional residual capacity and consequently atelectasis, increased airways resistance and closure, and ventilation/perfusion mismatch.[98,99] Although these changes likely underlie obesity-associated delays in liberation

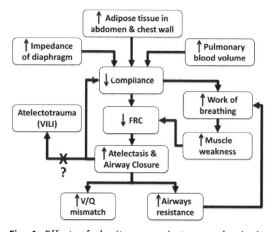

Fig. 1. Effects of obesity on respiratory mechanics in acute respiratory distress syndrome (ARDS). Obesity prolongs the duration of mechanical ventilation in ARDS through numerous effects on respiratory compliance and airways resistance. Yet, despite seeming to increase the risk of atelectrauma, the development of ventilator-induced lung injury may be reduced in this setting for unclear reasons.

from mechanical ventilation, how such alterations might be protective in ARDS are unclear.

It is possible that the combination of lower respiratory system compliance and higher airways resistance, which yield atelectasis and higher static and dynamic airway pressures for a given tidal volume, may prompt clinicians to selectively increase positive end-expiratory pressure and decrease tidal volumes in the obese, thus mimicking or accentuating a protective low tidal volume strategy. However, it has been shown that obese ARDS patients are typically ventilated at higher tidal volumes (mL/kg ideal body weight [IBW]) than normal weight patients,[17,18] indicating that, in light of comparable to improved survival in the obese, mechanical ventilation (even at higher tidal volumes) may be better tolerated in these patients. Furthermore, although overall mortality in the randomized control trial (RCT) of low tidal volume ventilation in ARDS was not different between lean and obese patients,[17] data from this study suggest that obese patients may have tolerated higher tidal volumes (12 mL/kg IBW) better than did lean patients. The relative reduction in mortality attributable to lower tidal volumes (6 mL/kg IBW) in the overall cohort was 30%, yet when stratified into normal, overweight, and obese BMI categories, the relative reductions in mortality between high and low tidal volume arms of the study were 42%, 27%, and 12%, respectively, although this finding did not attain significance. Thus, obese patients may be less susceptible to ventilator-induced lung injury. Whether this might be related to the mechanical interaction between obese patients and ventilation or an additional manifestation of attenuated inflammatory response in obese ARDS patients has yet to be examined.

In reviewing the literature describing the many effects of obesity and the metabolic syndrome, it is important to emphasize that both human and, with rare exceptions, animal studies examining "discrete" elements of obesity and the metabolic syndrome have not examined these in isolation of obesity or the other facets of the syndrome. For instance, only one of the reported clinical studies on diabetes and ARDS included BMI as a confounding variable, and the *db/db* mouse model, although used in various studies to specifically examine leptin resistance, diabetes, or obesity, is also noted to be extremely dyslipidemic. Furthermore, until the recent study of Yu and colleagues,[63] none of the published studies examining the effects of diabetes on ARDS risk included BMI as a potential confounding factor, and none has yet to include measures of dyslipidemia. Thus, it remains unclear which elements of obesity and the metabolic syndrome may be operative in the majority of reported findings, but several are plausible (**Fig. 2**).

Clinical Recommendations on Caring for Obese Acute Respiratory Distress Syndrome Patients

Caring for critically ill obese and severely obese patients in a clinical setting can be challenging. Like all ICU patients, special attention should be paid to prevention of infection with measures, such as the use of a checklist during central line insertion to prevent central line–associated blood stream infection[100] and semirecumbent positioning to prevent ventilator-associated pneumonia.[101] Prior studies have also suggested that obese patients who are mechanically ventilated receive tidal volumes early in their ICU course substantially greater than the 6 mL/kg predicted body weight shown to improve survival.[18,25,102] ICU clinicians should therefore be conscientious when choosing tidal volumes in obese patients. Furthermore, the recumbent position leads to increased atelectasis and greater mechanical loading of the diaphragm in obesity, contributing to hypoxia and difficulty weaning. Therefore, consideration should be given to positioning obese patients as upright (45°) as safely as possible and transitioning to chair during weans, both of which have been shown to improve

mechanics in these patients.[103] Last, the pharmacokinetics and pharmacodynamics of many drugs commonly used in critical illness are substantially altered in obese and severely obese patients compared with those of normal weight (eg, heparin and benzodiazepines); attention to detail when using these medicines is important (**Box 2**).

Summary: Obesity and Acute Respiratory Distress Syndrome

Survival in the general population is J-shaped, with increased mortality in underweight people, lowest mortality in patients with a BMI near 25 kg/m², and increasing mortality rates in overweight, obese, and extremely obese patients.[1,104] Evidence in critically ill patients, however, suggests that overweight, obese, and extremely obese patients have lower mortality compared with normal weight patients. The limited studies of obese patients published to date show that increasing BMI may increase the risk for the development of ARDS, but paradoxically does not increase mortality from this disease, and may in fact be protective. Health professionals may assume that obese patients have worse survival and morbidity owing to presumed difficulties of caring for such critically ill patients including transport, body positioning, intravascular access, diagnostic imaging, and ventilator weaning. Although the literature does

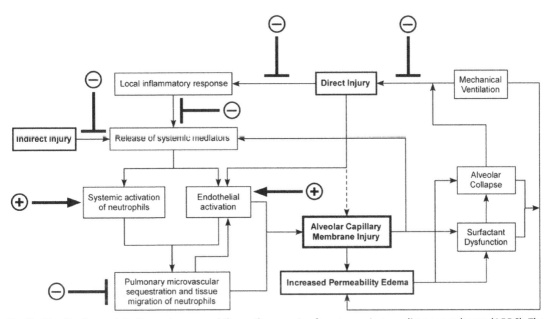

Fig. 2. Obesity, the metabolic syndrome, and the pathogenesis of acute respiratory distress syndrome (ARDS). The paradox of obesity-associated increased risk for the development of ARDS, yet associated improvement in ARDS outcomes is schematically summarized. ↑, possible synergistic effects of obesity on ARDS pathogenesis; ⊥, possible inhibitory effects (see text). (*Adapted from* Suratt BT, Parsons PE. Mechanisms of acute lung injury/acute respiratory distress syndrome. Clin Chest Med 2006;27(4):587; with permission.)

Box 2
Management recommendations for obese acute respiratory distress syndrome (ARDS) patients

- Low tidal volume (6 mL/kg) ventilation based on *ideal body weight*
- Drug dosing based on appropriate body weight (actual, ideal, lean)
- Semirecumbent positioning and wean upright (45°)
- Anticipate slow wean from mechanical ventilation
- Proper gastrointestinal and deep venous thrombosis prophylaxis and skin care

---

suggest that obese patients may have greater durations of ventilation and ICU LOS, their survival is at least as good as normal weight patients. This information is important for clinicians to recognize when discussing prognosis and expectations with critically ill patients and their families.

NUTRITION IN PATIENTS WITH ACUTE RESPIRATORY DISTRESS SYNDROME

Critical illness, and more specifically the ARDS, is a catabolically stressed state where patients demonstrate a systemic inflammatory response, multiple organ dysfunction, hypermetabolism, infectious complications, and malnutrition.[105] Malnutrition is coupled with impairment of immune function and increased morbidity and mortality in critically ill patients.[106] Over the past decade or more, as we have come to better understand immunologic effects of nutrition in critical illness, nutrition has begun to be thought of as therapeutic, rather than purely supportive. Additionally, the concept of pharmaconutrition, or the delivery of specific nutrients with potential immunomodulating properties, has emerged. Fortunately, several recent large studies about nutrition in critical care, with some investigations specifically in patients with ARDS, have provided valuable new evidence (**Table 2**).

Enteral Versus Parenteral Nutrition

Enteral nutrition (EN) is the standard of care in patients with ARDS and should be initiated preferentially over parenteral nutrition (PN), unless there is a known contraindication to EN such as ischemic bowel, intestinal obstruction, severe malabsorption, or severe short gut syndrome. Several RCTs have compared EN with PN in critically ill patients with an intact gastrointestinal (GI) tract, and when these data were aggregated in metaanalyses,

there was no difference in survival.[107–109] However, EN is associated with a significant reduction in infectious complications (RR, 0.58; 95% CI, 0.41–0.80), in addition to being less expensive than PN. Data also suggest that lack of use of the GI tract rapidly leads to atrophy of gut lumenal mucosa, and this may increase bacterial translocation across the wall of the gut into the bloodstream.[110] Even small amounts of EN, called trophic feedings, increase blood flow to the GI tract and preserve GI epithelium, and EN may also improve overall immune function by supporting gut-associated lymphoid tissue.[111]

Early Versus Delayed Nutrition

Early EN is most often defined as being initiated within 48 hours of ICU admission. Many prior RCTs have compared early EN versus delayed nutrient intake in mechanically ventilated critically ill patients, and when these results were metaanalyzed, early EN was associated with a trend toward mortality reduction (relative risk [RR], 0.75; 95% CI, 0.50–1.04; $P = .08$) and a significant reduction in infectious complications (RR, 0.81; 95% CI, 0.68–0.97; $P = .02$).[112] The provision of early EN does not seem to be associated with duration of mechanical ventilation or ICU LOS. There have been 6 studies that have investigated EN versus no EN or intravenous fluids alone, and when these data are aggregated, the trends in reduction of mortality (RR, 0.62; 95% CI, 0.37–1.05; $P = .08$) and infectious complications (RR, 0.70; 95% CI, 0.48–1.02; $P = .06$) hold. Thus, these data suggest that EN should be initiated in critically ill patients with ARDS within 48 hours of ICU admission unless there is an absolute contraindication to EN.

Ischemic bowel has been reported as a very rare complication of EN in critically ill patients and can be fatal. Recent guidelines therefore recommend that EN be avoided when patients are in shock or being actively resuscitated, when vasopressors are being initiated, or when vasopressor doses are increasing.[113] However, a recent, well-done, large, observational study of 1174 mechanically ventilated patients receiving vasopressors found that early EN (initiated <48 hours after ICU admission) was associated with reduced hospital mortality (odds ratio, 0.65; 95% CI, 0.48–0.89) and hazard of death (HR = 0.70; 95% CI, 0.56–0.88) after adjustment for severity of illness (APACHE score), age, sex, standardized mortality ratio, race, source of admission, and admitting diagnosis.[114] After propensity matching, hospital mortality remained significantly lower in the early EN group. These new data suggest that initiating EN early is safe,

Table 2
Nutrition in ARDS/critical illness: summary of the evidence

Intervention	Evidence
EN vs PN	In mechanically ventilated critically ill patients, EN is associated with fewer infectious complications but no change in survival.
Early vs delayed EN	Among mechanically ventilated critically ill patients, early EN compared with delayed nutrient intake is associated with a trend toward mortality reduction and significant reduction in infectious complications, but no change in DMV or ICU LOS. Among 6 studies investigating EN vs no EN or intravenous fluids alone, trends in reduction of mortality and infectious complications hold.
Caloric prescription of EN	In patients with ARDS, there are no differences in VFDs, OFFDs, mortality, infectious complications, or long-term outcomes between patients receiving full or trophic enteral feeding for the first 6 d of their ICU course.
Supplementation of calories with PN	Among general critically ill patients, early supplemental PN to meet calculated caloric goals does not change mortality or functional status at discharge, but does lead to longer ICU LOS, more infectious complications, longer DMV and renal replacement therapy, and higher costs. Among critically ill patients with a relative short-term contraindication to EN, early supplemental PN does not affect mortality, ICU LOS, or hospital LOS.
Glutamine	Controversial, but recent data suggest that glutamine should not be administered at higher doses in mechanically ventilated patients with multiple organ failure (increased 28-day and 6-month mortality).
Antioxidants	In mechanically ventilated critically ill patients, no clear benefit of antioxidants including selenium, as well as enteral zinc, β-carotene, and vitamins C and E.
Omega-3 fatty acids	Controversial, with studies of an enteral feeding formula containing omega-3s demonstrating benefits and studies of bolus enteral fish oil finding no benefit.

Abbreviations: ARDS, acute respiratory distress syndrome; EN, enteral nutrition; ICU, intensive care unit; LOS, length of stay; OFFDs, organ failure–free days; PN, parenteral nutrition; VFDs, ventilator-free days.

even in patients receiving vasopressors, but that care should be taken in patients who are in shock and being aggressively resuscitated.

Caloric Prescription of Enteral Nutrition

These data suggest that EN, preferentially over PN, should be started early in critically ill patients with ARDS, but they do not inform the questions of how many calories patients should receive or whether supplemental PN should be used to meet caloric requirement. Fortunately, several large RCTs in critically ill patients discussed herein have shed more light on these issues. Energy expenditure is variable and depends on age, gender, body mass, and type and severity of illness. In critically ill patients, total energy expenditure can be measured with indirect calorimetry. However, in clinical practice, resting energy expenditure is usually estimated using a variety of available equations and is then multiplied by a "stress factor" of

1.0 to 2.0 to estimate total energy expenditure (and therefore caloric requirements). Roughly 25 kcal/kg IBW is frequently the standard practice, and other equations such as Harris-Benedict, Ireton-Jones, and Weir are commonly used. Predictive equations, however, tend to be inaccurate,[115] and furthermore, data do not suggest that precise estimation of caloric need is associated with improved outcomes.

The National Heart Lung and Blood Institute's ARDS Network recently published a large RCT of trophic enteral feeding versus full enteral feeding.[116] Before this study, literature on hypocaloric feeding in critically ill patients had been largely observational and found contradictory results. For example, 1 study found that a greater cumulative caloric deficit was associated with worse clinical outcomes,[117] whereas another observational study demonstrated that ICU patients who received from 33% to 66% of their caloric goal had better clinical outcomes than those patients who received 67%

to 100% of their goal.[118] In the ARDS Network trophic feeding study, 1000 adults with ARDS for less than 48 hours were randomized to receive either 10 to 20 kcal/h or full calorie enteral feeding for the first 6 days after enrollment, followed by full enteral feeding in all patients. Participants were relatively young (mean age, 52 years) and obese (mean BMI, approximately 30 kg/m^2). The trophic group received approximately 400 kcal/d for the first 6 days, whereas the full feeding group received 1300 kcal/d. There were no differences in the primary outcome of ventilator-free days between the trophic and full feeding groups (14.9 [95% CI, 13.9–15.9] and 15.0 [95% CI, 14.1–15.9]; $P = .81$). Mortality at 60 days (23.3% vs 22.2%; $P = .77$), organ failure–free days, and infectious complications were also not different between the 2 groups.

In addition to participants in this trophic feeding study being relatively young and well-nourished, 1 additional criticism of this trial was that it did not examine long-term outcomes, so any deleterious effect of trophic feeding after hospitalization are unknown. In response, 2 studies examining long-term outcomes in surviving participants of the trophic feeding trial have recently been published, and both suggest that trophic feeding in these patients has no long-term untoward effects. In the first study, the authors used several survey instruments administered over the phone or by mail to assess physical function, mental health, quality of life, anxiety, depression, posttraumatic stress disorder, cognition, and employment at 6 ($n = 525$) and 12 ($n = 508$) months after randomization in the trophic feeding RCT.[119] Patients who were cognitively impaired at baseline, homeless, non–English speaking, or younger than 18 years were excluded. There was no difference in survival at 12 months (65% of trophic group vs 63% of full feeding group; $P = .63$). Physical function at 12 months (the primary outcome) was not different between the trophic and full feeding groups, and the vast majority of hypothesis-generating secondary outcome analyses also found no difference between groups. Because self-reported outcomes may differ from those actually measured, in the second study the same authors also examined a smaller sample of 174 surviving participants of the trophic feeding trial to determine their in-person physical and cognitive performance.[120] Six-minute walk test, 4-minute timed walk speed, manual muscle testing, hand grip strength, maximum inspiratory pressure, forced expiratory volume in the first second of expiration, forced vital capacity, BMI, arm anthropometrics, and a battery of cognitive tests evaluating executive function, language, memory, verbal reasoning, and attention were all measured at 6 and 12 months after ARDS onset by blinded research personnel. None of the physical or cognitive outcomes measured at 6 and 12 months were different between participants in the trophic and full feeding groups, even after adjustment for nonsignificant baseline differences in multivariable analyses. These studies of early trophic versus full enteral feedings in patients with ARDS suggest that either approach is reasonable in patients who are relatively well-nourished and young. Data on caloric prescription for malnourished patients are sparse, and these patients should probably receive full calorie feedings until further research is available.

Monitoring Enteral Nutrition

Given the frequency of gastric dysmotility in critically ill patients, it became common practice over the past several decades to frequently monitor tolerance of enteral feeding by checking gastric residual volumes (GRV), especially in the first few days after initiating enteral feedings. However, lower GRV thresholds result in delivery of less EN owing to frequent interruptions and are not associated with less vomiting, aspiration, or pneumonias.[121–123] Thus, many institutions have increased their GRV thresholds for stopping enteral feedings up to 500 mL, as per current guidelines.[113]

Importantly, a recent RCT investigated the effect of not monitoring GRV at all. In this noninferiority study, 452 mechanically ventilated adults receiving EN within 36 hours of initiation of ventilation were randomized to either undergo no GRV monitoring or to undergo GRV monitoring every 6 hours with adjustment in the EN delivery rate if the GRV exceeded 250 mL.[124] Patients whose GRV were not being monitored did experience more vomiting. However, rates of ventilator-associated pneumonia were similar between the nonmonitored and monitored groups (16.7% vs 15.8%; difference, 0.9%; 90% CI, −4.8% to 6.7%) and were within the 10% specified noninferiority margin. Additional clinical outcomes, including infectious complications, duration of mechanical ventilation, ICU and hospital LOS, and mortality, were also similar between the 2 groups. These new data should prompt clinicians and institutions to consider changing practice to not routinely monitor GRV.

Supplementing Calories with Parenteral Nutrition

Practices with using PN in critically ill patients differ greatly between North America and Europe. European guidelines suggest that PN should be started within the first 2 days of critical illness in patients who cannot be adequately fed with EN, whereas American guidelines recommend against using PN unless there is an absolute contraindication to EN.[113,125] To investigate this controversy, a group of European investigators randomized 4640 critically ill adults to receive PN initiated early (within the first 48 hours of ICU admission) or late (not until day 8).[126] All patients received early EN per protocol. Approximately 22% of patients were admitted with sepsis, and slightly more than 41% of patients were emergency admissions. Mortality at 90 days was similar in both groups (11.2% in both; $P = 1.00$), and functional status was not different between the groups at discharge. ICU LOS was shorter in the late initiation group than in the early initiation group (3 [interquartile range, 2–7] vs 4 days [interquartile range, 2–9]; $P = .02$). Patients in the late initiation group also had fewer new infections, shorter durations of mechanical ventilation and renal replacement therapy, and a reduction in overall health care costs.

Subsequently, the Australia New Zealand Intensive Care Society Clinical Trials Group investigated the use of PN in patients with contra-indications to EN.[127] In this RCT, 1372 patients with short-term relative contraindications to EN were randomized to receive early PN or standard care. In the standard care group, time to EN or PN was a mean of 2.8 days, whereas participants in the early PN group because receiving their PN an average of 44 minutes after randomization. In this study, 65% of participants were surgery patients. Only approximately 15% were admitted with either sepsis or a primary respiratory diagnosis, and the proportion of patients with ARDS in this study is not clear. There was no difference in 60-day mortality between the groups (21.5% of early PN vs 22.8% of standard care participants; $P = .60$). Patients receiving early PN did have an average of one half less day of mechanical ventilation (7.73 vs 7.26 days; $P = .01$), but their ICU and hospital LOS were not different than patients receiving standard care. Taken together, these 2 recent large RCTs, although not restricted to patients with ARDS, indicate that there is likely no benefit in supplementing with PN early in the ICU course to meet caloric goals in a general ICU population that included surgical patients, nor is there a clear benefit to initiating PN early in patients who have short-term relative contraindications to receiving EN. These results are not generalizable to malnourished patients, and current guidelines recommend the consideration of early PN in patients who are unable to receive EN and who are malnourished.[113]

Provision of Macronutrients and Micronutrients in Patients with Acute Respiratory Distress Syndrome

There are few data available to inform the macronutrient composition of enteral feedings. In general, guidelines suggest that critically ill patients should receive an amount of protein daily between 1.5 and 2.0 g/kg IBW. The use of whole protein, or polymeric, formulas is recommended because there are insufficient data to support the routine use of peptide-based formulas in most patients.[113] In most enteral formulas, approximately 25% to 30% of calories are from fat. Similar to protein, there is insufficient evidence in the literature to support the routine use of high-fat or low-fat enteral formulas.

Several individual micronutrients have been examined over the past decade for their potential benefit in patients with ARDS and in critically ill patients in general. Recent data suggest that glutamine, antioxidants, and omega-3 fatty acids are not beneficial in critically ill patients.

Glutamine

Glutamine is a ubiquitous amino acid that plays a large role in protein synthesis, and literature has suggested that it may be beneficial in terms of maintaining integrity of the GI lumen. A 2002 systematic review of glutamine supplementation in critically ill patients suggested that it was associated with a reduction in mortality and infectious complications, and that these effects were generally limited to parenteral higher dose glutamine.[128] Although a concentrated dipeptide formulation of intravenous glutamine is available outside of North America and is commonly administered, intravenous glutamine is only available in a formulation in Canada and the United States that has limited solubility and requires excess fluid administration.

In contradiction, a recent blinded 2×2 factorialized trial glutamine and antioxidants suggests that supplemental glutamine may be harmful in critically ill patients with organ failure.[129] In this RCT, 1223 critically ill adults who were mechanically ventilated with at least 2 organ failures were randomized to receive enteral and parenteral glutamine or placebo (and were also randomized to receive enteral and parental antioxidants or placebo). Approximately 30% of the participants were admitted with a respiratory disorder, and another 30% had sepsis. Mortality at 28 days among those who received glutamine was 32.4% versus 27.2% among those receiving placebo ($P = .05$), and mortality at 6 months was also greater in the glutamine group. Additionally, glutamine had no effect on infectious complications or rates of organ failure. Although this study was not specifically conducted in patients with ARDS, these recent data indicate that glutamine should not be administered to mechanically ventilated patients with more than 1 organ failure.

Antioxidants

Because oxidative stress plays a prominent role in critical illness and may contribute to worsening systemic inflammation and organ failure, it has been hypothesized that supplementation with antioxidants may improve clinical outcomes. More than 20 trials have investigated antioxidants and minerals in critically ill patients, including various combinations of selenium, zinc, copper, manganese, β-carotene, and vitamins C and E. When the results of these studies were meta-analyzed, antioxidants were associated with a reduction in mortality (RR, 0.82; 95% CI, 0.72–0.93; P = .002), as well as reduction in duration of mechanical ventilation (0.67 fewer days; 95% CI, −1.22 to −0.13; P = .02), and a trend toward a reduction in infections (RR, 0.88; 95% CI, 0.76–1.02; P = .08).[130]

Subsequent to this metaanalysis in 2013, the large 2 × 2 factorialized trial of glutamine and antioxidants was published.[129] The 1223 mechanically ventilated critically ill adults with more than 1 organ failure were randomized to receive placebo or to receive both intravenous and enteral selenium, as well as enteral zinc, β-carotene, and vitamins C and E. Mortality at 28 days was not different between the antioxidant and control groups (30.8% vs 28.8%; P = .48). Secondary outcomes including hospital mortality, 6-month mortality, hospital LOS, ICU LOS, organ failure, and infectious complications were also not different between the 2 groups. Again, although this large RCT was not conducted specifically in patients with ARDS, this study population was similar to ARDS patients in that they were all mechanically ventilated with more than 1 organ failure. The lack of benefit with combined antioxidant supplementation indicates that there is a limited role for antioxidant delivery at the doses given.

Omega-3 fatty acids

Through several mechanisms, including alteration of inflammatory cell membrane phospholipid composition, omega-3 fatty acids can modify eicosanoid inflammatory profiles, and delivery has therefore been investigated as a therapy for ARDS and sepsis. The use of feeding formulas containing omega-3 fatty acids (fish oil) in patients with ARDS and sepsis is currently controversial. Three prior trials comparing an enteral feeding formula containing omega-3 fatty acids, borage oil (γ-linolenic acid), and antioxidants to placebo found benefit, but the control group in those studies received a high-fat feeding formula that is not standard of care.[131–133] However, 2 additional recent randomized trials of omega-3 fatty acids found no benefit. The first study was a phase II RCT that investigated enteral liquid fish oil versus saline placebo in 90 patients with ARDS and found no difference in biologic (various systemic and circulating markers of inflammation and injury) or clinical endpoints.[134] The second study was a large ARDS Network RCT of a twice daily enteral supplement containing fish oil, γ-linolenic acid, and antioxidants compared with an isocaloric control. This study was stopped early for futility after enrollment of 272 patients. Results demonstrated that participants receiving the omega-3 supplement had fewer ventilator-free days (14.0 vs 17.2; P = .02), ICU-free days (14.0 vs 16.7; P = .04), and organ failure-free days (12.3 vs 15.5; P = .02) than participants in the control group. Additionally, 60-day mortality was greater in the omega-3 group (26.6% vs 16.3%; P = .054). Explanations for the contradictory finding between these studies are unclear and may include fat and protein content of the control group supplement as well as potential differences with continuous versus bolus delivery of omega-3 fats. More research is needed in this area to provide definitive recommendations, but given the results of the ARDS Network study that was stopped for futility, there is concern for potential harm with these supplements.

Summary: Nutrition in Acute Respiratory Distress Syndrome

Over the past several years, much research on nutrition in critical illness and ARDS has been performed. Key questions such as the amount of protein that should be delivered remain unanswered, but important information has been obtained. Aggregated data suggest that patients with ARDS should preferentially receive EN, and this should be started early (within 48 hours of ICU admission) to preserve GI lumen integrity and prevent infectious complications. New research demonstrates that in well-nourished, relatively young patients with ARDS, provision of both full calorie or trophic enteral feedings during the first 6 days of the ICU course, followed by full calorie feedings, is reasonable and does not affect long-term outcomes. After patients with shock are resuscitated and hemodynamically stable, they can safely receive EN even if they are receiving stable lower doses of vasopressors. Additionally,

Box 3
Clinical nutrition in critically ill patients with acute respiratory distress syndrome (ARDS)

- Enteral nutrition, rather than parenteral nutrition, should be used in the vast majority of ARDS patients and should be started within 48 hours of ICU admission.
- Either full feeding or trophic feeding for the first few days of a patient's ICU stay is reasonable.
- After patients with shock are resuscitated and hemodynamically stable, they can safely receive enteral nutrition even if they are receiving stable lower doses of vasopressors.
- Consideration should be given to not monitor gastric residual volumes in most critically ill patients, because new evidence suggests this is safe and does not lead to worse outcomes.
- In reasonably well-nourished critically ill patients, there is no role for parenteral nutrition either as a caloric supplement to enteral nutrition early during the ICU course or in patients who have a short-term relative contraindication to enteral nutrition. The optimal role of parenteral nutrition in malnourished patients is currently being investigated.
- New data suggest that glutamine, antioxidants, and omega-3 fatty acids may not be beneficial in critically ill patients.

Abbreviation: ICU, intensive care unit.

a recent study found that not monitoring GRV in most critically ill patients is safe and does not lead to worse outcomes; thus, it is reasonable for clinicians to devise enteral feeding protocols for their ARDS patients that do not involve routine monitoring of GRV. Two recent international RCTs of PN concluded that it is not beneficial as either a caloric supplement to EN or an alternative in patients who have a short-term relative contraindication to EN. Finally, additional newly published RCTS have found that glutamine and antioxidants, as well as omega-3 fatty acids, are of no benefit in critically ill patients with at least 2 organ failures and with ARDS, respectively (**Box 3**).

REFERENCES

1. Adams KF, Schatzkin A, Harris TB, et al. Overweight, obesity, and mortality in a large prospective cohort of persons 50 to 71 years old. N Engl J Med 2006;355(8):763–78.
2. Flegal KM, Carroll MD, Ogden CL, et al. Prevalence and trends in obesity among US adults, 1999-2008. JAMA 2010;303(3):235–41.
3. Moss M, Guidot DM, Steinberg KP, et al. Diabetic patients have a decreased incidence of acute respiratory distress syndrome. Crit Care Med 2000;28(7):2187–92.
4. Diaz E, Rodriguez A, Martin-Loeches I, et al. Impact of obesity in patients infected with 2009 influenza A(H1N1). Chest 2011;139(2):382–6.
5. Gong MN, Bajwa EK, Thompson BT, et al. Body mass index is associated with the development of acute respiratory distress syndrome. Thorax 2010;65(1):44–50.
6. Soto GJ, Frank AJ, Christiani DC, et al. Body mass index and acute kidney injury in the acute respiratory distress syndrome. Crit Care Med 2012;40(9):2601–8.
7. Finkielman JD, Gajic O, Afessa B. Underweight is independently associated with mortality in postoperative and non-operative patients admitted to the intensive care unit: a retrospective study. BMC Emerg Med 2004;4(1):3.
8. Garrouste-Orgeas M, Troche G, Azoulay E, et al. Body mass index. An additional prognostic factor in ICU patients. Intensive Care Med 2004;30(3):437–43.
9. Aldawood A, Arabi Y, Dabbagh O. Association of obesity with increased mortality in the critically ill patient. Anaesth Intensive Care 2006;34(5):629–33.
10. O'Brien JM Jr, Phillips GS, Ali NA, et al. Body mass index is independently associated with hospital mortality in mechanically ventilated adults with acute lung injury. Crit Care Med 2006;34(3):738–44.
11. Peake SL, Moran JL, Gholani DR, et al. The effect of obesity on 12-month survival following admission to intensive care: a prospective study. Crit Care Med 2006;34(12):2929–39.
12. Martino JL, Stapleton RD, Wang M, et al. Extreme obesity and outcomes in critically ill patients. Chest 2011;140(5):1198–206.
13. Marik P, Doyle H, Varon J. Is obesity protective during critical illness? an analysis of a National ICU database. Crit Care Shock 2003;6:156–62.
14. Tremblay A, Bandi V. Impact of body mass index on outcomes following critical care. Chest 2003;123(4):1202–7.
15. Smith RL, Chong TW, Hedrick TL, et al. Does body mass index affect infection-related outcomes in the intensive care unit? Surg Infect (Larchmt) 2007;8(6):581–8.
16. Newell MA, Bard MR, Goettler CE, et al. Body mass index and outcomes in critically injured blunt trauma patients: weighing the impact. J Am Coll Surg 2007;204(5):1056–61 [discussion: 1062–4].
17. O'Brien JM Jr, Welsh CH, Fish RH, et al. Excess body weight is not independently associated with outcome in mechanically ventilated patients with acute lung injury. Ann Intern Med 2004;140(5):338–45.

18. Morris AE, Stapleton RD, Rubenfeld GD, et al. The association between body mass index and clinical outcomes in acute lung injury. Chest 2007;131(2): 342–8.

19. Alban RF, Lyass S, Margulies DR, et al. Obesity does not affect mortality after trauma. Am Surg 2006;72(10):966–9.

20. Brown CV, Rhee P, Neville AL, et al. Obesity and traumatic brain injury. J Trauma 2006;61(3):572–6.

21. Ciesla DJ, Moore EE, Johnson JL, et al. Obesity increases risk of organ failure after severe trauma. J Am Coll Surg 2006;203(4):539–45.

22. Ray DE, Matchett SC, Baker K, et al. The effect of body mass index on patient outcomes in a medical ICU. Chest 2005;127(6):2125–31.

23. Pickkers P, de Keizer N, Dusseljee J, et al. Body mass index is associated with hospital mortality in critically ill patients: an observational cohort study. Crit Care Med 2013;41(8):1878–83.

24. Sakr Y, Elia C, Mascia L, et al. Being overweight or obese is associated with decreased mortality in critically ill patients: a retrospective analysis of a large regional Italian multicenter cohort. J Crit Care 2012;27(6):714–21.

25. Stapleton RD, Dixon AE, Parsons PE, et al. The association between BMI and plasma cytokine levels in patients with acute lung injury. Chest 2010;138(3):568–77.

26. Akinnusi ME, Pineda LA, El Solh AA. Effect of obesity on intensive care morbidity and mortality: a meta-analysis. Crit Care Med 2008;36(1):151–8.

27. Hogue CW Jr, Stearns JD, Colantuoni E, et al. The impact of obesity on outcomes after critical illness: a meta-analysis. Intensive Care Med 2009;35(7): 1152–70.

28. Oliveros H, Villamor E. Obesity and mortality in critically ill adults: a systematic review and meta-analysis. Obesity (Silver Spring) 2008;16(3):515–21.

29. Clinical guidelines on the identification, evaluation, and treatment of overweight and obesity in adults– the Evidence Report. National Institutes of Health. Obes Res 1998;6(Suppl 2):51S–209S.

30. McCallister JW, Adkins EJ, O'Brien JM Jr. Obesity and acute lung injury. Clin Chest Med 2009;30(3): 495–508, viii.

31. Knaus WA, Draper EA, Wagner DP, et al. APACHE II: a severity of disease classification system. Crit Care Med 1985;13(10):818–29.

32. Le Gall JR, Lemeshow S, Saulnier F. A new Simplified Acute Physiology Score (SAPS II) based on a European/North American multicenter study. JAMA 1993;270(24):2957–63.

33. O'Brien JM Jr, Philips GS, Ali NA, et al. The association between body mass index, processes of care, and outcomes from mechanical ventilation: a prospective cohort study. Crit Care Med 2012; 40(5):1456–63.

34. Maxwell MH, Waks AU, Schroth PC, et al. Error in blood-pressure measurement due to incorrect cuff size in obese patients. Lancet 1982;2(8288):33–6.

35. Walz JM, Zayaruzny M, Heard SO. Airway management in critical illness. Chest 2007;131(2):608–20.

36. Konter J, Baez E, Summer RS. Obesity: "priming" the lung for injury. Pulm Pharmacol Ther 2013; 26(4):427–9.

37. Bustamante AF, Repine JE. The obesity ARDS paradox: "a pre-conditioning cloud". J Pulm Respir Med 2012;2(8):e122.

38. Ware LB, Matthay MA. The acute respiratory distress syndrome. N Engl J Med 2000;342(18): 1334–49.

39. Suratt BT, Parsons PE. Mechanisms of acute lung injury/acute respiratory distress syndrome. Clin Chest Med 2006;27(4):579–89 [abstract: viii].

40. Kim JA, Park HS. White blood cell count and abdominal fat distribution in female obese adolescents. Metabolism 2008;57(10):1375–9.

41. Desai MY, Dalal D, Santos RD, et al. Association of body mass index, metabolic syndrome, and leukocyte count. Am J Cardiol 2006;97(6):835–8.

42. Ramos EJ, Xu Y, Romanova I, et al. Is obesity an inflammatory disease? Surgery 2003;134(2):329–35.

43. Yudkin JS. Adipose tissue, insulin action and vascular disease: inflammatory signals. Int J Obes Relat Metab Disord 2003;27(Suppl 3):S25–8.

44. Cottam DR, Schaefer PA, Fahmy D, et al. The effect of obesity on neutrophil Fc receptors and adhesion molecules (CD16, CD11b, CD62L). Obes Surg 2002;12(2):230–5.

45. Cottam DR, Schaefer PA, Shaftan GW, et al. Effect of surgically-induced weight loss on leukocyte indicators of chronic inflammation in morbid obesity. Obes Surg 2002;12(3):335–42.

46. Nijhuis J, Rensen SS, Slaats Y, et al. Neutrophil activation in morbid obesity, chronic activation of acute inflammation. Obesity (Silver Spring) 2009; 17(11):2014–8.

47. Blann AD, Bushell D, Davies A, et al. von Willebrand factor, the endothelium and obesity. Int J Obes Relat Metab Disord 1993;17(12):723–5.

48. van Harmelen V, Eriksson A, Astrom G, et al. Vascular peptide endothelin-1 links fat accumulation with alterations of visceral adipocyte lipolysis. Diabetes 2008;57(2):378–86.

49. Pontiroli AE, Frige F, Paganelli M, et al. In morbid obesity, metabolic abnormalities and adhesion molecules correlate with visceral fat, not with subcutaneous fat: effect of weight loss through surgery. Obes Surg 2009;19(6):745–50.

50. Shore SA. Obesity and asthma: lessons from animal models. J Appl Physiol (1985) 2007;102(2): 516–28.

51. Ikejima S, Sasaki S, Sashinami H, et al. Impairment of host resistance to Listeria monocytogenes

infection in liver of db/db and ob/ob mice. Diabetes 2005;54(1):182–9.

52. Hsu A, Aronoff DM, Phipps J, et al. Leptin improves pulmonary bacterial clearance and survival in ob/ob mice during pneumococcal pneumonia. Clin Exp Immunol 2007;150(2):332–9.

53. Mancuso P, Gottschalk A, Phare SM, et al. Leptin-deficient mice exhibit impaired host defense in Gram-negative pneumonia. J Immunol 2002; 168(8):4018–24.

54. Wright JK, Nwariaku FN, Clark J, et al. Effect of diabetes mellitus on endotoxin-induced lung injury. Arch Surg 1999;134(12):1354–8 [discussion: 1358–9].

55. Bellmeyer A, Martino JM, Chandel NS, et al. Leptin resistance protects mice from hyperoxia-induced acute lung injury. Am J Respir Crit Care Med 2007;175(6):587–94.

56. Barazzone-Argiroffo C, Muzzin P, Donati YR, et al. Hyperoxia increases leptin production: a mechanism mediated through endogenous elevation of corticosterone. Am J Physiol Lung Cell Mol Physiol 2001;281(5):L1150–6.

57. Shore SA, Lang JE, Kasahara DI, et al. Pulmonary responses to subacute ozone exposure in obese vs. lean mice. J Appl Physiol (1985) 2009;107(5): 1445–52.

58. Kordonowy LL, Burg E, Lenox CC, et al. Obesity is associated with neutrophil dysfunction and attenuation of murine acute lung injury. Am J Respir Cell Mol Biol 2012;47(1):120–7.

59. Lu FL, Johnston RA, Flynt L, et al. Increased pulmonary responses to acute ozone exposure in obese db/db mice. Am J Physiol Lung Cell Mol Physiol 2006;290(5):L856–65.

60. Johnston RA, Theman TA, Lu FL, et al. Diet-induced obesity causes innate airway hyperresponsiveness to methacholine and enhances ozone-induced pulmonary inflammation. J Appl Physiol (1985) 2008;104(6):1727–35.

61. Gong MN, Thompson BT, Williams D, et al. Clinical predictors of and mortality in acute respiratory distress syndrome: potential role of red cell transfusion. Crit Care Med 2005;33(6):1191–8.

62. Iscimen R, Cartin-Ceba R, Yilmaz M, et al. Risk factors for the development of acute lung injury in patients with septic shock: an observational cohort study. Crit Care Med 2008;36(5):1518–22.

63. Yu S, Christiani DC, Thompson BT, et al. Role of diabetes in the development of acute respiratory distress syndrome. Crit Care Med 2013;41(12): 2720–32.

64. Boichot E, Sannomiya P, Escofier N, et al. Endotoxin-induced acute lung injury in rats. Role of insulin. Pulm Pharmacol Ther 1999;12(5):285–90.

65. Alba-Loureiro TC, Martins EF, Landgraf RG, et al. Role of insulin on PGE2 generation during LPS-induced lung inflammation in rats. Life Sci 2006;78(6):578–85.

66. de Oliveira Martins J, Meyer-Pflug AR, Alba-Loureiro TC, et al. Modulation of lipopolysaccharide-induced acute lung inflammation: role of insulin. Shock 2006;25(3):260–6.

67. Alba-Loureiro TC, Munhoz CD, Martins JO, et al. Neutrophil function and metabolism in individuals with diabetes mellitus. Braz J Med Biol Res 2007; 40(8):1037–44.

68. Moreno-Navarrete JM, Fernandez-Real JM. Antimicrobial-sensing proteins in obesity and type 2 diabetes: the buffering efficiency hypothesis. Diabetes Care 2011;34(Suppl 2):S335–41.

69. Moutschen MP, Scheen AJ, Lefebvre PJ. Impaired immune responses in diabetes mellitus: analysis of the factors and mechanisms involved. Relevance to the increased susceptibility of diabetic patients to specific infections. Diabete Metab 1992;18(3): 187–201.

70. Huang ZS, Chien KL, Yang CY, et al. Peripheral differential leukocyte counts in humans vary with hyperlipidemia, smoking, and body mass index. Lipids 2001;36(3):237–45.

71. Giugliano G, Brevetti G, Lanero S, et al. Leukocyte count in peripheral arterial disease: a simple, reliable, inexpensive approach to cardiovascular risk prediction. Atherosclerosis 2010;210(1):288–93.

72. Gomes AL, Carvalho T, Serpa J, et al. Hypercholesterolemia promotes bone marrow cell mobilization by perturbing the SDF-1:CXCR4 axis. Blood 2010;115(19):3886–94.

73. Drechsler M, Megens RT, van Zandvoort M, et al. Hyperlipidemia-triggered neutrophilia promotes early atherosclerosis. Circulation 2010;122(18): 1837–45.

74. Hansson GK, Libby P. The immune response in atherosclerosis: a double-edged sword. Nat Rev Immunol 2006;6(7):508–19.

75. Kopprasch S, Leonhardt W, Pietzsch J, et al. Hypochlorite-modified low-density lipoprotein stimulates human polymorphonuclear leukocytes for enhanced production of reactive oxygen metabolites, enzyme secretion, and adhesion to endothelial cells. Atherosclerosis 1998;136(2):315–24.

76. Lehr HA, Krombach F, Munzing S, et al. In vitro effects of oxidized low density lipoprotein on CD11b/CD18 and L-selectin presentation on neutrophils and monocytes with relevance for the in vivo situation. Am J Pathol 1995;146(1):218–27.

77. Palvinskaya T, Antkowiak M, Burg E, et al. Effects of acute and chronic low density lipoprotein exposure on neutrophil function. Pulm Pharmacol Ther 2013; 26(4):405–11.

78. Porreca E, Sergi R, Baccante G, et al. Peripheral blood mononuclear cell production of interleukin-8 and IL-8-dependent neutrophil function in

hypercholesterolemic patients. Atherosclerosis 1999;146(2):345–50.

79. Stragliotto E, Camera M, Postiglione A, et al. Functionally abnormal monocytes in hypercholesterolemia. Arterioscler Thromb 1993;13(6):944–50.

80. Madenspacher JH, Draper DW, Smoak KA, et al. Dyslipidemia induces opposing effects on intrapulmonary and extrapulmonary host defense through divergent TLR response phenotypes. J Immunol 2010;185(3):1660–9.

81. Fantuzzi G. Adipose tissue, adipokines, and inflammation. J Allergy Clin Immunol 2005;115(5):911–9 [quiz: 920].

82. La Cava A, Matarese G. The weight of leptin in immunity. Nat Rev Immunol 2004;4(5):371–9.

83. Umemoto Y, Tsuji K, Yang FC, et al. Leptin stimulates the proliferation of murine myelocytic and primitive hematopoietic progenitor cells. Blood 1997;90(9):3438–43.

84. Claycombe K, King LE, Fraker PJ. A role for leptin in sustaining lymphopoiesis and myelopoiesis. Proc Natl Acad Sci U S A 2008;105(6):2017–21.

85. Moore SI, Huffnagle GB, Chen GH, et al. Leptin modulates neutrophil phagocytosis of Klebsiella pneumoniae. Infect Immun 2003;71(7):4182–5.

86. Caldefie-Chezet F, Poulin A, Tridon A, et al. Leptin: a potential regulator of polymorphonuclear neutrophil bactericidal action? J Leukoc Biol 2001;69(3):414–8.

87. Bruno A, Conus S, Schmid I, et al. Apoptotic pathways are inhibited by leptin receptor activation in neutrophils. J Immunol 2005;174(12):8090–6.

88. Ottonello L, Gnerre P, Bertolotto M, et al. Leptin as a uremic toxin interferes with neutrophil chemotaxis. J Am Soc Nephrol 2004;15(9):2366–72.

89. Caldefie-Chezet F, Poulin A, Vasson MP. Leptin regulates functional capacities of polymorphonuclear neutrophils. Free Radic Res 2003;37(8):809–14.

90. Montecucco F, Bianchi G, Gnerre P, et al. Induction of neutrophil chemotaxis by leptin: crucial role for p38 and Src kinases. Ann N Y Acad Sci 2006;1069:463–71.

91. Ubags ND, Vernooy JH, Burg E, et al. The role of leptin in the development of pulmonary neutrophilia in infection and acute lung injury. Crit Care Med 2014;42(2):e143–51.

92. Bruno A, Chanez P, Chiappara G, et al. Does leptin play a cytokine-like role within the airways of COPD patients? Eur Respir J 2005;26(3):398–405.

93. Vernooy JH, Drummen NE, van Suylen RJ, et al. Enhanced pulmonary leptin expression in patients with severe COPD and asymptomatic smokers. Thorax 2009;64(1):26–32.

94. Torpy DJ, Bornstein SR, Chrousos GP. Leptin and interleukin-6 in sepsis. Horm Metab Res 1998;30(12):726–9.

95. Arnalich F, Lopez J, Codoceo R, et al. Relationship of plasma leptin to plasma cytokines and human survival in sepsis and septic shock. J Infect Dis 1999;180(3):908–11.

96. Yousef AA, Amr YM, Suliman GA. The diagnostic value of serum leptin monitoring and its correlation with tumor necrosis factor-alpha in critically ill patients: a prospective observational study. Crit Care 2010;14(2):R33.

97. Jain M, Budinger GR, Lo A, et al. Leptin promotes fibroproliferative acute respiratory distress syndrome by inhibiting peroxisome proliferator-activated receptor-gamma. Am J Respir Crit Care Med 2011;183(11):1490–8.

98. Gattinoni L, Chiumello D, Carlesso E, et al. Bench-to-bedside review: chest wall elastance in acute lung injury/acute respiratory distress syndrome patients. Crit Care 2004;8(5):350–5.

99. Hess DR, Bigatello LM. The chest wall in acute lung injury/acute respiratory distress syndrome. Curr Opin Crit Care 2008;14(1):94–102.

100. Berenholtz SM, Pronovost PJ, Lipsett PA, et al. Eliminating catheter-related bloodstream infections in the intensive care unit. Crit Care Med 2004;32(10):2014–20.

101. Drakulovic MB, Torres A, Bauer TT, et al. Supine body position as a risk factor for nosocomial pneumonia in mechanically ventilated patients: a randomised trial. Lancet 1999;354(9193):1851–8.

102. Ventilation with lower tidal volumes as compared with traditional tidal volumes for acute lung injury and the acute respiratory distress syndrome. The Acute Respiratory Distress Syndrome Network. N Engl J Med 2000;342(18):1301–8.

103. Burns SM, Egloff MB, Ryan B, et al. Effect of body position on spontaneous respiratory rate and tidal volume in patients with obesity, abdominal distension and ascites. Am J Crit Care 1994;3(2):102–6.

104. Adams DH, Snedden DP. How misconceptions among elderly patients regarding survival outcomes of inpatient cardiopulmonary resuscitation affect do-not-resuscitate orders. J Am Osteopath Assoc 2006;106(7):402–4.

105. Cerra FB, Benitez MR, Blackburn GL, et al. Applied nutrition in ICU patients. A consensus statement of the American College of Chest Physicians. Chest 1997;111(3):769–78.

106. Correia MI, Waitzberg DL. The impact of malnutrition on morbidity, mortality, length of hospital stay and costs evaluated through a multivariate model analysis. Clin Nutr 2003;22(3):235–9.

107. Heyland DK, Dhaliwal R, Drover JW, et al. Canadian clinical practice guidelines for nutrition support in mechanically ventilated, critically ill adult patients. JPEN J Parenter Enteral Nutr 2003;27(5):355–73. Available at: www.criticalcarenutrition.com. for updated data.

108. Gramlich L, Kichian K, Pinilla J, et al. Does enteral nutrition compared to parenteral nutrition result in

better outcomes in critically ill adult patients? A systematic review of the literature. Nutrition 2004; 20(10):843–8.

109. Canadian Critical Care Nutrition Clinical Practice Guidelines: The Use of Enteral Nutrition vs. Parenteral Nutrition. Available at: http://criticalcarenutrition.com/docs/cpgs2012/1.0.pdf. Accessed March 4, 2014.

110. Groos S, Hunefeld G, Luciano L. Parenteral versus enteral nutrition: morphological changes in human adult intestinal mucosa. J Submicrosc Cytol Pathol 1996;28(1):61–74.

111. Li J, Kudsk KA, Gocinski B, et al. Effects of parenteral and enteral nutrition on gut-associated lymphoid tissue. J Trauma 1995;39(1):44–51 [discussion: 51–2].

112. Canadian critical care nutrition clinical practice guidelines: early vs. delayed nutrient intake. Available at: http://criticalcarenutrition.com/docs/cpgs2012/2.0.pdf. Accessed March 4, 2014.

113. McClave SA, Martindale RG, Vanek VW, et al. Guidelines for the provision and assessment of nutrition support therapy in the adult critically ill patient: Society of Critical Care Medicine (SCCM) and American Society for Parenteral and Enteral Nutrition (A.S.P.E.N.). JPEN J Parenter Enteral Nutr 2009;33(3):277–316.

114. Khalid I, Doshi P, DiGiovine B. Early enteral nutrition and outcomes of critically ill patients treated with vasopressors and mechanical ventilation. Am J Crit Care 2010;19(3):261–8.

115. Kross EK, Sena M, Schmidt K, et al. A comparison of predictive equations of energy expenditure and measured energy expenditure in critically ill patients. J Crit Care 2012;27(3):321.e5–12.

116. Rice TW, Wheeler AP, Thompson BT, et al. Initial trophic vs full enteral feeding in patients with acute lung injury: the EDEN randomized trial. JAMA 2012;307(8):795–803.

117. Villet S, Chiolero RL, Bollmann MD, et al. Negative impact of hypocaloric feeding and energy balance on clinical outcome in ICU patients. Clin Nutr 2005; 24(4):502–9.

118. Krishnan JA, Parce PB, Martinez A, et al. Caloric intake in medical ICU patients: consistency of care with guidelines and relationship to clinical outcomes. Chest 2003;124(1):297–305.

119. Needham DM, Dinglas VD, Bienvenu OJ, et al. One year outcomes in patients with acute lung injury randomised to initial trophic or full enteral feeding: prospective follow-up of EDEN randomised trial. BMJ 2013;346:f1532.

120. Needham DM, Dinglas VD, Morris PE, et al. Physical and cognitive performance of patients with acute lung injury 1 year after initial trophic versus full enteral feeding. EDEN trial follow-up. Am J Respir Crit Care Med 2013;188(5):567–76.

121. McClave SA, Sexton LK, Spain DA, et al. Enteral tube feeding in the intensive care unit: factors impeding adequate delivery. Crit Care Med 1999; 27(7):1252–6.

122. McClave SA, Lukan JK, Stefater JA, et al. Poor validity of residual volumes as a marker for risk of aspiration in critically ill patients. Crit Care Med 2005;33(2):324–30.

123. Montejo JC, Minambres E, Bordeje L, et al. Gastric residual volume during enteral nutrition in ICU patients: the REGANE study. Intensive Care Med 2010;36(8):1386–93.

124. Reignier J, Mercier E, Le Gouge A, et al. Effect of not monitoring residual gastric volume on risk of ventilator-associated pneumonia in adults receiving mechanical ventilation and early enteral feeding: a randomized controlled trial. JAMA 2013;309(3): 249–56.

125. Singer P, Berger MM, Van den Berghe G, et al, ESPEN. ESPEN guidelines on parenteral nutrition: intensive care. Clin Nutr 2009;28(4):387–400.

126. Casaer MP, Mesotten D, Hermans G, et al. Early versus late parenteral nutrition in critically ill adults. N Engl J Med 2011;365(6):506–17.

127. Doig GS, Simpson F, Sweetman EA, et al. Early parenteral nutrition in critically ill patients with short-term relative contraindications to early enteral nutrition: a randomized controlled trial. JAMA 2013; 309(20):2130–8.

128. Novak F, Heyland DK, Avenell A, et al. Glutamine supplementation in serious illness: a systematic review of the evidence. Crit Care Med 2002;30(9):2022–9.

129. Heyland D, Muscedere J, Wischmeyer PE, et al. A randomized trial of glutamine and antioxidants in critically ill patients. N Engl J Med 2013; 368(16):1489–97.

130. Manzanares W, Dhaliwal R, Jiang X, et al. Antioxidant micronutrients in the critically ill: a systematic review and meta-analysis. Crit Care 2012;16(2):R66.

131. Gadek JE, DeMichele SJ, Karlstad MD, et al. Effect of enteral feeding with eicosapentaenoic acid, gamma-linolenic acid, and antioxidants in patients with acute respiratory distress syndrome. Enteral Nutrition in ARDS Study Group. Crit Care Med 1999;27(8):1409–20.

132. Singer P, Theilla M, Fisher H, et al. Benefit of an enteral diet enriched with eicosapentaenoic acid and gamma-linolenic acid in ventilated patients with acute lung injury. Crit Care Med 2006;34(4): 1033–8.

133. Pontes-Arruda A, Aragao AM, Albuquerque JD. Effects of enteral feeding with eicosapentaenoic acid, gamma-linolenic acid, and antioxidants in mechanically ventilated patients with severe sepsis and septic shock. Crit Care Med 2006;34(9):2325–33.

134. Stapleton RD, Martin TR, Weiss NS, et al. A phase II randomized placebo-controlled trial of omega-3 fatty acids for the treatment of acute lung injury. Crit Care Med 2011;39(7):1655–62.

Beyond Single-Nucleotide Polymorphisms

Genetics, Genomics, and Other 'Omic Approaches to Acute Respiratory Distress Syndrome

Nuala J. Meyer, MD, MS

KEYWORDS

- Acute respiratory distress syndrome • Genomic • Proteomic • Metabolomic • Gene expression
- Complex trait

KEY POINTS

- Numerous candidate gene-association studies and protein investigations have been used in acute respiratory distress syndrome (ARDS) to moderate success, but large-scale genomic, proteomic, or metabolomic studies have not yet been undertaken. There exists significant opportunity to apply 'omic platforms to advance the understanding of ARDS pathophysiology.
- Although small proteomic and metabolomics investigations into ARDS have proven feasibility, to date there has been limited mechanistic follow-up of compelling candidates and questions remain regarding the optimal target tissue and the best analytical strategy for ARDS.
- Future studies could leverage 'omic experience gained evaluating other non-ARDS complex traits, and could explore unbiased analytical strategies for class distinction or network analysis.
- The success of high-throughput discovery 'omic investigations derives from tracing observations in human populations back to their mechanistic underpinnings.

Acute respiratory distress syndrome (ARDS) inflicts considerable morbidity and mortality among critically ill patients and lacks any specific pharmacologic therapy.[1,2] Because clinical factors alone fail to explain which patients with ARDS risk factors will develop the syndrome, or to accurately predict which patients will die as a result of ARDS, there is great interest to understand whether one could leverage new biologic techniques to better characterize risk and prognosis. With major advances in the fields of genomics, mass spectroscopy, and bioinformatics, there are numerous approaches that can now be applied to a complex trait like ARDS, yet the benefit of these is uncertain (**Table 1**). This article reviews the state of knowledge of genetic contributions to ARDS risk and mortality, reviews broader applications of genomics to ARDS pathogenesis, and considers examples from non-ARDS fields whereby genomic approaches have yielded major advances. Applying similar approaches to ARDS may deepen our understanding and offer new therapeutic paradigms for patients with ARDS.

SHIFTING THE PARADIGM: WHAT CAN GENOMICS TEACH ABOUT A TRAIT LIKE ACUTE RESPIRATORY DISTRESS SYNDROME?

Many investigators associate the word "genomic" with inherited conditions that obviously cluster among families. Because there are no reported families in whom ARDS has affected multiple

The author has no disclosures relevant to this publication.

Pulmonary, Allergy, and Critical Care Medicine, University of Pennsylvania, Perelman School of Medicine, 3600 Spruce Street, 5039 Maloney Building, Philadelphia, PA 19104, USA

E-mail address: nuala.meyer@uphs.upenn.edu

Clin Chest Med 35 (2014) 673–684
http://dx.doi.org/10.1016/j.ccm.2014.08.006

Table 1
Potential applications of different 'omic technologies to a complex trait like ARDS

Analyte Field	Infer Mechanism	Candidate Marker Validation	Candidate Marker Discovery	Identify Subclasses	Risk Stratify	Improve Diagnosis	Identify Therapeutic Targets
DNA Genomics	x	x	x		x		x
DNA methylation or acetylation Epigenomics	x	x			x		x
mRNA miRNA ncRNA Transcriptomics	x	x	x	x	x		x
Proteins Proteomics	x	x	x	x	x	x	x
Metabolites Metabolomics	x	x	x	x	x	x	x
Systems Interactome	x			x	x		x
Microbiota Microbiome	x	x	x	x	x	x	x

Abbreviations: mRNA, messenger RNA; miRNA, micro RNA; ncRNA, noncoding RNA.
For each application, the tested analyte is named and the most likely potential applications are highlighted with an X.

members, one might conclude that genomics would offer little to the understanding of ARDS. However, an alternative perspective is to consider ARDS as a pattern of response to injury, be it pneumonia, sepsis, or trauma. As a trait, the response to injury has significant heritability.[3–7] In fact, death from infection was the most heritable condition when studied in a large Danish registry of adoptees, with a much stronger heritability than vascular disease or cancer.[8] Rather than acting as monogenetic, or Mendelian, traits, whereby a single genetic variation explains the bulk of the observed phenotype, ARDS risk and severity are likely influenced by multiple genetic variants that each contribute to a modest degree. Small effect sizes of each contributing gene variant mandate large study populations for detection. In addition, ARDS is ripe for the use of intermediate traits and the identification of endotypes, or subtypes, which may demonstrate a more homogeneous genetic background.

SURVEYING THE LANDSCAPE OF ACUTE RESPIRATORY DISTRESS SYNDROME GENOMICS

Numerous candidate gene-association studies have been reported in ARDS, and several reproducible associations have emerged. Although a complete review of the genetic associations with ARDS risk or ARDS mortality is beyond the scope of this article, comprehensive reviews recently have been published.[9–11] The best replicated genetic variants for ARDS risk represent the present understanding of ARDS pathophysiology; proinflammatory and anti-inflammatory cytokine gene polymorphisms are well represented (*IL6, IL10, IL1RN, MBL2*),[12–18] as are vascular injury markers (*VEGFA, ANGPT2, ACE, MYLK*),[19–24] innate immunity pathway members (*IRAK3, TLR1, NFKB1, NFKBIA, FAS, PI3*),[5,25–28] and markers of respiratory epithelial injury (*SFTPB*).[29,30] Although each of these associations has been associated with ARDS risk or outcome in at least two populations, none influences ARDS risk or severity to a degree that warrants genetic testing of at-risk populations. Instead, the main contribution of ARDS genetic associations to date has been to focus attention on molecular pathways at play in causing or perpetuating the syndrome.

Furthermore, it is tempting to speculate that genetic associations may highlight potential therapeutic targets to either prevent ARDS or to improve outcomes once it has developed. For example, the association of variants in the angiopoietin-2 gene (*ANGPT2*) with ARDS risk in mixed intensive care unit population and trauma populations,[22,23] coupled with strong animal evidence that antagonizing angiopoietin-2 protein (ANG2) or augmenting its counterpart, angiopoietin-1 (ANG1), results in decreased mortality[31–34] suggests that it may be helpful to block this protein in humans at risk for ARDS. Given numerous failed trials to prevent or treat ARDS, however, it may be that investigators should seek a molecular marker, such as high ANG2 plasma protein level or carriage of an *ANGPT2* genetic variant, to enrich a clinical trial population for subjects likely to respond. A similar case could be made for the use of human neutrophil elastase inhibitors, already used in Japan to treat ARDS albeit with scant evidence of efficacy,[35–37] because the gene pre-elafin (*PI3*) is dysregulated among patients who fail to resolve ARDS[38] and functional promoter variants in *PI3* associate with ARDS,[27,28] and because plasma levels of its gene product elafin are reduced in patients with ARDS.[39] Perhaps patients with low elafin levels or high human neutrophil elastase activity would be more likely to respond to human neutrophil elastase inhibitors. The angiotensin-converting enzyme (ACE) gene also may suggest a therapeutic strategy, because *ACE* gene variants that increase ACE1 levels have been associated with ARDS mortality[24,40–43] and the counterregulatory ACE2 enzyme seems to decrease lung injury.[44,45]

ACUTE RESPIRATORY DISTRESS SYNDROME ENTERS THE GENOMIC AGE

The earliest contributions of genomics to the understanding of ARDS successfully leveraged animal models, quantitative traits, and bioinformatics. Grigoryev and colleagues[46] used bioinformatic approaches to find overlap in the gene expression or messenger RNA (mRNA) levels from human cells or animal lung tissue subjected to repeated mechanical stress or models of ventilator-induced injury. Orthologues, or genes with common structure and function across different species, that behaved in a reproducible manner across numerous models of injury were subsequently investigated through mouse knockout models or gene silencing. In this manner, Ye and colleagues[47,48] identified pre–B cell colony-enhancing factor, also known by the gene symbol *NAMPT*, as a regulator of inflammatory cytokines, which in turn cause epithelial and endothelial permeability.[49] In addition, independent groups have now replicated the association between promoter variants in *NAMPT* and the development of ARDS.[50] New candidate genes can also arise from screening multiple rodent species for differential susceptibility to lung injury, as Leikauf and colleagues[51–53] performed using inhalational injury models. When translating animal and in vitro work to human populations, however, the choice of experimental model is highly relevant. Dos Santos and colleagues[54] demonstrated that the gene expression response to ventilator-induced lung injury is distinct from endotoxin models of sepsis, which is consonant with findings in human populations that gene variants associated with ARDS may be specific to ARDS risk factor.[55]

In the first published human genome-wide association study (GWAS) for ARDS susceptibility, Christie and colleagues[56] identified a novel locus, *PPFIA1* or liprin alpha, as a replicable risk factor for ARDS following trauma. Although little was known about how liprin alpha would contribute to lung injury at the time of discovery, subsequent work has implicated liprin alpha as a binding partner and downregulator of mammalian homolog of diaphanous, a Rho effector that mediates stress fiber formation.[57] Just as nonmuscle myosin light-chain kinase is a critical regulator of the endothelial cytoskeleton with implications for ARDS,[58,59] liprin alpha may also prove to have relevance for barrier enhancement.

As future GWAS are published, new candidates will undoubtedly emerge and meta-analysis will be possible to harness the power of multiple populations. At the same time, however, GWAS may prove more fruitful if the heterogeneity of ARDS is acknowledged a priori, and analyses are conducted within more homogenous subtypes. For instance, Tejera and coworkers[55] demonstrated that the genetic risk factors for extrapulmonary ARDS and pulmonary ARDS were distinct, a finding echoed by most reviews.[9,41] In addition to ARDS precipitant, such factors as ancestry,[12] gender,[60] age, or comorbidity[17] may be important. Furthermore, given the notable heterogeneity of ARDS, there are almost certainly additional subtypes that may become apparent with additional data, as elegantly proved by Calfee and colleagues[61] applying latent class analysis to two populations from the National Heart Lung Blood Institute ARDS network. Because the unbiased model suggested two classes of patients with ARDS, one characterized by higher inflammatory cytokine plasma levels, lower plasma bicarbonate, and a tendency for shock, and because the two subclasses had dramatically different outcomes and response to a high positive end-expiratory pressure, it may be that leveraging GWAS within each subclass would yield important insights about processes driving each type of ARDS.

ADVANCES FROM GENE EXPRESSION

In addition to the animal studies mentioned previously, several human investigations have explored the use of gene expression to identify novel candidate genes in ARDS. Gene expression analysis can be advantageous, because the output of the analysis is a quantitative trait that offers strong statistical power relative to a dichotomous trait, such as the presence or absence of ARDS. In addition, because mRNA reflects the mature transcript that will be translated into protein, changes in transcript abundance are likely to be functional and thus offer strong evidence for involvement in a trait. Finally, multidimensional analysis of global gene expression changes is possible using microarray technology, whereby a small amount of starting mRNA can be assessed for roughly 20,000 transcripts simultaneously. This technique is not only a very efficient way to assess gene expression level, but also allows multidimensional analytical strategies to define patterns of expression. Two general types of analyses can be performed: a supervised, or hierarchical analysis, in which samples are assigned to their class by the investigator; or an unbiased or machine-learning analysis, whereby the analysis seeks to detect unobserved patterns from unlabeled data. An early example of the hierarchical analysis involved the demonstration that gene expression changes between acute myelogenous leukemia bone marrow mononuclear cells were distinct from acute lymphogenous leukemia cells.[62] A subsequent group performed a similar genome-wide expression analysis of acute lymphogenous leukemia blast cells in an unsupervised manner, identifying six major molecular subtypes that reflected different biologic mechanisms and suggested differential response to treatment.[63] Expression patterns of specific factors in tumor tissue are now routinely assayed in hematologic and solid organ malignancies to personalize therapy.[64,65]

Research in ARDS transcriptomics is hampered by the lack of available lung tissue on which to perform microarray analysis, because only the minority of patients (<10%) progress to lung biopsy.[66] Without lung tissue, most investigations have relied on gene expression of either specific blood cell populations or white blood cells collected from whole blood. Although whole blood is a relatively convenient way to sample RNA, this collection method may introduce variability and will never reflect the expression pattern of lung endothelium or epithelium, because gene expression is cell-specific (**Fig. 1**).[67] In one of the first descriptions of applying microarray technology to human ARDS, Howrylak and colleagues[68] reported the global whole-blood gene expression of 13 patients with sepsis and ARDS compared with 20 with sepsis alone, and reported that differential expression of eight transcripts distinguished patients with ARDS. The most dysregulated transcript encoded for the heavy subunit of ferritin, which is interesting given the role of iron in catalyzing reactive oxygen species and the potential contribution of reactive oxygen species toward lung injury.[69–72] A novel approach was applied by Wang and colleagues[38] to compare the whole-blood gene expression profile of patients during

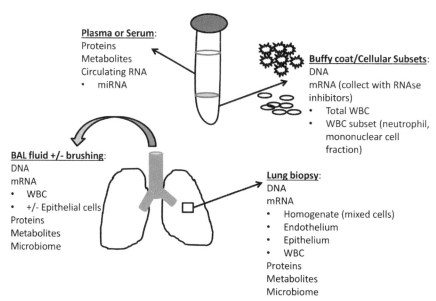

Plasma or Serum:
Proteins
Metabolites
Circulating RNA
• miRNA

Buffy coat/Cellular Subsets:
DNA
mRNA (collect with RNAse inhibitors)
• Total WBC
• WBC subset (neutrophil, mononuclear cell fraction)

BAL fluid +/- brushing:
DNA
mRNA
• WBC
• +/- Epithelial cells
Proteins
Metabolites
Microbiome

Lung biopsy:
DNA
mRNA
• Homogenate (mixed cells)
• Endothelium
• Epithelium
• WBC
Proteins
Metabolites
Microbiome

Fig. 1. Biospecimens available for 'omic applications in ARDS. WBC, white blood cell.

acute ARDS and convalescence, which used each patient as his or her own control and thus filtered much of the background variability between expression across individuals. Using this approach, the investigators identified the peptidase inhibitor 3 gene *PI3*, encoding elafin, as downregulated in ARDS. Functional promoter variants in *PI3* associate with lower cytokine-induced transcriptional activity and greater sepsis-associated ARDS, potentially acting through more durable binding of pre-elafin to extracellular matrix proteins.[27]

To date, there has been no large systematic application of gene expression in human samples with ARDS. Furthermore, it remains unclear whether the signature obtained from whole blood or from circulating leukocytes will provide relevant answers for a condition of alveolar epithelial and endothelial dysfunction. Although questions remain about the suitability of studying whole blood to gain insights into a lung-centric condition, advances have been made by applying this approach in sepsis, generally considered a systemic vascular disorder. Wong and colleagues[73] performed unbiased clustering analysis to whole-blood gene expression of approximately 100 children with sepsis and identified three subclasses that correlated with differential mortality. The highest mortality subclass was characterized by significant downregulation of genes annotated to glucocorticoid signaling, the adaptive immune system, and zinc-related biology. The investigators were able to extend their findings by analyzing the secreted protein products of some of the most dysregulated genes in the high-mortality group, resulting in a five-biomarker decision tool that reliably identifies a higher-risk group for death when applied to children and adults with septic shock.[74,75] Thus, despite limitations of whole blood or even leukocyte gene expression to inform about lung tissue expression, large-scale peripheral blood gene expression may yield advances in ARDS.

UNTAPPED POTENTIAL: TRANSCRIPTOMICS OF THE FUTURE

Although transcriptomics to date has been dominated by microarray studies quantifying mRNA, the transcriptome encompasses all forms of RNA, including transfer RNA, ribosomal RNA, and many forms of noncoding RNA. The science of noncoding RNA molecules has exploded in the past 10 years, with the identification of multiple new classes of non–protein-coding entities[76] and emerging understanding of their complex roles in regulating gene expression.[77] Advances in next-generation sequencing capabilities, coupled with improved bioinformatic support and efficiencies of scale, have fueled high-throughput sequencing of RNA in targeted and genome-wide approaches.[78] Because the technology of RNA sequencing is so nascent, there are few published reports applying these methods to a complex trait like ARDS. However, applications of RNA-seq to cancer and cardiovascular traits may exemplify useful approaches for the future. MicroRNA (miRNA), only described in 1993,[79] are now understood to be small, roughly 22-nucleotide RNA sequences that typically bind the 3′ untranslated region of target mRNA and inhibit translation or promote mRNA degradation.[80,81] Candidate genes influencing ARDS, including *MYLK* and *PBEF/NAMPT*, are regulated by miRNA,[82,83] which raises the possibility that engineered miRNA or their antagonists may be a therapeutic strategy in the future. In cancer, circulating miRNA profiles in plasma are being investigated as biomarkers with diagnostic or prognostic utility,[84] approaches that may prove fruitful in ARDS.

Another underexplored aspect of genomic regulation of ARDS is whether epigenetic modifications influence disease susceptibility or outcome. Epigenetic changes are classically construed as heritable changes in gene expression, function, or activity that occur without a change in DNA sequence, such as might occur because of changes in DNA methylation, histone modification, gene silencing, or imprinting.[85,86] Epigenetic mechanisms are attractive explanations for severe gene-by-environment interactions, and thus may be relevant to a complex trait like ARDS, which only manifests in the setting of a severe environmental insult, such as mechanical ventilation, systemic infection, or severe trauma. Much of the understanding surrounding DNA methylation and histone modification comes from cancer biology. Tumor-suppressor gene hypermethylation leads to transcriptional silencing, promoting tumorigenesis.[87,88] Histones are dynamically regulated by processes including acetylation, methylation, phosphorylation, and ubiquitinylation, resulting in dynamic effects on gene expression and chromatin structure.[88,89] Differential epigenetic regulation can be assessed in either targeted or unbiased, genome-wide approaches by leveraging bisulfite sequencing (for methylation) and/or mass spectrometry to detect posttranslational histone modification.[88] Given evidence from the Encyclopedia of DNA Elements project highlighting vast complexity of genome regulation,[77,90,91] future studies should explore the role of epigenomic variation in the context of ARDS and potentially for distinct ARDS precipitants.

PROTEOMICS AND METABOLOMICS: SEARCHING FOR THE KEY PLAYERS

Although it was once assumed that gene expression would adequately describe the state of expressed proteins in a body site or cellular compartment, the correlation between mRNA and protein profiles is surprisingly poor.[92–94] Understanding the differential regulation of proteins relative to gene expression has enabled a better understanding of alternative splicing and posttranslational regulation, whereas focusing on the expressed proteins has aided the identification of biomarkers for diagnosis, prognosis, and potentially, mechanistic importance. Proteomic approaches are generally conceived as large-scale analyses, going beyond individual or even multiplex protein quantification by enzyme-linked immunosorbent assay or bead-based immunoassays. Parallel to the explosion in next-generation sequencing technology to analyze the genome have been advances in matrix-assisted laser desorption/ionization time-of-flight (MALDI-TOF) mass spectrometry to analyze high-dimensional protein populations, including the identification of unknown proteins. More than 10 years ago, Bowler and colleagues[95] performed two-dimensional electrophoresis followed by mass spectrometry on edema fluid from 16 subjects with ARDS compared with 12 healthy control subjects. Compared with healthy subjects, alveolar fluid albumin, transferrin, IgG, and clusterin were increased, and surfactant protein A and α_1-antitrypsin were decreased in patients with ARDS.[95] In addition, several proteins detectable in the alveolar fluid of subjects with ARDS demonstrated significant posttranslational modifications.[95] Schnapp and a group from the University of Washington applied liquid chromatography–tandem mass spectrometry proteomics to three bronchoalveolar lavage (BAL) samples from subjects with ARDS, and analyzed almost 900 resulting unique proteins.[96] Focusing on secreted proteins, the authors identified increased insulin-like growth factor–binding protein-3 and its ligand insulin growth factor 1 (IGF) early in ARDS and suggested that IGF contributes to fibroblast survival in ARDS.[96] Several investigators have since reported the identification of increased BAL apolipoproteins,[97] S100 calcium-binding proteins,[97–99] and inflammatory proteins including acute-phase proteins and cytokines (tumor necrosis factor-α, interleukin-1β).[96,99] Investigating the plasma compartment, Chen and colleagues[100] identified 16 proteins as differentially expressed in patients with ARDS compared with healthy control subjects, with ARDS subjects showing significantly downregulated plasma apolipoproteins (apo A-I,

A-IV, B-100, C-II, and CIII) and complement factor H, with upregulated complement C9, serum amyloid A, and C-reactive protein. Consonant with the individual protein findings, the most dysregulated pathways were annotated as acute-phase signaling, complement system, interleukin-12 signaling, and production of nitric oxide and reactive oxygen species.[100]

A complementary approach to proteomics is to examine the small molecule metabolite profile of either the blood or lung compartment to gain more information about the physiologic processes occurring in that compartment. Metabolites, the intermediate products of metabolism, can be endogenous or exogenous, and can be peptides but also lipids, carbohydrates, amino acids, nucleotides, hormones, vitamins, or foreign chemical substrates as from a drug, diet, or other exposure. Metabolites are first separated with gas and/or liquid chromatography and then quantified with mass spectrometry or isotope-labeled nuclear magnetic resonance spectroscopy (^{1}H-NMR or ^{13}C-NMR).[101,102] Stringer and colleagues[103] at the University of Michigan first reported on ^{1}H-NMR–identified metabolites in the plasma of 13 sepsis-associated subjects with ARDS compared with six healthy control subjects. Forty metabolites were identified, and ARDS plasma was characterized by higher adenosine, glutathione, sphingomyelin, and phoshatidylserine, and pathway annotation analysis suggested that each metabolite participated in a unique metabolic network.[103] Because sepsis-associated ARDS samples were compared with healthy control subjects' plasma, it remained unclear whether the analytes identified were specific to ARDS or whether they might reflect alterations from sepsis. To study ARDS-specific metabolites requires a study with non-ARDS subjects with sepsis as control subjects.

Metabolomic profiling of plasma has been applied more commonly to sepsis. Seymour and coworkers[104] identified numerous differences in the initial emergency department plasma sample of sepsis survivors versus nonsurvivors after matching subjects on clinical characteristics and procalcitonin level. Metabolism of bile acids, sterols, amino acids, nucleotides, and energy were among the most dysregulated pathways in nonsurvivors.[104] Langley and colleagues[105] performed multiple analyses, comparing sepsis survivors with noninfected subjects presenting with noninfectious systemic inflammatory response syndrome, and also sepsis survivors with nonsurvivors. There was a progressive decline in glycerophosphocholine and glycerophosphoethanolamine esters among subjects with sepsis that was more pronounced among nonsurvivors, and increased lactate and increased carnitine esters, products of fatty acid metabolism, in nonsurvivors.[105] One of the limitations of metabolomic investigations is the lack of consensus for analytical strategy using multiple layers of large data. This fact is highlighted by a second metabolomic investigation in the same populations as the Langley study, but done in reverse order and with a different analytical strategy. Rogers and colleagues[106] first identified and then validated individual metabolites associated with death during critical illness, and then developed an iterative bayesian network to risk stratify for mortality. Compared with the Langley study, which identified four critical metabolites, two clinical variables (age and hematocrit), and lactate in a predictive model, the Rogers model identified no clinical data but seven metabolites, all of them distinct from those chosen by the Langley model.[105,106] In a pediatric septic population, Mickiewicz and coworkers[107] applied ^{1}H-NMR spectroscopy to serum samples and demonstrated with principal components analysis that the metabolic profile of septic shock differed from that in healthy children or those with systemic inflammatory response syndrome, and septic shock was characterized by increased levels of metabolites associated with muscle turnover, amino acid oxidation, and decreased energy supply. Metabolomics seems ripe for the development of consensus recommendations governing analytical approach, need for independent replication, and to prompt both meta-analysis and application of unsupervised learning methodologies for class prediction.

BAL fluid has posed a challenge for metabolomics because of the fluid's high protein and salt content, and relatively low concentration of most metabolites.[108] However, Evans and colleagues[103] recently overcame these limitations by testing BAL fluid on multiple high-performance liquid chromatography platforms, and determining that the optimal performance was with reversed-phase and hydrophilic interaction chromatography before mass spectrometry. Consonant with proteomic studies of ARDS BAL fluid that demonstrated reduced surfactant proteins, Evans and coworkers[109] reported measuring reduced phosphatidylcholine, the major phospholipid of pulmonary surfactant, in BAL fluid among subjects with ARDS. Alveolar fluid from subjects with ARDS also demonstrated higher levels of products associated with energy metabolism (lactate, citrate, creatine, and creatinine), all of which were similarly increased in the plasma of patients with ARDS.[103,109] As novel findings, several guanosine network metabolites were increased in ARDS BAL fluid, prompting re-examination of xanthine oxidase activity in lung injury models.[109]

INTRODUCING THE INTERACTOME: A SYSTEMS BIOLOGY APPROACH

The common thread through this review of various 'omic approaches has been the exponential growth in complex data fueled by major technologic advances. The explosion of data has created new challenges for computing power and analysis, but similarly new opportunities to describe how multiple aspects of human data fit together. Groundbreaking examples of integrative thinking paired whole-genome genotyping to tissue-specific gene expression and identified not only the genetic determinants of specific traits, but used annotation and enrichment analysis to determine which transcription factors were critical to obesity[110] or coronary artery disease.[111] This approach, sometimes termed "network biology," is particularly successful when it helps to prioritize further mechanistic study, translating observations in human populations back to the laboratory for testing of causality. In one notable example, Rader and colleagues[111] built on the demonstration that one genetic variant strongly associated with coronary artery disease, low-density lipoprotein cholesterol levels, and hepatic expression of the sortilin gene *SORT1*. The investigators then performed fine mapping of the single-nucleotide polymorphism's linkage disequilibrium block to identify the functional variant, replicated the genetic association in populations of different ancestral background, and used overexpression and knockdown experiments in mice to prove that *SORT1* expression modifies plasma low-density lipoprotein and a novel pathway of low-density lipoprotein regulation was identified.[112,113] Thus the network analysis integrating multiple threads of data not only suggested putative candidates for mechanistic follow-up, but helped to prioritize the functional candidate and suggested the causal pathway through which it acted. Network science is most effective with multiple platforms of systematic data acquisition, thus it has been leveraged successfully with several cancer networks[114] and common traits, such as coronary artery disease.[115] As investigators begin gathering ARDS-specific systematic data, a network-based approach may prove feasible in the future.

Further complexity may be added to the system by considering not only the human interactome, but also the interaction between the human host and resident microbial flora. Although not yet widely applied to lung injury models, careful examination of gut microbiota in animal models of metabolic syndrome has demonstrated the critical interaction between inflammasome signaling and gut microflora.[116] Not only have microbes shaped genetic architecture of global populations through natural selection,[117] but they may be dynamic partners in the evolution of a complex phenotype like ARDS.[118] Next-generation sequencing technology makes it possible to characterize the lung microbiome,[119] which may yield important insights in the future.

SUMMARY

ARDS is a complex trait poised to benefit from the application of high-throughput technologies to assay DNA, mRNA, proteins, metabolites, microbiomes, and systems. Although hindered by infrequent access to lung tissue, researchers have made important advances in the early application of multiple 'omic applications. As clinicians apply lessons from non-ARDS phenotypes highlighting the potential for these techniques to expand the pathophysiologic understanding, new discoveries in ARDS await.

REFERENCES

1. Rubenfeld GD, Caldwell E, Peabody E, et al. Incidence and outcomes of acute lung injury. N Engl J Med 2005;353(16):1685–93.
2. Ranieri VM, Rubenfeld GD, Thompson BT, et al. Acute respiratory distress syndrome: the Berlin definition. JAMA 2012;307(23):2526–33.
3. Ferguson J, Patel P, Shah R, et al. Race and gender variation in response to evoked inflammation. J Transl Med 2013;11(1):63.
4. Mehta NN, Heffron SP, Patel PN, et al. A human model of inflammatory cardio-metabolic dysfunction: a double blind placebo-controlled crossover trial. J Transl Med 2012;10:124.
5. Wurfel MM, Gordon AC, Holden TD, et al. Toll-like receptor 1 polymorphisms affect innate immune responses and outcomes in sepsis. Am J Respir Crit Care Med 2008;178(7):710–20.
6. Zabaleta J, Schneider B, Ryckman K, et al. Ethnic differences in cytokine gene polymorphisms: potential implications for cancer development. Cancer Immunol Immunother 2008;57(1):107–14.
7. Pillay V, Gaillard MC, Halkas A, et al. Differences in the genotypes and plasma concentrations of the INTERLEUKIN-1 receptor antagonist in black and white South African asthmatics and control subjects. Cytokine 2000;12(6):819–21.
8. Sorensen TI, Nielsen GG, Andersen PK, et al. Genetic and environmental influences on premature death in adult adoptees. N Engl J Med 1988; 318(12):727–32.
9. Meyer NJ, Christie JD. Genetic heterogeneity and risk for ARDS. Semin Respir Crit Care Med 2013; 34(4):459–74.
10. Acosta-Herrera M, Pino-Yanes M, Perez-Mendez L, et al. Assessing the quality of studies supporting genetic susceptibility and outcomes of ARDS. Front Genet 2014;5:20.
11. Gao L, Barnes KC. Recent advances in genetic predisposition to clinical acute lung injury. Am J Physiol Lung Cell Mol Physiol 2009;296(5):L713–25.
12. Meyer NJ, Daye ZJ, Rushefski M, et al. SNP-set analysis replicates acute lung injury genetic risk factors. BMC Med Genet 2012;13(1):52.
13. O'Mahony DS, Glavan BJ, Holden TD, et al. Inflammation and immune-related candidate gene associations with acute lung injury susceptibility and severity: a validation study. PLoS One 2012;7(12):e51104.
14. Flores C, Ma SF, Maresso K, et al. IL6 gene-wide haplotype is associated with susceptibility to acute lung injury. Transl Res 2008;152(1):11–7.
15. Marshall RP, Webb S, Hill MR, et al. Genetic polymorphisms associated with susceptibility and outcome in ARDS. Chest 2002;121(Suppl 3):68S–9S.
16. Gong MN, Zhou W, Williams PL, et al. Polymorphisms in the mannose binding lectin-2 gene and acute respiratory distress syndrome. Crit Care Med 2007;35(1):48–56.
17. Gong MN, Thompson BT, Williams PL, et al. Interleukin-10 polymorphism in position -1082 and acute respiratory distress syndrome. Eur Respir J 2006;27(4):674–81.
18. Meyer NJ, Feng R, Li M, et al. IL1RN coding variant is associated with lower risk of acute respiratory distress syndrome and increased plasma IL-1 receptor antagonist. Am J Respir Crit Care Med 2013;187(9):950–9.
19. Medford AR, Godinho SI, Keen LJ, et al. Relationship between vascular endothelial growth factor + 936 genotype and plasma/epithelial lining fluid vascular endothelial growth factor protein levels in patients with and at risk for ARDS. Chest 2009; 136(2):457–64.
20. Medford AR, Millar AB. Vascular endothelial growth factor (VEGF) in acute lung injury (ALI) and acute respiratory distress syndrome (ARDS): paradox or paradigm? Thorax 2006;61(7):621–6.
21. Medford AR, Keen LJ, Bidwell JL, et al. Vascular endothelial growth factor gene polymorphism and acute respiratory distress syndrome. Thorax 2005;60(3):244–8.
22. Meyer NJ, Li M, Feng R, et al. ANGPT2 genetic variant is associated with trauma-associated acute lung injury and altered plasma angiopoietin-2 isoform ratio. Am J Respir Crit Care Med 2011;183: 1344–53.
23. Su L, Zhai R, Sheu CC, et al. Genetic variants in the angiopoietin-2 gene are associated with increased risk of ARDS. Intensive Care Med 2009;35:1024–30.
24. Marshall RP, Webb S, Bellingan GJ, et al. Angiotensin converting enzyme insertion/deletion

polymorphism is associated with susceptibility and outcome in acute respiratory distress syndrome. Am J Respir Crit Care Med 2002;166(5):646–50.

25. Pino-Yanes M, Ma SF, Sun X, et al. Interleukin-1 receptor-associated kinase 3 gene associates with susceptibility to acute lung injury. Am J Respir Cell Mol Biol 2011;45(4):740–5.

26. Pino-Yanes M, Corrales A, Casula M, et al. Common variants of TLR1 associate with organ dysfunction and sustained pro-inflammatory responses during sepsis. PLoS One 2010;5(10): e13759.

27. Tejera P, O'Mahony DS, Owen CA, et al. Functional characterization of polymorphisms in the PI3 (elafin) gene and validation of their contribution to risk of ARDS. Am J Respir Cell Mol Biol 2014; 51(2):262–72.

28. Tejera P, Wang Z, Zhai R, et al. Genetic polymorphisms of peptidase inhibitor 3 (elafin) are associated with acute respiratory distress syndrome. Am J Respir Cell Mol Biol 2009;41(6):696–704.

29. Lin Z, Thomas NJ, Wang Y, et al. Deletions within a CA-repeat-rich region of intron 4 of the human SP-B gene affect mRNA splicing. Biochem J 2005;389(Pt 2):403–12.

30. Lin Z, Pearson C, Chinchilli V, et al. Polymorphisms of human SP-A, SP-B, and SP-D genes: association of SP-B Thr131Ile with ARDS. Clin Genet 2000; 58(3):181–91.

31. David S, Mukherjee A, Ghosh CC, et al. Angiopoietin-2 may contribute to multiple organ dysfunction and death in sepsis. Crit Care Med 2012;40(11):3034–41. http://dx.doi.org/10.1097/CCM.3030b3013e31825fdc31831.

32. Kumpers P, Gueler F, David S, et al. The synthetic tie2 agonist peptide vasculotide protects against vascular leakage and reduces mortality in murine abdominal sepsis. Crit Care 2011;15(5):R261.

33. David S, Park JK, Meurs M, et al. Acute administration of recombinant angiopoietin-1 ameliorates multiple-organ dysfunction syndrome and improves survival in murine sepsis. Cytokine 2011; 55(2):251–9.

34. Alfieri A, Watson JJ, Kammerer RA, et al. Angiopoietin-1 variant reduces LPS-induced microvascular dysfunction in a murine model of sepsis. Crit Care 2012;16(5):R182.

35. Aikawa N, Ishizaka A, Hirasawa H, et al. Reevaluation of the efficacy and safety of the neutrophil elastase inhibitor, sivelestat, for the treatment of acute lung injury associated with systemic inflammatory response syndrome: a phase IV study. Pulm Pharmacol Ther 2011;24(5):549–54.

36. Iwata K, Doi A, Ohji G, et al. Effect of neutrophil elastase inhibitor (sivelestat sodium) in the treatment of acute lung injury (ALI) and acute respiratory distress syndrome (ARDS): a systematic review and meta-analysis. Intern Med 2010; 49(22):2423–32.

37. Zeiher BG, Artigas A, Vincent JL, et al. Neutrophil elastase inhibition in acute lung injury: results of the STRIVE study. Crit Care Med 2004;32(8): 1695–702.

38. Wang Z, Beach D, Su L, et al. A genome-wide expression analysis in blood identifies pre-elafin as a biomarker in ARDS. Am J Respir Cell Mol Biol 2008;38(6):724–32.

39. Wang Z, Chen F, Zhai R, et al. Plasma neutrophil elastase and elafin imbalance is associated with acute respiratory distress syndrome (ARDS) development. PLoS One 2009;4(2):e4380.

40. Nakada TA, Russell JA, Boyd JH, et al. Association of angiotensin II type 1 receptor-associated protein gene polymorphism with increased mortality in septic shock. Crit Care Med 2011;39(7):1641–8.

41. Flores C, Pino-Yanes Mdel M, Villar J. A quality assessment of genetic association studies supporting susceptibility and outcome in acute lung injury. Crit Care 2008;12(5):R130.

42. Adamzik M, Frey U, Sixt S, et al. ACE I/D but not AGT (-6)A/G polymorphism is a risk factor for mortality in ARDS. Eur Respir J 2007;29(3):482–8.

43. Jerng JS, Yu CJ, Wang HC, et al. Polymorphism of the angiotensin-converting enzyme gene affects the outcome of acute respiratory distress syndrome. Crit Care Med 2006;34(4):1001–6.

44. Kuba K, Imai Y, Rao S, et al. A crucial role of angiotensin converting enzyme 2 (ACE2) in SARS coronavirus-induced lung injury. Nat Med 2005; 11(8):875–9.

45. Nicholls J, Peiris M. Good ACE, bad ACE do battle in lung injury, SARS. Nat Med 2005;11(8):821–2.

46. Grigoryev DN, Ma SF, Irizarry RA, et al. Orthologous gene-expression profiling in multi-species models: search for candidate genes. Genome Biol 2004;5(5):R34.

47. Ye SQ, Simon BA, Maloney JP, et al. Pre-B-cell colony-enhancing factor as a potential novel biomarker in acute lung injury. Am J Respir Crit Care Med 2005;171(4):361–70.

48. Ye SQ, Zhang LQ, Adyshev D, et al. Pre-B-cell-colony-enhancing factor is critically involved in thrombin-induced lung endothelial cell barrier dysregulation. Microvasc Res 2005;70(3):142–51.

49. Liu P, Li H, Cepeda J, et al. Regulation of inflammatory cytokine expression in pulmonary epithelial cells by pre-B-cell colony-enhancing factor via a nonenzymatic and AP-1-dependent mechanism. J Biol Chem 2009;284(40):27344–51.

50. Bajwa EK, Yu CJ, Gong MN, et al. PBEF gene polymorphisms influence the risk of developing ARDS. Proc Am Thorac Soc 2006;3:A272.

51. Leikauf GD, Concel VJ, Liu P, et al. Haplotype association mapping of acute lung injury in mice

implicates activin a receptor, type 1. Am J Respir Crit Care Med 2011;183(11):1499–509.

52. Leikauf GD, Pope-Varsalona H, Concel VJ, et al. Functional genomics of chlorine-induced acute lung injury in mice. Proc Am Thorac Soc 2010; 7(4):294–6.

53. Leikauf GD, Concel VJ, Bein K, et al. Functional genomic assessment of phosgene-induced acute lung injury in mice. Am J Respir Cell Mol Biol 2013;49(3):368–83.

54. dos Santos CC, Okutani D, Hu P, et al. Differential gene profiling in acute lung injury identifies injury-specific gene expression. Crit Care Med 2008; 36(3):855–65.

55. Tejera P, Meyer NJ, Chen F, et al. Distinct and replicable genetic risk factors for acute respiratory distress syndrome of pulmonary or extrapulmonary origin. J Med Genet 2012;49(11):671–80.

56. Christie JD, Wurfel MM, Feng R, et al. Genome wide association identifies PPFIA1 as a candidate gene for acute lung injury risk following major trauma. PLoS One 2012;7(1):e28268.

57. Sakamoto S, Ishizaki T, Okawa K, et al. Liprin-α controls stress fiber formation by binding to mDia and regulating its membrane localization. J Cell Sci 2012;125(1):108–20.

58. Christie JD, Ma SF, Aplenc R, et al. Variation in the myosin light chain kinase gene is associated with development of acute lung injury after major trauma. Crit Care Med 2008;36(10):2794–800.

59. Gao L, Grant A, Halder I, et al. Novel polymorphisms in the myosin light chain kinase gene confer risk for acute lung injury. Am J Respir Cell Mol Biol 2006;34(4):487–95.

60. Sheu CC, Zhai R, Su L, et al. Sex-specific association of epidermal growth factor gene polymorphisms with acute respiratory distress syndrome. Eur Respir J 2009;33(3):543–50.

61. Calfee CS, Delucci K, Parsons PE, et al. Latent class analysis of ARDS subphenoypes: analysis of data from two randomized controlled trials. Lancet Respir Med 2014;2(8):611–20.

62. Golub TR, Slonim DK, Tamayo P, et al. Molecular classification of cancer: class discovery and class prediction by gene expression monitoring. Science 1999;286(5439):531–7.

63. Yeoh EJ, Ross ME, Shurtleff SA, et al. Classification, subtype discovery, and prediction of outcome in pediatric acute lymphoblastic leukemia by gene expression profiling. Cancer Cell 2002;1(2):133–43.

64. Kris MG, Johnson BE, Berry LD, et al. Using multiplexed assays of oncogenic drivers in lung cancers to select targeted drugs. JAMA 2014; 311(19):1998–2006.

65. Wolff AC, Hammond ME, Schwartz JN, et al. American Society of Clinical Oncology/College of American Pathologists guideline recommendations for human epidermal growth factor receptor 2 testing in breast cancer. J Clin Oncol 2006; 25(1):118–45.

66. Patel SR, Karmpaliotis D, Ayas NT, et al. The role of open-lung biopsy in ARDS. Chest 2004;125(1): 197–202.

67. Feezor RJ, Baker HV, Mindrinos MN, et al. Whole blood and leukocyte RNA isolation for gene expression analyses. Physiol Genomics 2004; 19(3):247–54.

68. Howrylak JA, Dolinay T, Lucht L, et al. Discovery of the gene signature for acute lung injury in patients with sepsis. Physiol Genomics 2009;37(2):133–9.

69. Lagan AL, Quinlan GJ, Mumby S, et al. Variation in iron homeostasis genes between patients with ARDS and healthy control subjects. Chest 2008; 133(6):1302–11.

70. Quinlan GJ, Chen Y, Evans TW, et al. Iron signalling regulated directly and through oxygen: implications for sepsis and the acute respiratory distress syndrome. Clin Sci 2001;100(2):169–82.

71. Connelly KG, Moss M, Parsons PE, et al. Serum ferritin as a predictor of the acute respiratory distress syndrome. Am J Respir Crit Care Med 1997;155(1):21–5.

72. Marzec JM, Christie JD, Reddy SP, et al. Functional polymorphisms in the transcription factor NRF2 in humans increase the risk of acute lung injury. FASEB J 2007;21(9):2237–46.

73. Wong HR, Cvijanovich N, Lin R, et al. Identification of pediatric septic shock subclasses based on genome-wide expression profiling. BMC Med 2009;7:34.

74. Wong HR, Lindsell CJ, Pettila V, et al. A multi-biomarker-based outcome risk stratification model for adult septic shock. Crit Care Med 2014;42(4): 781–9.

75. Wong H, Salisbury S, Xiao Q, et al. The pediatric sepsis biomarker risk model. Crit Care 2012; 16(5):R174.

76. Mattick JS, Makunin IV. Non-coding RNA. Hum Mol Genet 2006;15(Suppl 1):R17–29.

77. Morris KV, Mattick JS. The rise of regulatory RNA. Nat Rev Genet 2014;15(6):423–37.

78. Mercer TR, Gerhardt DJ, Dinger ME, et al. Targeted RNA sequencing reveals the deep complexity of the human transcriptome. Nat Biotechnol 2012; 30(1):99–104.

79. Lee RC, Feinbaum RL, Ambros V. The *C. elegans* heterochronic gene lin-4 encodes small RNAs with antisense complementarity to lin-14. Cell 1993; 75(5):843–54.

80. Lau NC, Lim LP, Weinstein EG, et al. An abundant class of tiny RNAs with probable regulatory roles in *Caenorhabditis elegans*. Science 2001;294(5543): 858–62.

81. Lee RC, Ambros V. An extensive class of small RNAs in *Caenorhabditis elegans*. Science 2001; 294(5543):862–4.

82. Adyshev DM, Moldobaeva N, Mapes B, et al. MicroRNA regulation of nonmuscle myosin light chain kinase expression in human lung endothelium. Am J Respir Cell Mol Biol 2013;49(1):58–66.

83. Adyshev DM, Elangovan VR, Moldobaeva N, et al. Mechanical stress induces pre-B-cell colony-enhancing factor/NAMPT expression via epigenetic regulation by miR-374a and miR-568 in human lung endothelium. Am J Respir Cell Mol Biol 2014;50(2): 409–18.

84. Schrauder MG, Strick R, Schulz-Wendtland R, et al. Circulating micro-RNAs as potential blood-based markers for early stage breast cancer detection. PLoS One 2012;7(1):e29770.

85. Bird A. Perceptions of epigenetics. Nature 2007; 447(7143):396–8.

86. Reik W. Stability and flexibility of epigenetic gene regulation in mammalian development. Nature 2007;447(7143):425–32.

87. Hanahan D, Weinberg RA. The hallmarks of cancer. Cell 2000;100(1):57–70.

88. Esteller M. Cancer epigenomics: DNA methylomes and histone-modification maps. Nat Rev Genet 2007;8(4):286–98.

89. Seligson DB, Horvath S, Shi T, et al. Global histone modification patterns predict risk of prostate cancer recurrence. Nature 2005;435(7046):1262–6.

90. ENCODE_project_consortium. An integrated encyclopedia of DNA elements in the human genome. Nature 2012;489(7414):57–74.

91. Djebali S, Davis CA, Merkel A, et al. Landscape of transcription in human cells. Nature 2012; 489(7414):101–8.

92. Ideker T, Thorsson V, Ranish JA, et al. Integrated genomic and proteomic analyses of a systematically perturbed metabolic network. Science 2001; 292(5518):929–34.

93. Chen G, Gharib TG, Huang CC, et al. Discordant protein and mRNA expression in lung adenocarcinomas. Mol Cell Proteomics 2002;1(4):304–13.

94. Rogers S, Girolami M, Kolch W, et al. Investigating the correspondence between transcriptomic and proteomic expression profiles using coupled cluster models. Bioinformatics 2008; 24(24):2894–900.

95. Bowler RP, Duda B, Chan ED, et al. Proteomic analysis of pulmonary edema fluid and plasma in patients with acute lung injury. Am J Physiol Lung Cell Mol Physiol 2004;286(6):L1095–104.

96. Schnapp LM, Donohoe S, Chen J, et al. Mining the acute respiratory distress syndrome proteome: identification of the insulin-like growth factor (IGF)/IGF-binding protein-3 pathway in acute lung injury. Am J Pathol 2006;169(1):86–95.

97. de Torre C, Ying SX, Munson PJ, et al. Proteomic analysis of inflammatory biomarkers in bronchoalveolar lavage. Proteomics 2006;6(13):3949–57.

98. Nguyen EV, Gharib SA, Palazzo SJ, et al. Proteomic profiling of bronchoalveolar lavage fluid in critically ill patients with ventilator-associated pneumonia. PLoS One 2013;8(3):e58782.

99. Chang DW, Hayashi S, Gharib SA, et al. Proteomic and computational analysis of bronchoalveolar proteins during the course of the acute respiratory distress syndrome. Am J Respir Crit Care Med 2008;178(7):701–9.

100. Chen X, Shan Q, Jiang L, et al. Quantitative proteomic analysis by iTRAQ for identification of candidate biomarkers in plasma from acute respiratory distress syndrome patients. Biochem Biophys Res Commun 2013;441(1):1–6.

101. Nicholson JK, Foxall PJD, Spraul M, et al. 750 MHz 1H and 1H-13C NMR spectroscopy of human blood plasma. Anal Chem 1995;67(5):793–811.

102. Dunn WB, Bailey NJ, Johnson HE. Measuring the metabolome: current analytical technologies. Analyst 2005;130(5):606–25.

103. Stringer KA, Serkova NJ, Karnovsky A, et al. Metabolic consequences of sepsis-induced acute lung injury revealed by plasma 1H-nuclear magnetic resonance quantitative metabolomics and computational analysis. Am J Physiol Lung Cell Mol Physiol 2011;300(1):L4–11.

104. Seymour C, Yende S, Scott M, et al. Metabolomics in pneumonia and sepsis: an analysis of the GenIMS cohort study. Intensive Care Med 2013;39(8). 1423–34.

105. Langley RJ, Tsalik EL, Velkinburgh JC, et al. An integrated clinico-metabolomic model improves prediction of death in sepsis. Sci Transl Med 2013; 5(195):195ra95.

106. Rogers AJ, McGeachie M, Baron RM, et al. Metabolomic derangements are associated with mortality in critically ill adult patients. PLoS One 2014;9(1): e87538.

107. Mickiewicz B, Vogel HJ, Wong HR, et al. Metabolomics as a novel approach for early diagnosis of pediatric septic shock and its mortality. Am J Respir Crit Care Med 2013;187(9):967–76.

108. Serkova NJ, Standiford TJ, Stringer KA. The emerging field of quantitative blood metabolomics for biomarker discovery in critical illnesses. Am J Respir Crit Care Med 2011;184(6):647–55.

109. Evans CR, Karnovsky A, Kovach MA, et al. Untargeted LC–MS metabolomics of bronchoalveolar lavage fluid differentiates acute respiratory distress syndrome from health. J Proteome Res 2014;13(2): 640–9.

110. Emilsson V, Thorleifsson G, Zhang B, et al. Genetics of gene expression and its effect on disease. Nature 2008;452(7186):423–8.

111. Schadt EE, Molony C, Chudin E, et al. Mapping the genetic architecture of gene expression in human liver. PLoS Biol 2008;6(5):e107.

112. Musunuru K, Strong A, Frank-Kamenetsky M, et al. From noncoding variant to phenotype via SORT1 at the 1p13 cholesterol locus. Nature 2010;466(7307): 714–9.

113. Strong A, Ding Q, Edmondson AC, et al. Hepatic sortilin regulates both apolipoprotein B secretion and LDL catabolism. J Clin Invest 2012;122(8):2807–16.

114. Jonsson PF, Bates PA. Global topological features of cancer proteins in the human interactome. Bioinformatics 2006;22(18):2291–7.

115. Chan SY, White K, Loscalzo J. Deciphering the molecular basis of human cardiovascular disease through network biology. Curr Opin Cardiol 2012; 27(3):202–9.

116. Henao-Mejia J, Elinav E, Jin C, et al. Inflammasome-mediated dysbiosis regulates progression of NAFLD and obesity. Nature 2012;482(7384): 179–85.

117. Karlsson EK, Kwiatkowski DP, Sabeti PC. Natural selection and infectious disease in human populations. Nat Rev Genet 2014;15(6):379–93.

118. Huang YJ, Charlson ES, Collman RG, et al. The role of the lung microbiome in health and disease. A National Heart, Lung, and Blood Institute workshop report. Am J Respir Crit Care Med 2013;187(12): 1382–7.

119. Charlson ES, Diamond JM, Bittinger K, et al. Lung-enriched organisms and aberrant bacterial and fungal respiratory microbiota after lung transplant. Am J Respir Crit Care Med 2012;186(6): 536–45.

Approach to the Patient with the Acute Respiratory Distress Syndrome

David R. Janz, MD, MSc[a], Lorraine B. Ware, MD[b],*

KEYWORDS

- Diagnosis • Evaluation • Acute respiratory distress syndrome • Risk

KEY POINTS

- Before meeting the formal criteria for the diagnosis of acute respiratory distress syndrome (ARDS), patients may exhibit signs that can be used to inform the bedside practitioner as to the risk of future development of ARDS and respiratory failure.
- Early implementation of therapies, such as lung protective ventilation, in the at-risk patient may prevent the development of ARDS.
- Noninvasive testing, such as the arterial oxygen saturation to fraction of inspired oxygen ratio and echocardiography, can be valuable in the bedside evaluation of a patient with respiratory failure and bilateral infiltrates.
- Once the diagnosis of ARDS is made, the bedside practitioner should begin a thorough search for the underlying cause of ARDS.
- In the absence of a direct or indirect risk factor for ARDS, the practitioner should also consider cardiac dysfunction and mimickers of ARDS in their differential diagnosis of respiratory failure and bilateral infiltrates on chest imaging.

INTRODUCTION

The acute respiratory distress syndrome (ARDS) is a common complication of a variety of illnesses and is associated with significant morbidity and mortality.[1,2] Early recognition of the patient at risk for or with ARDS and identification of the underlying cause allows more timely application of potentially life-saving therapies.[3–5] However, in a study by Ferguson and colleagues,[6] more than 50% of patients with ARDS went unrecognized by their physician and ARDS was only recognized at the time of autopsy. This underrecognition of ARDS can partly be related to the lack of sensitivity in the clinical definitions of this syndrome[6,7]; however regardless of the reasons, the underrecognition of ARDS likely leads to an underutilization of ARDS-specific therapies. For example, the benefit of lower tidal volume protective ventilator strategy has been established for more than 10 years,[3] but approximately 25% of patients worldwide with ARDS still do not receive this therapy.[8]

Therapies for ARDS have been reported to improve ARDS-related mortality by 8% to 16%.[3–5] Use of these therapies depends on the practitioner applying the definition of ARDS[7] at the bedside to make the diagnosis. However, the

Disclosures: The authors have no conflicts of interest to disclose.
Sources of Funding: Supported in part by the National Institutes of Health T32 HL087738 and UL1 RR024975-01.
[a] Section of Pulmonary and Critical Care Medicine, Department of Medicine, LSU School of Medicine, 1901 Perdido Street, Suite 3205, New Orleans, LA 70112, USA; [b] Department of Pathology, Microbiology and Immunology, Vanderbilt University School of Medicine, T-1218 MCN, 1161 21st Avenue South, Nashville, TN 37232-2650, USA
* Corresponding author.
E-mail address: lorraine.ware@vanderbilt.edu

Clin Chest Med 35 (2014) 685–696
http://dx.doi.org/10.1016/j.ccm.2014.08.007

clinical definition of ARDS neither identifies patients at risk for later development of ARDS, consider other conditions that can mimic ARDS, nor does it take into account the respiratory dysfunction that exists before meeting ARDS criteria that might benefit from early implementation of therapy. Illustrated with case-based presentations, this article aims to describe a bedside approach to the early identification of critically ill patients at risk of developing ARDS as well as a practical approach to diagnosis and evaluation for the underlying cause in patients with ARDS.

IDENTIFYING PATIENTS AT RISK OF DEVELOPING ACUTE RESPIRATORY DISTRESS SYNDROME

A 65-year-old woman with a history of diabetes mellitus presents with an acute abdomen, fever, tachycardia, leukocytosis, and hypotension. She is found to have a perforated diverticulum with an intra-abdominal abscess that is effectively drained in the operating room. Post-operatively and despite fluid resuscitation and broad-spectrum antibiotics, she arrives in the intensive care unit (ICU) hypotensive and mechanically ventilated. Vasoactive medications are initiated for blood pressure support. Her chest radiograph shows no pulmonary infiltrates (Fig. 1), and she has an arterial oxygen saturation of 95% on mechanical ventilation with a fraction of inspired oxygen of 0.40. What is the subsequent risk of this patient developing ARDS during his course in the ICU?

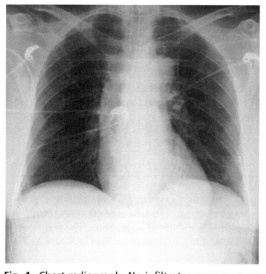

Fig. 1. Chest radiograph. No infiltrates were seen on the chest radiograph of the intubated and mechanically ventilated patient in this case presentation.

Recently, increased attention has been given to the critically ill patient at risk of developing ARDS. With numerous studies showing a lack of benefit of pharmacologic interventions aimed at treating patients with established ARDS,[9–12] focus has shifted to identifying patients at risk of developing ARDS to provide earlier preventative therapies. As an example, early application of low tidal volume ventilation may prevent the development of ARDS in at-risk patients.[13,14] For this reason, clinical recognition of patients who are at risk of development of ARDS is critically important. Several strategies have been used to identify patient factors associated with the development of ARDS, including data that are collected both noninvasively and invasively.

Traditional Clinical Risk Factors and Risk Modifiers for Acute Respiratory Distress Syndrome

ARDS usually develops in the setting of an appropriate clinical risk factor. Awareness of these risk factors and other clinical factors that may increase or decrease risk can facilitate early diagnosis. The acutely injured lung is the end result of a pathologic process characterized by diffuse alveolar damage with influx of inflammatory cells and protein-rich pulmonary edema fluid into the alveolus.[15] Although the pathologic findings are similar regardless of the underlying cause, there are many different underlying diagnoses that put patients at risk for diffuse alveolar damage. Risk factors for the development of ARDS can be divided into diagnoses that induce direct injury to the lung and diagnoses that have an extrapulmonary origin, with ensuing systemic inflammation causing indirect lung injury. Among diagnoses that directly injure the alveolus, pneumonia (46%) and aspiration of gastric contents (11%) are the most common causes; severe sepsis of a nonpulmonary origin (33%) and trauma (7%) are the most common causes of indirect lung injury.[1] Distinct from risk factors, risk modifiers are patient characteristics that are not thought to cause ARDS but may make a risk factor (eg, sepsis) more or less likely to cause ARDS. Risk modifiers thought to decrease the risk of ARDS include diabetes mellitus,[16] whereas smoking,[17] alcohol use,[17] hypoalbuminemia,[18] oxygen therapy,[19] and chemotherapy[20] have all been reported to increase the risk of ARDS in the setting of an appropriate risk factor such as sepsis or severe trauma (**Table 1**).[21]

The Lung Injury Prediction Score

In addition to recognition of broad categories of clinical risk factors, bedside calculation of a risk

Table 1
Lung Injury Prediction score

	LIPS Points	Score	Positive-Predictive Value (Risk of the Future Development of ARDS), %
Predisposing Conditions		>3	14
Shock	2	>4	18
Aspiration	2	>5	23
Sepsis	1		
Pneumonia	1.5		
High-risk Surgery			
Orthopedic Spine	1		
Acute Abdomen	2		
Cardiac	2.5		
Aortic Vascular	3.5		
High-risk Trauma			
Traumatic Brain Injury	2		
Smoke Inhalation	2		
Near Drowning	2		
Lung Contusion	1.5		
Multiple Fractures	1.5		
Risk Modifiers			
Alcohol Abuse	1		
Obesity (BMI >30)	1		
Hypoalbuminemia	1		
Chemotherapy	1		
Fio_2 >0.35 (>4 L/min)	2		
Tachypnea (RR >30)	1.5		
SpO_2 <95%	1		
Acidosis (pH <7.35)	1.5		
Diabetes Mellitus	−1		

Abbreviations: BMI, body mass index; Fio_2, fraction of inspired oxygen; RR, respiratory rate; SpO_2, arterial oxygen saturation.

Data from Gajic O, Dabbagh O, Park PK, et al. Early identification of patients at risk of acute lung injury: evaluation of lung injury prediction score in a multicenter cohort study. Am J Respir Crit Care Med 2011;183(4):466.

prediction score may aid in identifying patients at highest risk of ARDS. Early in the study of ARDS it was recognized that certain clinical variables, such as ventilator settings, blood transfusions, and predisposing diagnoses, were associated with the subsequent development of ARDS.[1,22–26] Recent emphasis[27] has been placed on the use of these and other easily obtained clinical variables to predict the development of ARDS in critically ill patients to design clinical trials of interventions aimed at the prevention of ARDS. The Lung Injury Prediction Score (LIPS), first described in 2011[21] attempts to account for risk factors for the subsequent development of ARDS, such as sepsis, along with accounting for potential risk modifiers.

The LIPS was developed through an initial single-center, retrospective, and prospective observational cohort study[21] and a subsequent larger, multicenter validation study involving more than 5000 at-risk patients.[28] In the larger, multicenter study, clinical variables that included both known ARDS risk factors and risk modifiers were collected during the first 6 hours after presentation to an emergency department. Of 5584 at-risk patients enrolled, 277 (6.8%) subsequently developed ARDS, a median of 2 days after admission. After analyzing the association of both risk factors and risk modifiers with the future development of ARDS, points were assigned to each factor and modifier based on the strength of association in a regression model (see **Table 1**). Calculation of the

LIPS allows a percentage describing the risk of future development of ARDS to be assigned to each at-risk patient. For example, in the initial case presentation of a patient with a history of diabetes mellitus, sepsis, shock, Fio_2 greater than 0.35, and high-risk surgery, the calculated LIPS score is 6, corresponding to approximate 23% risk of future development of ARDS.

In the original study, an LIPS of greater than 4 was found to have good discriminatory power, in that 97% of patients with a score of less than or equal to 4 did not go on to develop ARDS, whereas 18% of patients with a score greater than 4 went on to develop ARDS. As such, clinical trials[29] aimed at preventing the development of ARDS in high-risk patients have used an LIPS greater than or equal to 4 to enrich patients to target for preventative interventions. Although the low positive predictive value of the LIPS[28] (see **Table 1**) is discouraging for the bedside practitioner in predicting which patient will develop ARDS, the LIPS remains the only validated scoring system available and involves almost no invasive testing.

While we await the results of preventative trials to guide the management of the at-risk patient, the bedside clinician can still use the LIPS and other tools[30] to identify patients at risk of ARDS and perform interventions that may decrease such risk. For example, a patient determined to be at high risk for development of ARDS may benefit from the earlier initiation of resuscitation and antibiotics for severe sepsis,[20] a more conservative fluid strategy early in their ICU course,[31] and lung-protective ventilation even in the absence of ARDS, an intervention that has been associated with improved clinical outcomes.[13,14,32] In the case presented earlier where the patient is in shock, has been volume resuscitated, treated with early antibiotics, and has an LIPS of 6, the addition of lung-protective ventilation may reduce the risk of pulmonary and extrapulmonary complications and shorten the patient's hospital stay.[14]

Plasma Biomarkers for the Risk Prediction of Acute Respiratory Distress Syndrome

ARDS is the culmination of multiple inflammatory and coagulopathic processes involving both the lung endothelium and epithelium that can produce measurable biomarkers before the development of bilateral pulmonary infiltrates on chest imaging.[33] As a biomarker of injury to the lung endothelium, plasma angiopoietin-2 (Ang-2) has received the most attention for prediction of the development of ARDS in at-risk patients.[34–36] In a recent study by Agrawal and colleagues,[36] plasma Ang-2 was measured in a heterogeneous group of 230

patients in the emergency department determined to be at risk for the development of ARDS based on planned admission to an ICU. Ang-2 was not only significantly higher in patients who went on to develop ARDS but also was at least as predictive of the development of ARDS as the LIPS (area under the receiver operating characteristic curve [AUC] of 0.74 and 0.74, respectively). Adding Ang-2 levels to the LIPS further improved discriminatory power (AUC 0.84) (**Fig. 2**). Although less studied, other plasma biomarkers such as club cell protein 16,[37] interleukin 8,[36] and tissue factor[38] have also shown promise in identifying at-risk patients.

The obvious limitations of using plasma biomarkers in risk prediction are cost, speed, and timing of measurement. None of the tests mentioned earlier are currently available for clinical use nor is it clear what the optimal time is for measurement. The Ang-2 study[36] was performed in the emergency department. However, it is unclear whether Ang-2 measurements would be useful in the already hospitalized patient, post-operative patients, or critically ill patients transferred from other ICU settings. As further data are collected on the predictive value of plasma biomarkers and the cost and time of measurement decreases, perhaps plasma biomarkers will be incorporated to improve the predictive power of other tools such as the LIPS.

DIAGNOSING ACUTE RESPIRATORY DISTRESS SYNDROME

*A 40-year-old woman who has been admitted to the ICU with community-acquired pneumonia is currently requiring 4 L of oxygen per minute to maintain an arterial oxygen saturation by pulse oximetry (SpO_2) of 88%, has a respiratory rate of 32, and has bilateral alveolar infiltrates on her chest radiograph (**Fig. 3**). Does this patient have ARDS and what is her risk of progressing to requiring mechanical ventilation?*

ARDS is a clinical syndrome that is diagnosed by application of clinical definitions that have been developed by expert consensus. The clinical definition of ARDS has undergone recent revision[7] (**Table 2**) from its original form.[39] The current definition's requirement of positive pressure ventilation, measurement of arterial blood gases, and evaluation of left ventricular function reduce the sensitivity to detect ARDS at the bedside in patients who may not fit these criteria (as in the case presentation), but are still at risk of progressive respiratory failure. Several strategies have been recently reported to address these shortcomings of the current definitions[7] in diagnosing ARDS at the bedside.

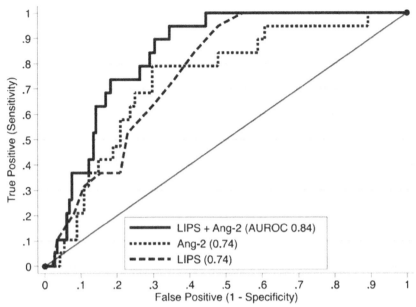

Fig. 2. Receiver operating characteristic curves for the prediction of the development of ARDS. When measured in the emergency department, Ang-2 was as predictive as the LIPS in determining which critically ill patients would go on to develop ARDS. The predictive power increased when Ang-2 was added to the LIPS. (*From* Agrawal A, Matthay MA, Kangelaris KN, et al. Plasma angiopoietin-2 predicts the onset of acute lung injury in critically ill patients. Am J Respir Crit Care Med 2013;187(7):740. Reprinted with permission of the American Thoracic Society. Copyright © 2013 American Thoracic Society. Official Journal of the American Thoracic Society.)

Early Acute Lung Injury

In autopsy studies, the sensitivity of the current definition of ARDS[7] is approximately 89%[40] when practitioners suspect the diagnosis and apply the criteria at the bedside. However, the sensitivity of this definition may be reduced by the requirement for either invasive or noninvasive positive pressure ventilation and measurement of arterial blood gases, along with dichotomizing ARDS as either being present or absent rather than recognizing that this syndrome encompasses a spectrum of severity of lung injury.

To address these concerns, Levitt and colleagues[41] recently performed a prospective cohort study to develop a definition of early acute lung injury (EALI) to alert the practitioner to patients who have acute lung injury that do not yet meet criteria for diagnosis of ARDS but who have high risk of progression to ARDS and need for invasive mechanical ventilation. Patients enrolled in this study had bilateral infiltrates on chest radiograph, were not mechanically ventilated, did not have a clinical suspicion of isolated left atrial hypertension, and did not have arterial blood gases available. In this group, a requirement of more than 2 L/minute of supplemental oxygen, a respiratory rate greater than or equal to 30 breaths per minute, and immune suppression were found to be independent risk factors for subsequent progression to ARDS with the need for mechanical ventilation. Patients with any 2 of these factors, termed an EALI score greater than 2 (as in the case presentation) had a 53% subsequent risk of progression to ARDS

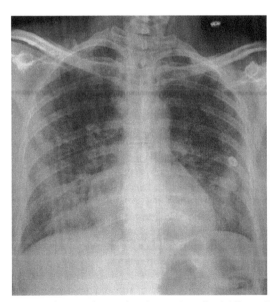

Fig. 3. Chest radiograph. The patient had bilateral alveolar infiltrates on chest radiograph, however was not currently requiring mechanical ventilation.

Table 2
The Berlin definition of acute respiratory distress syndrome

	Criteria	Notes
Timing	Within 1 wk of a known clinical risk factor	
Chest Imaging	Bilateral opacities (excluding effusions, atelectasis, and nodules)	
Cause of Edema	Respiratory failure not purely of cardiac origin	If no ARDS risk factor present, echocardiography or PAOP measurement to rule out cardiac causes
Oxygenation		
Mild ARDS	Pao_2/Fio_2 = 201–300 mm Hg and PEEP or CPAP $\geq$5 cm H_2O	Mild ARDS can be diagnosed even if the patient is receiving noninvasive ventilation
Moderate ARDS	Pao_2/Fio_2 = 101–200 mm Hg and PEEP $\geq$5 cm H_2O	
Severe ARDS	Pao_2/Fio_2 $\leq$100 mm Hg and PEEP $\geq$5 cm H_2O	

Abbreviations: CPAP, continuous positive airway pressure; PAOP, pulmonary artery occlusion pressure; PEEP, positive end-expiratory pressure.

Adapted from ARDS Definition Task Force, Ranieri VM, Rubenfeld GD, et al. Acute respiratory distress syndrome: the Berlin definition. JAMA 2012;307:2526–33. http://dx.doi.org/10.1001/jama.2012.5669.

with mechanical ventilation, a higher risk than calculated from concomitant LIPS scoring (33%). The median time from meeting criteria for EALI to need for positive pressure ventilation was 20 hours. The creation of this definition of EALI recognizes ARDS as a spectrum of illness and provides the bedside practitioner with a diagnostic tool to identify ARDS early in its progression, which may result in the early application of therapeutic interventions. For example, ICU admission for patients presenting to the emergency department with bilateral infiltrates on chest radiograph and an EALI score greater than or equal to 2 should strongly be considered given the high risk of rapid progression of respiratory failure requiring mechanical ventilation.

The Diagnosis of Acute Respiratory Distress Syndrome

Recent modifications in the definition of ARDS are worth noting, because they may affect application of the definitions at the bedside. The original American-European Consensus Conference (AECC) definition of ARDS[39] did not specify a timeframe as to what represented an "acute" onset of ARDS. The new Berlin definition[7] requires that the development of ARDS, including bilateral infiltrates on chest radiograph, occur within 1 week of a known precipitant. Secondly, patients receiving greater than or equal to 5

cmH_2O of continuous positive airway pressure via noninvasive positive pressure ventilation may now be diagnosed with mild ARDS without the need for invasive mechanical ventilation. The AECC definition of ARDS required that patients have pulmonary arterial occlusion pressure (PAOP), if measured, less than or equal to 18 mm Hg, whereas the current Berlin definition recognizes that elevated PAOP and ARDS can coexist[42,43] in patients receiving volume resuscitation with preexisting cardiac disease and elevated end-expiratory intrathoracic pressures. Currently, if a patient's respiratory failure cannot be explained fully by an ARDS risk factor, objective cardiac testing is needed, such as echocardiography or pulmonary artery catheterization. Finally, the term "acute lung injury" has been eliminated from the Berlin definition, and mild, moderate, and severe categories of ARDS have been created based on ratio of inspired to arterial oxygen (Pao_2/Fio_2). This clinical definition of ARDS is currently the primary diagnostic tool available at the bedside for practitioners to identify patients with ARDS.

Although both the AECC and Berlin definitions of ARDS require measurement of arterial Pao_2 to calculate the Pao_2/Fio_2 ratio, less invasive strategies for measurement of the oxygenation defect that use the arterial oxygen saturation measured by pulse oximetry (SpO_2) may be useful in diagnosing ARDS and are more continuously available.

In a derivation and validation study[44] of approximately 1000 patients and more than 4000 simultaneous measurements of Pao_2, SpO_2, and Fio_2, use of a SpO_2/Fio_2 ratio performed very well in comparison to a Pao_2/Fio_2 ratio in the diagnosis of ARDS. Specifically, SpO_2/Fio_2 ratios of 315 and 235 corresponded to Pao_2/Fio_2 ratios of 300 and 200, respectively. In pediatric patients where arterial blood sampling is more difficult than adults, the SpO_2/Fio_2 ratio may be useful in the diagnosis and prediction of respiratory failure requiring invasive mechanical ventilation in patients with ARDS.[45] Although use of a SpO_2/Fio_2 ratio is not accurate in the extremes of SpO_2 and Pao_2 given a nonlinear relationship at these levels (ie, when SpO_2 is $\geq 97\%$), the SpO_2/Fio_2 ratio represents a simple, noninvasive alternative to arterial blood gas measurement in diagnosing patients with ARDS.

Another challenge in diagnosing ARDS is the differentiation between ARDS and cardiogenic pulmonary edema.[46] Several indices on the chest radiograph may aid in this differentiation. Radiographic features of cardiogenic pulmonary edema include increased heart size, widened vascular pedicle width (>70 mm measured from the origin of the left subclavian artery from the aorta to the intersection of the right mainstem bronchus and superior vena cava),[47] centrally located edema, and pleural effusions.[48] Transthoracic echocardiography is also useful in this differentiation and has 86% agreement with pulmonary-artery catheters when diagnosing cardiac dysfunction.[49] Finally, if the diagnosis of ARDS or cardiogenic pulmonary edema is still in question after chest radiography and echocardiography, pulmonary artery catheterization may be necessary, while being mindful that the complication rate with this procedure in the critically ill has been reported as high as 9.5%.[50–52] Furthermore, a PAOP of greater than 18 mm Hg with a normal cardiac index was reported in 29% of patients with known ARDS.[43]

Taking into account the EALI definition[41] and the Berlin definition of ARDS,[7] the case patient presented earlier would be considered to have EALI but would not yet meet diagnostic criteria for ARDS. Evaluation of cardiac function would not be necessary to meet diagnostic criteria for ARDS as the patient's respiratory failure can be explained by the presence of pneumonia. Although the patient is receiving only a modest amount of oxygen, the patient has a 53% risk of the future development of ARDS and need for mechanical ventilation. Therefore, ICU-level monitoring is an appropriate disposition for this patient.

EVALUATION OF THE PATIENT WITH ACUTE RESPIRATORY DISTRESS SYNDROME

*A 24-year-old woman with no past medical history but who recently started smoking tobacco is admitted to the ICU with fever, cough, dyspnea, and rapidly progressive hypoxemic respiratory failure. She requires invasive mechanical ventilation with an initial Pao_2/Fio_2 of 80 mm Hg. Chest radiography shows bilateral alveolar infiltrates (**Fig. 4**), and there are no signs of left ventricular dysfunction. Despite treatment with broad-spectrum antibiotics for community-acquired pneumonia she fails to improve over the subsequent 3 days. Results of bacterial cultures of the sputum on presentation are negative. Would any additional testing be beneficial in the evaluation of this patient with ARDS?*

It cannot be overemphasized that ARDS is a syndrome that indicates an underlying diagnosis. Without recognition and treatment of the underlying diagnosis, ARDS is unlikely to improve. Potential underlying diagnoses may not be readily apparent in the critically ill, sedated or comatose patient who is unable to provide a complete history. For example, intra-abdominal processes such as pancreatitis, cholecystitis, or viscus perforation may be occult unless clinical suspicion leads to appropriate testing. Atypical infectious processes such as fungal pneumonias, psittacosis, or tick-borne illness will not respond to usual antibiotic therapy for community-acquired pneumonia and may be missed if an appropriate history and testing are not obtained. Drug overdose can also lead to ARDS either directly or due to consequent aspiration and may be missed

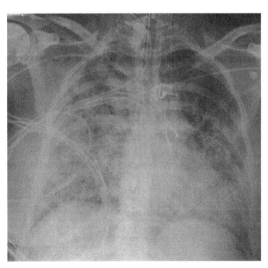

Fig. 4. Chest radiograph. Bilateral alveolar infiltrates were seen on the patient's chest radiograph during her critical illness.

unless appropriate toxicology tests are ordered. For this reason, the diagnosis of ARDS should be viewed as a starting point in the diagnostic evaluation rather than the endpoint, and the underlying diagnosis leading to ARDS[15] should always be thoroughly investigated, including the consideration of more unusual causes of ARDS.[53,54] The importance of a thorough history cannot be overstated and if the patient is unable to provide a history (as is often the case), every effort should be made to contact family or friends to obtain a complete description of the antecedent illness and any exposures.

Mimickers of Acute Respiratory Distress Syndrome

The approach to the differential diagnosis in patients with ARDS should also include mimickers of ARDS. Although the definitions of ARDS[7,39] include parameters that should reduce the possibility of misclassifying pure cardiogenic pulmonary edema and chronic lung diseases as ARDS, there are other conditions that can present acutely with hypoxemia, bilateral alveolar infiltrates, and no evidence of left ventricular dysfunction. Diagnoses such as diffuse alveolar hemorrhage, pulmonary alveolar proteinosis, acute interstitial pneumonia, cryptogenic organizing pneumonia, acute eosinophilic pneumonia, and acute exacerbations of idiopathic pulmonary fibrosis may meet the diagnostic criteria for ARDS (**Table 3**); however, these syndromes are not a result of the same inflammatory mechanisms that underlie the direct and indirect causes of ARDS and treatment may vary widely based on the diagnosis. Careful attention should be paid to the possibility of an alternative diagnosis in patients with ARDS, particularly when no apparent underlying cause for ARDS is readily identified.

Invasive Evaluation of Acute Respiratory Distress Syndrome

Invasive sampling of the lung, in the absence of a diagnosis after noninvasive testing, may aid in determining the cause of ARDS. Flexible bronchoscopy with bronchoalveolar lavage may play a role in determining the cause of ARDS and evaluating for mimickers of ARDS. In the setting of pneumonia as the cause of ARDS, bronchoalveolar lavage may have a sensitivity as high as 60%

Table 3
Mimickers of acute respiratory distress syndrome

	Chest Imaging Characteristics	Diagnostic Tests	Potential Changes in Therapy
Diffuse Alveolar Hemorrhage	Bilateral alveolar and ground-glass infiltrates	Bronchoscopy with bronchoalveolar lavage	Glucocorticoids, transfusion, immunosuppressive therapy
Pulmonary Alveolar Proteinosis	Central and lower lung zone alveolar infiltrates, "batwing" appearance, "crazy paving" on CT	High-resolution computed tomography (CT), bronchoscopy with bronchoalveolar lavage	Whole lung lavage, granulocyte macrophage colony-stimulating factor
Acute Interstitial Pneumonia	Bilateral alveolar and ground-glass infiltrates, septal thickening, traction bronchiectasis	No alternative cause of ARDS identified, open or thoracoscopic lung biopsy	Glucocorticoids
Cryptogenic Organizing Pneumonia	Peripheral distribution of alveolar infiltrates, migratory infiltrates	Bronchoscopy with Transbronchial lung biopsy	Glucocorticoids
Acute Exacerbation of Idiopathic Pulmonary Fibrosis	Ground-glass opacities superimposed on peripheral, basilar fibrotic changes	CT	Glucocorticoids
Acute Eosinophilic Pneumonia	Bilateral alveolar and ground-glass infiltrates	Bronchoscopy with bronchoalveolar lavage	Glucocorticoids

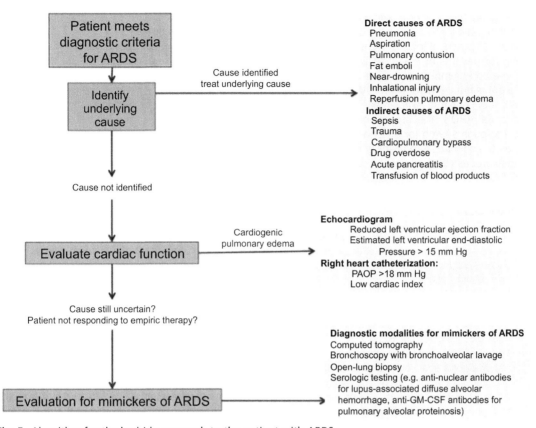

Fig. 5. Algorithm for the bedside approach to the patient with ARDS.

for identification of a specific pathogen.[55] Bronchoscopy may also be helpful in the patient with persistent ARDS given that new, superimposed ventilator-associated pneumonia diagnosed by bronchoalveolar lavage occurs in approximately 36% of patients with ARDS[56] and may prolong the patient's recovery from the initial diagnosis. In the case presented earlier, the patient underwent flexible bronchoscopy and was found to have a differential cell count of 48% eosinophils on bronchoalveolar lavage and was diagnosed with acute eosinophilic pneumonia. Once this diagnosis was made, she was treated with glucocorticoids leading to extubation 3 days later.[57] This case of acute eosinophilic pneumonia mimicking ARDS emphasizes the point that if an underlying cause of ARDS is not identified and the patient is not improving with empirical therapy for common causes of ARDS, invasive testing may be useful for specific diagnosis and treatment.

Open lung biopsy may also play a similar role in patients with undifferentiated ARDS and has produced an alternative diagnosis and change in therapy in up to 60% of patients, with few major complications.[58,59] In one study, even in the setting of marked hypoxemic respiratory failure (mean Pao_2/Fio_2 = 145 mm Hg, SD ± 61), major complications occurred in only 7% of patients with no procedure-related deaths.[59] In fact, a study by Papazian and colleagues[58] showed that there was no significant change in arterial blood gas values pre- and post-procedure, whereas there was an increase in the Pao_2/Fio_2 ratio after the procedure. From the total of 93 cases of open lung biopsy described in these 2 studies, it can be conclude that in a selected patient population with ARDS and no identified underlying cause, the risks of open lung biopsy may be acceptable given that this procedure may provide additional information that may change therapy.

SUMMARY

Given the high incidence and mortality of ARDS in critically ill patients, every practitioner needs a bedside approach (**Fig. 5**) both for early identification of patients at risk for ARDS and for the appropriate evaluation of patients who meet the diagnostic criteria of ARDS. Recent advances such as the Lung Injury Prediction score, the Early

Acute Lung Injury score, and validation of the SpO_2/Fio_2 ratio for assessing the degree of hypoxemia are all practical tools to aid the practitioner in caring for patients at risk of ARDS and will likely become more important in the future because more preventative therapies for ARDS are investigated. For patients who meet the diagnostic criteria for ARDS, the practitioner should focus on a thorough search for an underlying cause as well as the concurrent possibility of an underlying disease process that mimics the clinical syndrome of ARDS.

REFERENCES

1. Rubenfeld GD, Caldwell E, Peabody E, et al. Incidence and outcomes of acute lung injury. N Engl J Med 2005;353(16):1685–93. http://dx.doi.org/10.1056/NEJMoa050333.

2. Herridge MS, Tansey CM, Matté A, et al. Functional disability 5 years after acute respiratory distress syndrome. N Engl J Med 2011;364(14):1293–304. http://dx.doi.org/10.1056/NEJMoa1011802.

3. Ventilation with lower tidal volumes as compared with traditional tidal volumes for acute lung injury and the acute respiratory distress syndrome. The Acute Respiratory Distress Syndrome Network. N Engl J Med 2000;342(18):1301–8. http://dx.doi.org/10.1056/NEJM200005043421801.

4. Guérin C, Reignier J, Richard JC, et al. Prone positioning in severe acute respiratory distress syndrome. N Engl J Med 2013;368(23):2159–68. http://dx.doi.org/10.1056/NEJMoa1214103.

5. Papazian L, Forel JM, Gacouin A, et al. Neuromuscular blockers in early acute respiratory distress syndrome. N Engl J Med 2010;363(12):1107–16. http://dx.doi.org/10.1056/NEJMoa1005372.

6. Ferguson ND, Frutos-Vivar F, Esteban A, et al. Acute respiratory distress syndrome: underrecognition by clinicians and diagnostic accuracy of three clinical definitions. Crit Care Med 2005;33(10):2228–34.

7. ARDS Definition Task Force, Ranieri VM, Rubenfeld GD, et al. Acute respiratory distress syndrome: the Berlin Definition. JAMA 2012;307:2526–33. http://dx.doi.org/10.1001/jama.2012.5669.

8. Esteban A, Frutos-Vivar F, Muriel A, et al. Evolution of mortality over time in patients receiving mechanical ventilation. Am J Respir Crit Care Med 2013;188(2):220–30. http://dx.doi.org/10.1164/rccm.201212-2169OC.

9. Ketoconazole for early treatment of acute lung injury and acute respiratory distress syndrome: a randomized controlled trial. The ARDS Network. JAMA 2000;283(15):1995–2002.

10. Steinberg KP, Hudson LD, Goodman RB, et al. Efficacy and safety of corticosteroids for persistent acute respiratory distress syndrome. N Engl J Med 2006;354(16):1671–84. http://dx.doi.org/10.1056/NEJMoa051693.

11. National Heart, Lung, and Blood Institute Acute Respiratory Distress Syndrome (ARDS) Clinical Trials Network, Matthay MA, Brower RG, et al. Randomized, placebo-controlled clinical trial of an aerosolized β_2-agonist for treatment of acute lung injury. Am J Respir Crit Care Med 2011;184(5):561–8. http://dx.doi.org/10.1164/rccm.201012-2090OC.

12. Rice TW, Wheeler AP, Thompson BT, et al. Enteral omega-3 fatty acid, gamma-linolenic acid, and antioxidant supplementation in acute lung injury. JAMA 2011;306(14):1574–81. http://dx.doi.org/10.1001/jama.2011.1435.

13. Determann RM, Royakkers A, Wolthuis EK, et al. Ventilation with lower tidal volumes as compared with conventional tidal volumes for patients without acute lung injury: a preventive randomized controlled trial. Crit Care 2010;14(1):R1. http://dx.doi.org/10.1186/cc8230.

14. Futier E, Constantin JM, Paugam-Burtz C, et al. A trial of intraoperative low-tidal-volume ventilation in abdominal surgery. N Engl J Med 2013;369(5):428–37. http://dx.doi.org/10.1056/NEJMoa1301082.

15. Ware LB, Matthay MA. The acute respiratory distress syndrome. N Engl J Med 2000;342(18):1334–49. http://dx.doi.org/10.1056/NEJM200005043421806.

16. Moss M, Guidot DM, Steinberg KP, et al. Diabetic patients have a decreased incidence of acute respiratory distress syndrome. Crit Care Med 2000;28(7):2187–92.

17. Iribarren C, Jacobs DR, Sidney S, et al. Cigarette smoking, alcohol consumption, and risk of ARDS: a 15-year cohort study in a managed care setting. Chest 2000;117(1):163–8.

18. Mangialardi RJ, Martin GS, Bernard GR, et al. Hypoproteinemia predicts acute respiratory distress syndrome development, weight gain, and death in patients with sepsis. Ibuprofen in Sepsis Study Group. Crit Care Med 2000;28(9):3137–45.

19. Levitt JE, Bedi H, Calfee CS, et al. Identification of early acute lung injury at initial evaluation in an acute care setting prior to the onset of respiratory failure. Chest 2009;135(4):936–43. http://dx.doi.org/10.1378/chest.08-2346.

20. Iscimen R, Cartin-Ceba R, Yilmaz M, et al. Risk factors for the development of acute lung injury in patients with septic shock: an observational cohort study. Crit Care Med 2008;36(5):1518–22. http://dx.doi.org/10.1097/CCM.0b013e31816fc2c0.

21. Trillo-Alvarez C, Cartin-Ceba R, Kor DJ, et al. Acute lung injury prediction score: derivation and validation in a population-based sample. Eur Respir J 2011;37(3):604–9. http://dx.doi.org/10.1183/09031936.00036810.

22. Matthay MA, Zimmerman GA, Esmon C, et al. Future research directions in acute lung injury: summary

of a National Heart, Lung, and Blood Institute working group. Am J Respir Crit Care Med 2003;167(7): 1027–35. http://dx.doi.org/10.1164/rccm.200208-966WS.

23. Gong MN. Genetic epidemiology of acute respiratory distress syndrome: implications for future prevention and treatment. Clin Chest Med 2006;27(4): 705–24. http://dx.doi.org/10.1016/j.ccm.2006.07. 001 [abstract x].

24. Gajic O, Frutos-Vivar F, Esteban A, et al. Ventilator settings as a risk factor for acute respiratory distress syndrome in mechanically ventilated patients. Intensive Care Med 2005;31(7):922–6. http://dx.doi.org/10.1007/s00134-005-2625-1.

25. Khan H, Belsher J, Yilmaz M, et al. Fresh-frozen plasma and platelet transfusions are associated with development of acute lung injury in critically ill medical patients. Chest 2007;131(5):1308–14. http://dx.doi.org/10.1378/chest.06-3048.

26. Janz DR, Zhao Z, Koyama T, et al. Longer storage duration of red blood cells is associated with an increased risk of acute lung injury in patients with sepsis. Ann Intensive Care 2013;3(1):33. http:// dx.doi.org/10.1186/2110-5820-3-33.

27. Spragg RG, Bernard GR, Checkley W, et al. Beyond mortality: future clinical research in acute lung injury. Am J Respir Crit Care Med 2010;181: 1121–7. http://dx.doi.org/10.1164/rccm.201001-0024WS.

28. Gajic O, Dabbagh O, Park PK, et al. Early identification of patients at risk of acute lung injury: evaluation of lung injury prediction score in a multicenter cohort study. Am J Respir Crit Care Med 2011; 183(4):462–70. http://dx.doi.org/10.1164/rccm. 201004-0549OC.

29. Kor DJ, Talmor DS, Banner-Goodspeed VM, et al. Lung Injury Prevention with Aspirin (LIPS-A): a protocol for a multicentre randomised clinical trial in medical patients at high risk of acute lung injury. BMJ Open 2012;2(5). http://dx.doi.org/10.1136/bmjopen-2012-001606.

30. Schmickl CN, Shahjehan KK, Li GG, et al. Decision support tool for early differential diagnosis of acute lung injury and cardiogenic pulmonary edema in medical critically ill patients. Chest 2012;141(1): 43–50. http://dx.doi.org/10.1378/chest.11-1496.

31. Park PK, Birkmeyer NO, Gentile NT, et al. Early cumulative fluid balance and development of acute lung injury. Am J Respir Crit Care Med 2011;183:A5592.

32. Serpa Neto A, Cardoso SO, Manetta JA, et al. Association between use of lung-protective ventilation with lower tidal volumes and clinical outcomes among patients without acute respiratory distress syndrome: a meta-analysis. JAMA 2012;308(16): 1651–9. http://dx.doi.org/10.1001/jama.2012.13730.

33. Janz DR, Ware LB. Biomarkers of ALI/ARDS: pathogenesis, discovery, and relevance to clinical trials. Semin Respir Crit Care Med 2013;34(4):537–48. http://dx.doi.org/10.1055/s-0033-1351124.

34. van der Heijden M, van Nieuw Amerongen GP, Koolwijk P, et al. Angiopoietin-2, permeability oedema, occurrence and severity of ALI/ARDS in septic and non-septic critically ill patients. Thorax 2008;63(10):903–9. http://dx.doi.org/10.1136/thx. 2007.087387.

35. Gallagher DC, Parikh SM, Balonov K, et al. Circulating angiopoietin 2 correlates with mortality in a surgical population with acute lung injury/adult respiratory distress syndrome. Shock 2008;29(6):656–61. http://dx.doi.org/10.1097/shk.0b013e31815dd92f.

36. Agrawal A, Matthay MA, Kangelaris KN, et al. Plasma angiopoietin-2 predicts the onset of acute lung injury in critically ill patients. Am J Respir Crit Care Med 2013;187(7):736–42. http://dx.doi. org/10.1164/rccm.201208-1460OC.

37. Determann RM, Millo JL, Waddy S, et al. Plasma CC16 levels are associated with development of ALI/ARDS in patients with ventilator-associated pneumonia: a retrospective observational study. BMC Pulm Med 2009;9:49. http://dx.doi.org/10. 1186/1471-2466-9-49.

38. Fuchs-Buder T, de Moerloose P, Ricou B, et al. Time course of procoagulant activity and D dimer in bronchoalveolar fluid of patients at risk for or with acute respiratory distress syndrome. Am J Respir Crit Care Med 1996;153(1):163–7. http://dx. doi.org/10.1164/ajrccm.153.1.8542111.

39. Bernard GR, Artigas A, Brigham KL, et al. The American-European Consensus Conference on ARDS. Definitions, mechanisms, relevant outcomes, and clinical trial coordination. Am J Respir Crit Care Med 1994;149:818–24. http://dx.doi.org/ 10.1164/ajrccm.149.3.7509706.

40. Thille AW, Esteban A, Fernández-Segoviano P, et al. Comparison of the Berlin definition for acute respiratory distress syndrome with autopsy. Am J Respir Crit Care Med 2013;187(7):761–7. http:// dx.doi.org/10.1164/rccm.201211-1981OC.

41. Levitt JE, Calfee CS, Goldstein BA, et al. Early acute lung injury: criteria for identifying lung injury prior to the need for positive pressure ventilation. Crit Care Med 2013. http://dx.doi.org/10.1097/ CCM.0b013e31828a3d99.

42. Ferguson ND, Meade MO, Hallett DC, et al. High values of the pulmonary artery wedge pressure in patients with acute lung injury and acute respiratory distress syndrome. Intensive Care Med 2002; 28(8):1073–7. http://dx.doi.org/10.1007/s00134-002-1354-y.

43. National Heart, Lung, and Blood Institute Acute Respiratory Distress Syndrome (ARDS) Clinical Trials Network, Wheeler AP, Bernard GR, et al. Pulmonary-artery versus central venous catheter to guide treatment of acute lung injury. N Engl J

Med 2006;354(21):2213–24. http://dx.doi.org/10.1056/NEJMoa061895.

44. Rice TW, Wheeler AP, Bernard GR, et al. Comparison of the SpO2/FIO2 ratio and the PaO2/FIO2 ratio in patients with acute lung injury or ARDS. Chest 2007;132(2):410–7. http://dx.doi.org/10.1378/chest.07-0617.

45. Mayordomo-Colunga J, Pons M, López Y, et al. Predicting non-invasive ventilation failure in children from the SpO$_2$/FiO$_2$ (SF) ratio. Intensive Care Med 2013;39(6):1095–103. http://dx.doi.org/10.1007/s00134-013-2880-5.

46. Ware LB, Matthay MA. Clinical practice. Acute pulmonary edema. N Engl J Med 2005;353(26):2788–96. http://dx.doi.org/10.1056/NEJMcp052699.

47. Ely EW, Haponik EF. Using the chest radiograph to determine intravascular volume status: the role of vascular pedicle width. Chest 2002;121(3):942–50.

48. Aberle DR, Wiener-Kronish JP, Webb WR, et al. Hydrostatic versus increased permeability pulmonary edema: diagnosis based on radiographic criteria in critically ill patients. Radiology 1988;168(1):73–9. http://dx.doi.org/10.1148/radiology.168.1.3380985.

49. Kaul S, Stratienko AA, Pollock SG, et al. Value of two-dimensional echocardiography for determining the basis of hemodynamic compromise in critically ill patients: a prospective study. J Am Soc Echocardiogr 1994;7(6):598–606.

50. Harvey S, Harrison DA, Singer M, et al. Assessment of the clinical effectiveness of pulmonary artery catheters in management of patients in intensive care (PAC-Man): a randomised controlled trial. Lancet 2005;366(9484):472–7. http://dx.doi.org/10.1016/S0140-6736(05)67061-4.

51. Binanay C, Califf RM, Hasselblad V, et al. Evaluation study of congestive heart failure and pulmonary artery catheterization effectiveness: the ESCAPE trial. JAMA 2005;294(13):1625–33. http://dx.doi.org/10.1001/jama.294.13.1625.

52. Shah MR, Hasselblad V, Stevenson LW, et al. Impact of the pulmonary artery catheter in critically ill patients: meta-analysis of randomized clinical trials. JAMA 2005;294(13):1664–70. http://dx.doi.org/10.1001/jama.294.13.1664.

53. Morgan WK. "Zamboni disease". Pulmonary edema in an ice hockey player. Arch Intern Med 1995;155(22):2479–80.

54. Abdulla KA, Davidson NM. A woman who collapsed after painting her soles. Lancet 1996;348(9028):658. http://dx.doi.org/10.1016/S0140-6736(96)04506-0.

55. Meduri GU, Reddy RC, Stanley T, et al. Pneumonia in acute respiratory distress syndrome. A prospective evaluation of bilateral bronchoscopic sampling. Am J Respir Crit Care Med 1998;158(3):870–5. http://dx.doi.org/10.1164/ajrccm.158.3.9706112.

56. Markowicz P, Wolff M, Djedaïni K, et al. Multicenter prospective study of ventilator-associated pneumonia during acute respiratory distress syndrome. Incidence, prognosis, and risk factors. ARDS Study Group. Am J Respir Crit Care Med 2000;161(6):1942–8. http://dx.doi.org/10.1164/ajrccm.161.6.9909122.

57. Janz DR, O'Neal HR, Ely EW. Acute eosinophilic pneumonia: a case report and review of the literature. Crit Care Med 2009;37(4):1470–4. http://dx.doi.org/10.1097/CCM.0b013e31819cc502.

58. Papazian L, Thomas P, Bregeon F, et al. Open-lung biopsy in patients with acute respiratory distress syndrome. Anesthesiology 1998;88(4):935–44.

59. Patel SR, Karmpaliotis D, Ayas NT, et al. The role of open-lung biopsy in ARDS. Chest 2004;125(1):197–202.

Invasive Diagnostic Strategies in Immunosuppressed Patients with Acute Respiratory Distress Syndrome

Juan F. Sanchez, MD, Shekhar A. Ghamande, MD,
John K. Midturi, DO, MPH, Alejandro C. Arroliga, MD*

KEYWORDS

- Immunocompromised • Organ transplant • Hematopoietic stem cell transplant
- Human immunodeficiency virus • Acute respiratory distress syndrome • Pulmonary infection
- Fiber-optic bronchoscopy • Open lung biopsy

KEY POINTS

- Acute respiratory distress syndrome (ARDS) in immunocompromised patients represents a diagnostic dilemma, and early invasive diagnosis affects treatment.
- Fiber-optic bronchoscopy is an important tool in solid-organ transplant recipients with ARDS of infectious and noninfectious cause.
- In hematopoietic stem cell transplants with ARDS, bronchoscopy is safe and results in a good yield but is more effective when performed early. Evidence for mortality benefit is mixed. Transbronchial biopsy should be performed in selected cases.
- In patients infected with human immunodeficiency virus with ARDS, bronchoscopy is safe and provides an excellent yield. Transbronchial biopsy complements bronchoalveolar lavage when cytomegalovirus, aspergillosis, or other fungal infections are suspected. Open lung biopsy has a role in selected cases.

Immunosuppression increases the likelihood of developing pulmonary infections that may result in the development of the acute respiratory distress syndrome (ARDS)

This review focuses on the different invasive diagnostic modalities in the etiologic diagnosis of ARDS based on the available literature. Given the scant information about ARDS in certain subsets of immunosuppressed hosts, literature is also considered that reports on multilobar pulmonary infiltrates in different populations of immunosuppressed patients, such as hematologic and solid-organ transplants, immunosuppression related to human immunodeficiency virus (HIV) infection, and chemotherapy or immunosuppressive therapy in the setting of cancer or collagen vascular disease.[1]

ACUTE RESPIRATORY DISTRESS SYNDROME IN THE SOLID-ORGAN TRANSPLANT RECIPIENT

Predisposing Factors

In solid-organ transplants, multiple risk factors predispose to ARDS, such as pulmonary and

Disclosure statements: the authors have no disclosures.
Pulmonary and Critical Care Medicine Division, Baylor Scott and White Healthcare, 2401 South 31st street, Temple, TX 76508, USA
* Corresponding author. Internal Medicine Department, Baylor Scott & White Health, 2401 South 31st Street, Temple, TX 76508.
E-mail address: aarroliga@sw.org

extrapulmonary infections, crystalloid overload, transfusion of blood and blood products, prolonged surgical times, gastric aspiration, and ischemia-reperfusion injury of the transplanted organ.[2–4]

Pulmonary infections can lead to respiratory failure and ARDS.[5] There are many reasons why the lung is commonly affected. Some of these factors that predispose to infection include use of induction agents during the surgical procedure, diminished cough reflex, altered mucociliary clearance, transient diaphragmatic dysfunction (which occurs after some transplants, such as lung and liver), infections transmitted by the donor organ or harbored by the recipient, and augmented immunosuppression for acute rejection.[6–8] Platelet transfusions after orthotopic liver transplantation (OLT) are another important risk factor for early ARDS and are associated with high postoperative mortality.

Epidemiology, Risk Factors, and Outcomes of Acute Respiratory Distress Syndrome in Solid-Organ Transplant Recipients

The reported incidence of ARDS after OLT ranges between 4.5% and 16.3%, with mortality that has been reported to exceed 80%.[9] Most of the patients developed ARDS within the first 24 hours, with blood product transfusion, prolonged surgical time, intraoperative fluid administration, sepsis, gastric aspiration, and use of intravenous cyclosporine identified as risk factors. Recently, in a cohort study of 212 consecutive liver transplant recipients, Levesque and colleagues[10] reported that the preoperative risk factors that independently predicted the development of pneumonia were a prolonged international normalized ratio and restrictive thoracic physiology in preoperative pulmonary function tests.[11]

In kidney transplant recipients, the reported annualized rate of ARDS ranges between 8.3 and 51 cases per 100,000 patients per year.[12,13] In a retrospective analysis of the national registry for end-stage renal disease in the United States, Shorr and colleagues[12] reported a prevalence of 0.2% with 28-day mortality (52.1%). At 3 years, the survival of those patients who developed ARDS was 57.8% compared with 88.9% for those who did not develop the condition. ARDS was the strongest mortality predictor at 3 years, with a hazard ratio of 3.94. The use of antilymphocyte globulin and graft failure were the only risk factors found to be associated with ARDS.[13]

In lung transplant recipients, Pietrantoni and colleagues[14] reported a 39% incidence of ARDS in a retrospective study of intensive care unit (ICU) readmissions after the first month post transplantation, with 66% mortality. When ARDS and acute lung injury criteria were combined, the incidence increased to 58.6% and the mortality was 39%, with ARDS, shock, and systemic inflammatory response syndrome predicting increased mortality.

Diagnosis of Acute Respiratory Distress Syndrome in Solid-Organ Transplant Recipients

ARDS is diagnosed clinically, with ancillary studies performed to exclude potential mimickers and modify therapy that can alter the natural history of the disease. Clinically, the diagnosis is made by rapid progression to respiratory failure, bilateral alveolar infiltrates on chest radiograph or computed tomography scan in the absence of heart failure or volume overload. Severity is classified based on the oxygenation impairment severity measured by the Pa_{O_2}/Fi_{O_2} ratio, with an 89% sensitivity and 63% specificity when compared with autopsy results of patients who died of ARDS.[15]

DIAGNOSTIC STRATEGIES
Fiber-Optic Bronchoscopy in Solid-Organ Transplant Recipients

Fiber-optic bronchoscopy (FOB) is a minimally invasive procedure that allows deep and targeted pulmonary sampling by different techniques, including bronchoalveolar lavage (BAL), protected specimen brush, and direct histopathologic examination of transbronchial biopsy (TBB) samples. These methods facilitate sampling of distal airways, reducing contamination with proximal respiratory flora or airway colonizers and allowing the real source of distal airway infections or other processes responsible for respiratory failure and pulmonary parenchymal infiltrates to be found.[16–20]

In the organ transplant recipient who presents with respiratory failure and pulmonary infiltrates, bronchoscopy allows for changing, narrowing, or discontinuing of antimicrobial therapy, according to the information obtained from the procedure. Changes in medical management have been reported between 20% and 70% after bronchoscopy.[21] Wallace and Kolbe[22] reported a change in therapy based on the BAL results in 61% of patients and showed that if only empirical management strategy was followed, 28% of the patients would have received incorrect treatment.

Pulmonary infections in organ transplant recipients are most commonly caused by bacterial pathogens. Bacterial pneumonia occurring during the first 30 days after transplant is caused by nosocomial pathogens, with *Pseudomonas*, *Staphylococcus aureus*, and *Acinetobacter* infections being most commonly isolated.[23] Community-acquired pathogens, including *Streptococcus pneumoniae* and *Mycoplasma pneumonia*, become more prevalent in late pneumonia in addition to gram negatives and *Staphylococcus aureus*.[24] After the immediate postoperative procedure and during the first 6 months after transplantation, the incidence of cytomegalovirus (CMV) pneumonitis, fungal infections, and *Pneumocystis jirovecii* pneumonia (PJP) increases.

In a retrospective study of 44 bronchoscopies with BAL performed in 35 heart transplant recipients with pulmonary infiltrates,[25] a specific microbiological diagnosis was established in 18 of 44 cases (41%), and therapy changes occurred in 32% of the cases based on the results of bronchoscopy. The period of highest yield occurred between the first and sixth month (73%), compared with the first month (18%) and after 6 months (28%).

Diagnostic Yield and Impact of the Results of Fiber-Optic Bronchoscopy

In solid-organ transplant recipients, FOB has a diagnostic yield that varies between 27% and 85%,[18,21,26–32] and the addition of TBB tends to increase the diagnostic yield compared with BAL alone. In a retrospective study of 104 immunosuppressed patients of whom 14.4% were solid-organ transplant recipients,[26] the combination of TBB and BAL increased the diagnostic yield to 70% when compared with BAL alone 38%.

Safety of Fiber-Optic Bronchoscopy on Mechanically Ventilated Patients

Two studies[33–35] found similar diagnostic yield with transbronchial biopsies as well as open lung biopsy (OLB), with a 21.2% overall complication rate. The main complications of FOB were bleeding (13.5%; 95% confidence interval [CI], 8–21), pneumothorax requiring drainage 0% to 16%,[36,37] hypotension and hypoxia with oxygen saturation less than 90% (9.6%; 95% CI, 6%–17%). There was no correlation between the presence of complications and the level of positive end-expiratory pressure, peak and plateau pressures, and number of TBB with the presence of pneumothorax.[38]

Open Lung Biopsy

The value of surgical lung biopsy in ARDS has been studied in several retrospective and prospective cohort series of mixed populations. Only a few patients included in those studies are organ transplant recipients. Several studies have shown

OLB to be safe even at levels of severe hypoxemia, with low procedure-related mortality.[39,40]

Only a few studies have addressed this question in a general immunosuppressed population.[41,42] Charbonney and colleagues[41] retrospectively studied 19 mechanically ventilated patients with ARDS after a median duration of mechanical ventilation of 5 days; only 1 solid-organ transplant recipient was included, and the mean Pao_2/Fio_2 ratio was 116.3 ($\pm$34.2) mm Hg. A specific diagnosis was obtained in 68% of patients, and unsuspected diagnosis was found in 47% of patients, prompting changes in treatment in 89%, including addition of new antimicrobial agent, addition of immunosuppressant, discontinuation of unnecessary antibiotics, discontinuation of corticosteroids, change in dose of corticosteroids, and discontinuation of supportive therapy.

Papazian and colleagues[43] studied the impact of a diagnostic OLB on survival of 100 patients with ARDS after 5 days of mechanical ventilation (only 4% were immunocompromised). A diagnosis that warranted change in therapy occurred in 78% of the patients, and survival was higher in patients in whom biopsy results allowed for treatment modification (67%) compared with (14%) for those patients who did not have change in therapy. The complication rate was 10%, including 2 pneumothoraces and 10 moderate air leaks. The only factor independently associated with complications was high minute ventilation.

Overall, the diagnostic yield of OLB, not specifically addressing immunocompromised patients, ranges between 44% and 80% and leads to changes in therapy in 44% to 91% of cases, with a reported complication rate between 7% and 52%, even in patients with severe oxygenation impairment (**Table 1**).[44–51]

ACUTE RESPIRATORY DISTRESS SYNDROME IN OTHER NON–HUMAN IMMUNODEFICIENCY VIRUS, NON–ORGAN TRANSPLANT POPULATIONS

Malignancies and rheumatologic diseases are conditions that warrant the use of cytotoxic therapy aimed at achieving control of neoplastic disease or antiinflammatory effect. Multiple agents with different mechanisms of action are being introduced and are associated with immunosuppression in the host,[52–54] which predisposes them to infections as well as direct toxicity on the lung parenchyma, which could lead to the development of acute respiratory failure with diffuse pulmonary infiltrates. Collectively, antineoplastic chemotherapy, conditioning and myeloablative regimens, alkylating chemotherapy agents

Table 1
OLB in ARDS

First Author and Reference	N	Immuno-compromised (%)	Pao$_2$/Fio$_2$ (mm Hg)	Diagnostic (%)	Treatment Change (%)	Complications (%)	Mortality (%)
Papazian[48]	37	3	118	80	91	—	—
Warner[51]	80	93	—	66	70	—	0
Flabouris[46]	24	29	—	46	75	—	0
Chuang[45]	17	12	—	47	60		0
Patel[50]	57	30	145 ± 61	60	60	39 minor 7 major	0
Kao[47]	41	41		44	73		
Papazian[43]	100	4		78	78		
Baumann[44]	27	67	188 ± 109	70	81	52 minor 7 major	
Charbonney[41]	19	19	116 ± 34.2	68	89	26	

and regimens containing cyclophosphamide, taxanes, busulfan, bleomycin, and FOLFOX can produce acute lung injury, including pulmonary edema, ARDS, and alveolar hemorrhage. In many of those patients, the specific cause can be difficult to identify.[55–60]

Biological agents, specifically tumor necrosis factor α inhibitors, have drastically improved the outlook of many rheumatologic conditions. However, there is strong evidence that therapy is associated with opportunistic infections, including tuberculosis (TB), and with autoimmunity. Using data collected from the Adverse Event Reporting System of the US Food and Drug Administration, Wallis and colleagues[61] reported rates of granulomatous infections of 239 per 100,000 patients receiving infliximab, 47 per 100,000 patients receiving etanercept, and a 3.25-fold increased risk of granulomatous infection in the patients receiving infliximab than in those receiving etanercept. Furthermore, ARDS has been reported in patients receiving this type of therapy.[62–66]

Fiber-Optic Bronchoscopy

In a prospective study quoted earlier,[19] 34% of patients with malignancy being treated with chemotherapy and 63% patients receiving chronic corticosteroids underwent bronchoscopy on mechanical ventilation, with positive diagnostic results in 81% of the patients compared with 41% for those who underwent noninvasive assessment with microbiological and serologic studies. FOB changed treatment in 46% of the studied patients. Furthermore, BAL and TBB were diagnostic in 63% of patients in a study of 38 patients on mechanical ventilation.[39] FOB changed treatment in

44% of the patients and was associated with a low rate of complication, including pneumothoraces (23%), low rate of bleeding (10%), and transient hypotension (5%). Jain and coworkers[33] reported a 70% diagnostic yield of combined BAL and TBB when compared with BAL alone (P<.001) in a cohort of immunocompromised patients, 40.4% of whom were immunocompromised non–organ transplant recipients. The complication rate was higher when TBB were performed during bronchoscopy (31% vs 13.6%; P = .036). The role of rapid on-site examination (ROSE) involves the immediate staining of cytologic and special stains, including fungal and mycobacterial, from BAL specimens in patients with ARDS. The role of ROSE was evaluated in 71 patients with ARDS (46% on invasive mechanical ventilation), 25 of whom (35%) were non-HIV, non–organ transplant immunocompromised patients. The diagnostic yield of ROSE of BAL was 41% for specific diagnosis, 39% were nonspecific diagnosis, and no diagnosis in 20%. The principal diagnoses were PJP, adenocarcinoma, hypersensitivity reaction to medications, cryptococcosis, and lymphoma.[67]

Open Lung Biopsy

OLB significantly affected treatment in 89% of the patients with ARDS, 58.8% of whom were immunocompromised non-HIV/non–organ transplant patients mainly on chronic steroid therapy, ranging from addition of new anti-infective therapy in 26%, addition of immunosuppressive therapy in 15.8%, discontinuation of antibiotics in 42%, discontinuation of corticosteroids in 15.8%, adjustment of corticosteroid dose in 21.1%, and discontinuation of support in 15.8%.[41]

ACUTE RESPIRATORY DISTRESS SYNDROME IN HEMATOPOIETIC STEM CELL TRANSPLANTATION

Infections are a major concern in patients with hematopoietic stem cell transplantation (HSCT), although noninfectious causes of acute respiratory failure contribute to morbidity and mortality (**Table 2**).[68] Among noninfectious causes, acute respiratory failure can occur as a result of cardiogenic pulmonary edema, transfusion-related acute lung injury, radiation pneumonitis, periengraftment respiratory distress syndrome (PERDS), idiopathic pneumonia syndrome (IPS), and diffuse alveolar hemorrhage (DAH) in the first 100 to 120 days after transplantation.[69] PERDS occurs in 7% to 11% of cases, usually after a median of 11 days (4–25 days) but generally seems to be responsive to corticosteroids.[70] IPS occurs less frequently with nonmyeloablative than conventional regimens (2.2% vs 8.4%), but when it develops, it results in severe acute hypoxic respiratory failure in most patients.[71] The diagnosis of IPS is made after excluding infections, cardiac failure, renal failure, and fluid overload in the setting of hypoxic respiratory failure with bilateral infiltrates. Acute respiratory failure is also frequent with DAH and is associated with high mortality.[72]

Late onset noninfectious pulmonary complications, such as bronchiolitis obliterans and cryptogenic organizing pneumonia (COP), occur in 7% to 10% of patients after transplantation and are associated with a low overall survival at 36 months.[73,74] Risk factors for the development of these noninfectious complications include graft-versus-host disease (GVHD), myeloablative conditioning, and allogeneic hematopoietic cell transplant for other than acute myelocytic leukemia or acute lymphocytic or blastic leukemia.[74]

During the pre-engraftment period when the patients are neutropenic, bacterial infections are predominant, including infections with gram-negative organisms and with an increasing trend for gram-positive cocci.[75] The cumulative incidences of infections are lower when reduced intensity preparation is used instead of myeloablative regimens. Other considerations include herpes viruses as well as *Aspergillus* spp and *Candida* spp.[76]

Administration of antifungal prophylaxis reduces but does not eliminate the risk. Even on antifungal prophylaxis, invasive fungal infections, especially aspergillosis or candidiasis, may occur in 5.1% of patients undergoing HSCT.[77] During the early postengraftment period (≤100 days), CMV and human herpesviruses are the major pathogens, with a median time to reactivation for CMV of 38 to

Table 2
Cause of acute respiratory failure in patients with HSCT

	Pre-engraftment 0–30 d	Early Postengraftment 31–100 d	Late Postengraftment >100 d
Infectious: bacterial	Gram-negative bacteria	*Legionella, Mycoplasma, Mycobacteria*	*Nocardia, Listeria*
	Gram-positive bacteria	Gram-positive bacteria	Encapsulated bacteria
Infectious: parasitic	*Strongyloides*	Toxoplasmosis	Toxoplasmosis
Infectious: viral	Herpes simplex	Herpes simplex CMV Human herpesvirus 6	Epstein-Barr virus CMV
	Seasonal respiratory viruses	Seasonal respiratory viruses	Seasonal respiratory viruses
Infectious: fungal	*Candida, Aspergillus,* atypical molds	*Candida, Aspergillus,* atypical molds, *Pneumocystis,* endemic fungi, *Cryptococcus*	*Candida, Aspergillus,* atypical molds, *Pneumocystis,* endemic fungi, *Cryptococcus*
Noninfectious	Heart failure, PERDS, radiation pneumonitis TRALI, DAH, IPS	Delayed pulmonary toxicity syndrome DAH, IPS, COP, pulmonary veno-occlusive disease	Delayed pulmonary toxicity syndrome BO/chronic GVHD, PTLD

Abbreviations: BO/GVHD, bronchiolitis obliterans/graft-versus-host disease; COP, cryptogenic organizing pneumonia; DAH, diffuse alveolar hemorrhage; IPS, idiopathic pneumonia syndrome; PERDS, periengraftment respiratory distress syndrome; PTLD, posttransplant lymphoproliferative disorder; TRALI, transfusion-related acute lung injury.

Data from Peter SG, Afessa B. Acute lung injury after hematopoietic stem cell transplantation. Clinics in Chest Medicine 2005;26:561–9; and Chi AK, Soubani AO, White AC. An update on pulmonary complications of hematopoietic stem cell transplantation. Chest 2013;144:1913–22.

47 days from transplantation.[75,76] Bacteria, *Aspergillus* spp, other invasive molds, and *Pneumocystis jirovecii* also need to be considered.[78] Early postengraftment diffuse pneumonias can be infectious or noninfectious in equal proportions. However, in the late postengraftment period ($\geq$100 days), chronic GVHD can delay immune reconstitution and contribute to impaired opsonization, enhancing the risk of infections with encapsulated bacteria and *Nocardia* spp. The risk of infections with *Aspergillus* spp, CMV, varicella zoster virus, Epstein-Barr virus, and PJP remains increased.[78]

Fiber-Optic Bronchoscopy in Hematopoietic Stem Cell Transplantation

FOB is the first invasive diagnostic modality used in immunocompromised patients with ARDS. BAL plays an important role in facilitating the correct diagnosis of these complex conditions. Advanced diagnostic techniques, including immunohistochemical staining, indirect fluorescent antibody testing, and polymerase chain reaction, have enhanced the diagnostic usefulness of BAL for opportunistic pathogens.

Timing for Fiber-Optic Bronchoscopy

Empirical antibiotic therapy can result in inadequate antimicrobial coverage, as determined by the microbiological results from subsequent FOB.[33] Early FOB confers a benefit; in a retrospective review of patients with pulmonary infiltrates in the first 100 days after HSCT,[79] FOB was 2.5 times more likely to establish a diagnosis when performed early (first 4 days) compared with late FOB (overall yield of 55%). This finding was even more striking if the FOB was performed in the first 24 hours after presentation (75% yield). Delaying the FOB beyond 4 days increased the possibility of culturing predominantly resistant organisms, which led to a higher mortality at 30 (6 vs 18%, $P = .0351$) days. The diagnostic yield decreased in the presence of GVHD, neutropenia, and diffuse infiltrates.

In an earlier study involving a cohort of immunocompromised patients with pulmonary infiltrates that included patients with HSCT,[19] when noninvasive diagnostic techniques combined with FOB established a diagnosis within the first 7 days versus beyond 7 days, the mortality improved (34% vs 53% $P = .017$), mostly as a result of change in antimicrobial treatment. However, FOB in patients with hypoxic respiratory failure can be fraught with risk for precipitating intubation.[80] The same group did not find a beneficial effect of early FOB compared with a noninvasive strategy

in a randomized control study in patients with cancer, including HSCT, who had acute hypoxic respiratory failure.[81]

Techniques

BAL is commonly performed during FOB in patients after HSCT, because it is safe and has superior diagnostic yield.[19,33] Protected specimen brush does not add substantially to BAL alone.[82] TBB are performed in selected patients if invasive fungal or viral disease is suspected. Although the yield seems to be similar to BAL alone, it increases the yield when BAL is combined with TBB in immunocompromised patients with pulmonary infiltrates[33] and should be strongly considered in the absence of contraindications.[83] A recent report corroborates the high (75.6%) yield in HSCT recipients, with a low complication rate using this approach.[84]

Yield and Impact of Bronchoalveolar Lavage or Fiber-Optic Bronchoscopy

The diagnostic yield depends on the underlying cause and is higher for infections. Based on retrospective case series, the diagnostic yield varies between 42% and 65%.[19,33,79,85–89] The yield is lower when the FOB is performed late, in patients with autologous HSCT, and in patients with GVHD and neutropenia.[79,88] FOB changes the management of patients 20% to 58% of the time,[19,79,85–89] which is mainly a change in antimicrobial agents. Overall, it does not seem to affect mortality in patients with HSCT,[86,88] with 1 study indicating a mortality benefit of early FOB.[79] However, in a randomized controlled trial of patients who have cancer with acute respiratory failure, which also included patients with HSCT, a strategy of early BAL (within 24 hours) compared with a noninvasive diagnostic strategy showed no mortality benefit to early BAL. The rate of intubation was similar in the 2 groups, and the diagnosis was obtained earlier with a noninvasive strategy, except for *Pneumocystis* pneumonia.[81] Galactomannan is a polysaccharide found in the cell wall of *Aspergillus* that is released during growth, such as with invasive disease. Detecting galactomannan using enzyme immunoassay can help in the diagnosis of invasive aspergillosis.[90] D'Haese and colleagues[91] evaluated the usefulness of BAL galactomannan retrospectively in 251 patients, 35% of whom had solid-organ or stem cell transplantation. These investigators found a BAL galactomannan optical density of 0.5 or greater to have a high sensitivity of 93.2%. So, a negative test virtually excludes invasive aspergillosis. A value of 0.8 or greater gave a diagnostic accuracy of 0.94 and a positive likelihood ratio of 9.29.[92]

Complications

FOB remains a safe procedure in patients with HSCT (**Table 3**). Major complications of bronchoscopy include respiratory failure, pneumothorax, arrhythmias, and major bleeding. Cardiac arrest occurs in less than 1% of cases, with a death rate of 0% to 0.04%.[93] Although the contraindications for a bronchoscopy are similar to the general population, a lower platelet count of 20,000/μL is not an absolute contraindication to FOB in transplant recipients.[87,94] In patients with HSCT, overall complications have been reported to be 2% to 21%.[19,79,86–89] Minor bleeding is more common and occurs in 7% to 15% of cases.[33,79,87] Major bleeding is less frequent but occurs in 0% to 9% of cases. This factor is particularly a concern when TBB is used. Pneumothorax in 0% to 4% and hypoxia are the other major complications, although intubation remains a major concern. The rate of intubation seems to be similar to a noninvasive strategy in the setting of acute respiratory failure.[81]

Open Lung Biopsy

OLB is performed infrequently in patients with HSCT. A specific diagnosis was obtained in 47% to 100%, depending on the series, with a complication rate of up to 13.3%.[19,33,88] Zihlif and colleagues[95] found a high diagnostic yield in 62 patients who underwent video-assisted thoracoscopy biopsy. A specific diagnosis was obtained in 60%, resulting in a change of therapy in 40%, with a complication rate of 11%. However, the mortality reported was high at 40%. Charbonney and colleagues[41] reported on 19 patients with severe ARDS on invasive mechanical ventilation in whom a bedside surgical lung biopsy was performed and well tolerated. These patients had a BAL and noninvasive diagnostic tests before the OLB. The procedure was associated with 1 death,

probably related to the procedure, and a complication rate of 26%, including bleeding and pneumothorax. In 89% of the cases, there was a change in management, including change in antimicrobials (68%), change in immunosuppression (53%), and withdrawal of care in 15.8%. A more recent retrospective review of video-assisted thoracoscopic (VATS) lung biopsy in pediatric immunosuppressed patients,[96] including 24% with HSCT, yielded a definite diagnosis in 50%, with 22% being caused by fungal disease. There was a change in management in 50% of patients, and the complication rate was 12% from need for chest tubes, air leaks, and respiratory failure in 2 patients. A VATS biopsy is useful in selected patients for achieving a diagnosis after initial procedure failure, primarily when an infectious cause is suspected.

ACUTE RESPIRATORY DISTRESS SYNDROME IN PATIENTS INFECTED WITH HUMAN IMMUNODEFICIENCY VIRUS

In the current era of antiretroviral therapy (ART), among patients with HIV, about 21% to 44% of ICU admissions are for AIDS-related illness, whereas at least half of admissions occur because of non–HIV-related diagnosis.[97,98] Acute respiratory failure has remained the most common cause for ICU admissions in patients with HIV, and pneumonia is the overall leading cause of ARDS.[99–101] Streptococcus pneumonia is the most frequent bacteria isolated, followed by Hemophilus influenzae and Staphylococcus aureus.[102] In addition, Pseudomonas aeruginosa and Enterobacteriaceae spp are important considerations.[103] TB and fungal diseases are infrequent causes of respiratory failure in the United States.[104] Among newly diagnosed patients with HIV or untreated patients, PJP is the most common cause of respiratory failure.[100,105] Other opportunistic infections

Table 3
Usefulness and complications of FOB in immunocompromised patients including HSCT

First Author and Reference	N	Diagnostic Yield (%)	Change Treatment (%)	Complications (%)	Bleeding (%)	Pneumothorax (%)	Mortality (%)
Jain[33]	104	56.2	—	21	13.5	4	0
Shannon[79]	501	55	51	12.3	—	0.6	0
Rano[19]	200	59	46	2.2	0.74	0.74	0
Feinstein[85]	61	42.1	31.6	3.9	—	3.9	34.3
Hofmeister[86]	78	49	20	8	6.5	3.3	—
Patel[88]	146	46	46.7	9	1.8	3	35

described causing acute respiratory failure include both tuberculous and other *Mycobacteria*, CMV, aspergillosis, histoplasmosis, cryptococcosis, and toxoplasmosis.[103,106] Viral infections account for much respiratory illness, particularly in those on ART. Influenza and human metapneumovirus top the list.[107] H1N1 influenza infection has been shown to cause substantial mortality in advanced HIV disease, and respiratory failure was more common when these patients also had opportunistic infections.[108]

Noninfectious Causes

COP can occur in the setting of PJP infection or with adenocarcinoma of the lung or in isolation and has been reported in previously diagnosed HIV infection.[109] TBB may not be diagnostic, and a VATS biopsy is needed. Another cause of acute respiratory failure in this patient population is hypersensitivity reaction to drugs, particularly with efavirenz and dapsone.[110,111] Here, temporal correlation with clinical history is important. Hypersensitivity to abacavir, leading to ARDS, is rare but should be in the differential diagnosis of ARDS.[112] A surgical biopsy is needed to establish this diagnosis.

Manifestations of the immune reconstitution inflammatory syndrome (IRIS) depends on underlying CD4 count when ART is instituted. Most IRIS can be managed with corticosteroids and does not lead to acute respiratory failure. except when IRIS is related to PJP infection.[113] This finding is characterized by significant worsening, leading to near fatality after early initiation of ART in patients with PJP. Mycobacterial IRIS tends to be milder and can be managed with corticosteroids.[114] Cryptococca/ IRIS predominantly affects the central nervous system but can affect the lungs and is associated with higher mortality.[115]

Prognosis of Acute Respiratory Distress Syndrome in Patients with Human Immunodeficiency Virus

Mendez-Tellez and colleagues[100] found that the short-term prognosis of ARDS in patients with HIV was not different from those without HIV. The presence of previous opportunistic infection was found to be associated with higher mortality in ARDS and HIV (odds ratio 6.4, 95% CI, 1.27–32.3; *P* = .025). However, in a more recent but smaller retrospective analysis,[116] there was a doubling of mortality in patients with HIV on mechanical ventilation compared with ventilated patients who did not have HIV. Only 15% of these patients were on ART. Similarly, a preliminary report on ARDS in HIV-infected patients[117]

indicated a higher mortality compared with non–HIV-infected patients with ARDS.

Diagnosis

Pulmonary infections remain one of the most important causes of morbidity and mortality in these patients; achieving an etiologic diagnosis rapidly is key, because of prognostic consequences. The CD4 count serves as a general guide to ascertain the susceptibility to opportunistic infections of patients with HIV and acute respiratory failure (**Table 4**). CD4 count less than 200 cells/mL increases the likelihood of bacterial pneumonia and bacteremia 5-fold, particularly with a high risk of bacteremia.[118] Ninety-five percent of PJP cases occur at CD4 count less than 200 cells/mL.[119] At counts less than 100 cells/mL, *Cryptococcus neoformans* should also be an important consideration. Cryptococcal pneumonia in patients with HIV is a disseminated disease that mimics PJP and has a high mortality. It has been reported to cause acute respiratory failure in 13.8% of patients with HIV with cryptococcosis. There is a frequent overlap with other opportunist infections, including nontuberculous mycobacteria, PJP, and bacterial pneumonia.[120] *Toxoplasma gondii* and Kaposi sarcoma are considerations at counts less than 100 cells/mL.[121,122] When the CD4 count decreases less than 50 cells/mL, the possibilities also include aspergillosis, CMV, and disseminated endemic fungal disease.[123] Histoplasmosis is the most common endemic mycoses in HIV-infected patients. Disseminated histoplasmosis carries a poor prognosis in HIV-infected patients, with their mortality being higher than those with other opportunistic infections in 1 study.[124] The odds of acute respiratory failure requiring mechanical ventilation in HIV-infected patients with disseminated histoplasmosis are 2.7 compared with other opportunistic infections in HIV-infected patients.

Fiber-Optic Bronchoscopy in Patients with Human Immunodeficiency Virus with Acute Respiratory Distress Syndrome

FOB with BAL is the most commonly used tool for the diagnosis of pulmonary infections in HIV-infected patients with respiratory failure, and TBB is used in selected cases. The overall yield of BAL in patients with pulmonary disease in HIV has been reported to be 51% to 91%.[125–129] TBB provided the exclusive diagnosis in 26% of patients with HIV and lung disease in 1 series.[130] The usefulness was particularly high in noninfectious causes and in infections other than PJP. Broaddus and colleagues[127] reported that the

Table 4
Cause of acute respiratory failure in patients infected with HIV

Infectious	CD4 >200	CD4 <200	CD4 <100	CD4 <50
Bacterial	*Streptococcus pneumonia, Hemophilus influenzae, Staphylococcus aureus*	Bacteremic pneumonia *Streptococcus pneumonia, Hemophilus influenzae, Staphylococcus aureus* *Moraxella catarrhalis*	Bacteremic pneumonia *Streptococcus pneumonia, Hemophilus influenzae, Staphylococcus aureus Pseudomonas aeruginosa, Legionella Moraxella catarrhalis*	Bacteremic pneumonia *Streptococcus pneumonia, Hemophilus influenzae, Staphylococcus aureus Pseudomonas aeruginosa, Legionella* *Rhodococcus equii, Nocardia*
Mycobacterial	*Mycobacterium tuberculosis*	Disseminated *Mycobacterium tuberculosis*	Disseminated *Mycobacterium tuberculosis*	Disseminated *Mycobacterium tuberculosis,* disseminated NTM
Fungal		PJP, endemic fungi, *Cryptococcus*	PJP, *Cryptococcus,* endemic fungi	*Aspergillus,* PJP, *Cryptococcus,* disseminated endemic fungi
Parasitic			Toxoplasmosis	Toxoplasmosis
Viral	Seasonal respiratory viruses	Seasonal respiratory viruses	Seasonal respiratory viruses Pulmonary Kaposi sarcoma	Seasonal respiratory viruses Cytomegalovirus Pulmonary Kaposi sarcoma
Noninfectious	COP, HP, LIP, sarcoid, drug toxicity	NSIP, NHL, PEL Multicentric Castleman disease, drug toxicity	NSIP, NHL, PEL Multicentric Castleman disease, drug toxicity	IRIS, NSIP, NHL, PEL Multicentric Castleman disease, drug toxicity

Abbreviations: HP, hypersensitivity pneumonitis; IRIS, immune reconstitution inflammatory syndrome; LIP, lymphocytic interstitial pneumonia; NHL, non-Hodgkin lymphoma; NSIP, nonspecific interstitial pneumonia; NTM, nontuberculous mycobacteria; PEL, primary effusion lymphoma.

Data from Tokman F, Huang L. Evaluation of respiratory disease. Clin Chest Med 2013;34:191–204; and Doffman SR, Miller RF. Interstitial lung disease in HIV. Clin Chest Med 2013;34:293–306.

yield of bronchoscopy increases to 96% with the addition of TBB. An older study from Rwanda[131] was an outlier, with a low yield on BAL of 26% but it increased to 72% with TBB. PJP was low in the diagnosed causes.

Pneumocystis jirovecii pneumonia

PJP is the most frequent opportunistic infection in HIV-infected patients in the United States and Europe. It cannot be cultured and FOB remains the gold standard in the diagnosis in ventilated patients.

BAL has a sensitivity of up to 98% for PJP.[132,133] A TBB is generally not required,[133]

but when TBB is added, the yield increases to 100% for PJP.[127] The yield with BAL in patients on pentamidine prophylaxis is as low as 62%.[134] Performing BAL in 2 lobes, including sampling at least 1 upper lobe and a second site guided by radiographic involvement, enhanced the sensitivity, especially in the setting of pentamidine prophylaxis.[135,136] Polymerase chain reaction (PCR) has been applied to augment the diagnostic yield in BAL, induced sputum, and oral wash specimens.[137] However, PCR does not distinguish between colonization and infection in HIV-infected patients. Maillet and colleagues[138] tested quantitative PCR (qPCR) assay in BAL and tracheobronchial aspirates in immunocompromised patients targeting the major surface glycoprotein gene as a way around this problem. The sensitivity and specificity of qPCR using a cutoff of 31,600 copies/mL were 80% and 100%, respectively; however, this finding requires further validation.

Mycobacterial infections

The usefulness of FOB in pulmonary TB in HIV is less well defined compared with PJP. Induced sputum has a reported sensitivity of 36% by smear and 60% by culture compared with BAL (40% and 60%, respectively).[139] In patients with negative smears, TBB increases the yield by 39%,[130] and it was the exclusive means of diagnosis in 16%. In a study from Latin America,[129] where TB is more endemic, the overall yield of FOB was 70.4%, with a BAL sensitivity of 37% for staining and 59% for culture. TBB had a sensitivity of 50%. In a large Swiss cohort of immunocompromised patients,[140] including HIV-infected patients, TB was found only in HIV-infected patients by BAL, and there was a decline in case detection over a decade. Rapid diagnosis of TB in HIV-infected patients can be achieved by using the World Health Organization recommended Xpert MTB/RIF assay on respiratory samples. This is an automated diagnostic molecular test that simultaneously detects TB and rifampin resistance in less than 2 hours. In culture-positive patients, the assay detected TB in 98% of sputum samples among smear-positive cases and 72.5% among smear-negative cases in 2 hours.[141] This situation may obviate bronchoscopy in many cases.

Fungal disease other than Pneumocystis jirovecii pneumonia

The diagnostic yield of sputum for cryptococcal disease is low and a bronchoscopy becomes necessary. The yield of BAL is 82%, and TBB does not add to the yield.[131] Because cryptococcal pneumonia is part of disseminated disease in HIV-infected patients, the serum cryptococcal antigen is positive in almost all patients.[142] A cerebrospinal fluid analysis is also required in these cases.

Endemic mycoses including histoplasmosis can reactivate and disseminate in HIV-infected patients. The diagnosis is established by identification on KOH smears from BAL, bone marrow, lymph node, liver, blood, or skin lesions along with the urine Histoplasma antigen test. In a case series,[143] the overall yield of bronchoscopy was 87%, which was mostly accounted for by positive histopathology from TBB in 69%. The yield of smear from BAL was only 14%.

FOB is useful for the diagnosis of blastomycosis. Although KOH smears from BAL were positive in 50% of patients compared with 17% with bronchial secretions, the culture was positive in 67% with BAL and 100% with bronchial washings. TBB had a low yield of 22%.[144]

The diagnosis of coccidioidomycosis can be established using BAL with a yield of 30% to 64%.[145,146] Cultures were positive in all cases but took a median of 25 days. On the other hand, TBB also yielded a 100% result in the few patients in whom it was performed.[145]

Invasive aspergillosis is relatively uncommon in HIV-infected patients until late in their disease, when the CD4 counts decreases less than 50. Although tissue invasion by biopsy is considered diagnostic, a positive stain and culture for Aspergillus spp correlates with histopathology in HIV-infected patients.[147] Although studies on BAL galactomannan assay are lacking in HIV-infected patients, this has been shown to have a sensitivity of 90% and specificity of 94% in invasive aspergillosis and is superior to serum galactomannan assay.[148] BAL Aspergillus PCR does not seem to have a good sensitivity or specificity (26% and 70%, respectively) for invasive aspergillosis.[149]

Cytomegalovirus

Establishing CMV as a cause for the respiratory failure even with a positive BAL result is difficult in HIV-infected patients, because the virus can be cultured from the lungs even in the absence of invasive disease. CMV often coexists with other opportunistic infections.[150–152] Cytomegalic inclusions from BAL and TBB in the absence of evidence of other opportunist infections strengthen the case for the diagnosis of CMV. However, the patchy nature of parenchymal disease with CMV might lead to false-negative TBB and frequently necessitate a VATS biopsy.[153]

Complications of Fiber-Optic Bronchoscopy

The complications reported in HIV-infected patients with FOB do not differ from bronchoscopy performed for general indications, and it seems to be a safe procedure overall.[140,154] Reported complications of TBB include a pneumothorax rate of 8% to 9%, of which a minority, 5.9%, require drainage. Minor complications include bleeding in 5%, fever, and new infiltrate.[127,131] An older series reported 22% complication rate[155] caused by pneumothorax and hemorrhage from using a TBB, but this has improved over the years.

Open Lung Biopsy in Patients with Human Immunodeficiency Virus with Acute Respiratory Distress Syndrome

There are few reports of surgical biopsy, which correlate clinical practice with the infrequent need to perform this procedure in HIV-infected patients. Miller and colleagues[156] described 23 patients who underwent an OLB for indications ranging from inadequate response to treatment as well as focal lesions with diagnostic dilemmas. Specific diagnosis was obtained in 95% of patients, including those with nonspecific interstitial pneumonia, Kaposi sarcoma, COP, and non-Hodgkin lymphoma, and induced a change in management in all patients. None of the patients died or required mechanical ventilation. An earlier report of OLB[157] showed a diagnostic yield of 70% with 2 deaths among 19 patients.

There may be a role for a VATS biopsy in selected patients who fail to improve and have nondiagnostic bronchoscopy or contraindication to TBB. The procedure is likely to be high yield and induce a change in management.

Considerations for invasive approach

In the immunosuppressed host, without clear contraindications, FOB is a safe diagnostic procedure, even on mechanical ventilation. BAL is highly useful in the setting of PJP and bacterial pneumonia. TBB in addition to BAL has shown benefits in increasing the yield when suspecting specific pathogens, such as viral and fungal infection. TBB should be performed in the absence of contraindications. It also helps to clarify a noninfectious cause of pulmonary infiltrates, such as organizing pneumonia, adenocarcinoma, and drug-induced pneumonitis.

OLB should be reserved for patients with nondiagnostic FOB in whom a specific diagnosis, most likely a noninfectious complication, is suspected.

REFERENCES

1. Ranieri VM, Rubenfeld GD, Thompson BT, et al. Acute respiratory distress syndrome: the Berlin Definition. J Am Med Assoc 2012;307:2526–33.
2. Camporota L, Ranieri VM. What's new in the "Berlin" definition of acute respiratory distress syndrome? Minerva Anestesiol 2012;78:1162–6.
3. De Boear MT, Christensen MC, Asmussen M, et al. The impact of intraoperative transfusion of platelets and red blood cells on survival after liver transplantation. Anesth Analg 2008;106:32–44.
4. Pareboom IT, de Boer MT, Haagsma EB, et al. Platelet transfusion during liver transplantation is associated with increased postoperative mortality due to acute lung injury. Anesth Analg 2009;108: 1083–91.
5. Estenssoro E, Dubin A, Laffaire E, et al. Incidence, clinical course, and outcome in 217 patients with acute respiratory distress syndrome. Crit Care Med 2002;30(11):2450–6.
6. Fishman JA. Infection in solid-organ transplant recipients. N Engl J Med 2007;357:2601–14.
7. Kotloff RM, Ahya VN, Crawford SW. Pulmonary complications of solid organ and hematopoietic stem cell transplantation. Am J Respir Crit Care Med 2004;170:22–48.
8. Speich R, van der Bij W. Epidemiology and management of infections after lung transplantation. Clin Infect Dis 2001;33:S58–65.
9. O'Brien JD, Ettinger NA. Pulmonary complications of liver transplantation. Clin Chest Med 1996;17: 99–114.
10. Levesque E, Hoti E, Azoulay D, et al. Pulmonary complications after elective liver transplantation: incidence, risk factors and outcome. Transplantation 2012;94:532–8.
11. Li GS, Ye QF, Xia SS, et al. Acute respiratory distress syndrome after liver transplantation: etiology, prevention and management. Hepatobiliary Pancreat Dis Int 2002;1:330–4.
12. Shorr AF, Abbott KC, Agadoa LY. Acute respiratory distress syndrome after kidney transplantation: epidemiology, risk factors and outcomes. Crit Care Med 2003;31:1325–30.
13. Thomsen GE, Morris AH. Incidence of adult respiratory distress syndrome in the state of Utah. Am J Respir Crit Care Med 1995;152:965–71.
14. Pietrantoni C, Minai OA, Yu NC, et al. Respiratory failure and sepsis are the major causes of ICU admissions and mortality in survivors of lung transplants. Chest 2003;123:504–9.
15. Thille AW, Esteban A, Fernandez-Segoviano P, et al. Comparison of the Berlin definition for acute respiratory distress syndrome with autopsy. Am J Respir Crit Care Med 2013;187:761–7.
16. Eriksson BM, Dahl H, Wang FZ. Diagnosis of pulmonary infections in immunocompromised patients by fiberoptic bronchoscopy with bronchoalveolar lavage and serology. Scand J Infect Dis 1996;28:479–85.
17. Martin WJ II, Smith TF, Sanderson DR, et al. Role of bronchoalveolar lavage in the assessment of opportunistic pulmonary infections: utility and complications. Mayo Clin Proc 1987;62:549–57.
18. Pisani RJ, Wright AJ. Clinical utility of bronchoalveolar lavage in immunocompromised hosts. Mayo Clin Proc 1992;67:221–7.
19. Rano A, Agusti C, Jumenez P, et al. Pulmonary infiltrates in non-HIV immunocompromised patients, a diagnostic approach using non-invasive and bronchoscopic procedures. Thorax 2001; 56:379–87.

20. Stover DE, Zaman MB, Hajdu SI. Bronchoalveolar lavage in the diagnosis of diffuse pulmonary infiltrates in the immunosuppressed host. Ann Intern Med 1984;101:1–7.

21. Chan CC, Abi-Saleh WJ, Arroliga AC, et al. Diagnostic yield and therapeutic impact of flexible bronchoscopy in lung transplant recipients. J Heart Lung Transplant 1996;15:196–205.

22. Wallace RH, Kolbe J. Fiberoptic bronchoscopy and bronchoalveolar lavage in the investigation of the immunocompromised lung. N Z Med J 1992;105:215–7.

23. Aguilar-Gisado M, Givalda J, Ussetti P, et al. Pneumonia after lung transplantation in the RESITRA cohort: a multicenter prospective study. Am J Transplant 2007;7:1989–96.

24. Nicholson V, Johnson PC. Infectious complications in solid organ transplant recipients. Surg Clin North Am 1994;74:1223–45.

25. Lehto JT, Anttila V, Lommi J, et al. Clinical usefulness of bronchoalveolar lavage in heart transplant recipients with suspected lower respiratory tract infection. J Heart Lung Transplant 2004;23:570–6.

26. Allen KA, Markin RS, Rennard SI. Bronchoalveolar lavage in liver transplant patients. Acta Cytol 1989;33:539–43.

27. Baz M, Layish DT, Govert JA. Diagnostic yield of bronchoscopies after isolated lung transplantation. Chest 1996;110:84–8.

28. Cazzadori A, Di Perri G, Todeschini G. Transbronchial biopsy in the diagnosis of pulmonary infiltrates in immunocompromised patients. Chest 1995;107:101–6.

29. Dummer JS. Infectious complications of transplantation. Cardiovasc Clin 1990;20:163–78.

30. Schulman LL, Smith CR, Drusin R. Utility of airway endoscopy in the diagnosis of respiratory complications of cardiac transplantation. Chest 1988;93:960–7.

31. Sibley RK, Berry GJ, Tazelaar HD. The role of transbronchial biopsies in the management of lung transplant recipients. J Heart Lung Transplant 1993;12:308–24.

32. Willcox PA, Bateman ED, Potgieter PD, et al. Experience with fiberoptic bronchoscopy in the diagnosis of pulmonary shadows in renal transplant recipients over a 12-year period. Respir Med 1990;84:297–302.

33. Jain P, Sandur S, Meli Y, et al. Role of flexible bronchoscopy in immunocompromised patients with lung infiltrates. Chest 2004;125:712–22.

34. O'Brien JD, Ettinger NA, Shelvin D, et al. Safety and yield of transbronchial biopsy in mechanically ventilated patients. Crit Care Med 1997;25:440–6.

35. Papin TA, Grum CM, Weg JG. Transbronchial biopsy during mechanical ventilation. Chest 1986;89:168–70.

36. Pincus PS, Kallenbach JM, Hurwitz MD. Transbronchial biopsy during mechanical ventilation. Crit Care Med 1987;15:1136–9.

37. Turner JS, Willcox PA, Hayhurst MD, et al. Fiberoptic bronchoscopy in the intensive care unit. A prospective study of 147 procedures in 107 patients. Crit Care Med 1994;22:259–64.

38. Martin C, Papazian L, Payan MJ, et al. Pulmonary fibrosis correlates with outcome in adult respiratory distress syndrome. A study in mechanically ventilated patients. Chest 1995;107:196–200.

39. Bulpa PA, Dive AM, Mertens L, et al. Combined bronchoalveolar lavage and transbronchial lung biopsy safety and yield in ventilated patients. Eur Respir J 2003;21:489–94.

40. Cockerill FR III, Wilson WR, Carpenter HA, et al. Open lung biopsy in immunocompromised patients. Arch Intern Med 1985;145:1398–404.

41. Charbonney E, Robert J, Pache JC, et al. Impact of bedside open lung biopsies on the management of mechanically ventilated immunocompromised patients with acute respiratory distress syndrome of unknown etiology. J Crit Care 2009;24:122–8.

42. McKenna RJ, Mountain CF, McMurtrey MJ. Open lung biopsy in immunocompromised patients. Chest 1984;86:671–4.

43. Papazian L, Doddoli C, Chetaille B, et al. A contributive result of open-lung biopsy improves survival in acute respiratory distress syndrome patients. Crit Care Med 2007;35:755–62.

44. Baumann HJ, Kluge S, Balke L, et al. Yield and safety of bedside open lung biopsy in mechanically ventilated patients with acute lung injury or acute respiratory distress syndrome. Surgery 2008;143:426–33.

45. Chuang ML, Lin IF, Tsai YH, et al. The utility of open lung biopsy in patients with diffuse pulmonary infiltrates as related to respiratory distress, its impact on decision making by urgent intervention, and the diagnostic accuracy based on the biopsy location. J Intensive Care Med 2003;18:21–8.

46. Flabouris A, Myburgh J. The utility of open lung biopsy in patients requiring mechanical ventilation. Chest 1999;115:811–7.

47. Kao KC, Tsai YH, Wu YK, et al. Open lung biopsy in early stage acute respiratory distress syndrome. Crit Care 2006;10:R106.

48. Papazian L, Thomas P, Bregeon F, et al. Open lung biopsy in patients with acute respiratory distress syndrome. Anesthesiology 1998;88:935–44.

49. Parambil JG, Myers JL, Aubry MC, et al. Causes and prognosis of diffuse alveolar damage diagnosed on surgical lung biopsy. Chest 2007;132:50–7.

50. Patel SR, Karmpaliotis D, Ayas NT, et al. The role of open lung biopsy in ARDS. Chest 2004;125:197–202.

51. Warner DO, Warner MA, Divertie MB. Open lung biopsy in patients with diffuse pulmonary infiltrates and acute respiratory failure. Am Rev Respir Dis 1988;137:90–4.

52. Barshes NR, Goodpastor SE, Goss JA. Pharmacologic immunosuppression. Front Biosci 2004;9:411–20.

53. Harris J, Sengar D, Stewart T, et al. The effect of immunosuppressive chemotherapy on immune function in patients with malignant disease. Cancer 1976;37(Suppl 2):1058–69.

54. Singh N, Rieder MJ, Tucker MJ. Mechanisms of glucocorticoid mediated anti-inflammatory and immunosuppressive action. Paediatric and Perinatal Drug Therapy 2004;6:107–15.

55. De Sanctis A, Taillade L, Vignot S, et al. Pulmonary toxicity related to systemic treatment of nonsmall cell lung cancer. Cancer 2011;117:3069–80.

56. Goligher EC, Cserti-Gazdewich C, Balter M, et al. Acute lung injury during antithymocyte globulin therapy for aplastic anemia. Can Respir J 2009; 16:e3–5.

57. Jung JI, Choi JE, Hahn ST, et al. Radiologic features of all-trans-retinoic acid syndrome. Am J Roentgenol 2002;178:475–80.

58. Minegishi Y, Takenaka J, Mizutani H, et al. Exacerbation of idiopathic interstitial pneumonias associated with lung cancer therapy. Intern Med 2009; 48:665–72.

59. Tamiya A, Okamoto I, Mioyazaki M, et al. Severe acute interstitial lung disease after crizotinib therapy in a patient with EML4-ALK-positive non-small cell lung cancer. J Clin Oncol 2013;31:e15–7.

60. Watanabe N, Taniguchi H, Kondoh Y, et al. Efficacy of chemotherapy for advanced nonsmall cell lung cancer with idiopathic pulmonary fibrosis. Respiration 2013;85:326–31.

61. Wallis RS, Broder MS, Wong JY, et al. Granulomatous infectious diseases associated with tumor necrosis factor antagonists. Clin Infect Dis 2004;38:1261–5.

62. Braun J, Brandt J, Listing J, et al. Treatment of active ankylosing spondylitis with infliximab: a randomised controlled multicentre trial. Lancet 2002;359:1187–93.

63. Courtney PA, Alderdice J, Whitehead EM. Comment on methotrexate pneumonitis after initiation of infliximab therapy for rheumatoid arthritis. Arthritis Rheum 2003;49:617.

64. Mutlu GM, Mutlu EA, Bellmeyer A, et al. Pulmonary adverse events of anti-tumor necrosis factor-alpha antibody therapy. Am J Med 2006;119:639–46.

65. Ostor AJ, Crisp AJ, Somerville MF, et al. Fatal exacerbation of rheumatoid arthritis associated fibrosing alveolitis in patients given infliximab. BMJ 2004;329:1266.

66. Peno-Green L, Lluberas G, Kingsley T, et al. Lung injury linked to etanercept therapy. Chest 2002; 122:1858–60.

67. Ravaglia C, Gurioli C, Casoni G, et al. Diagnostic role of rapid on-site cytologic examination (ROSE) of broncho-alveolar lavage in ALI/ARDS. Pathologica 2013;104:65–9.

68. Soubani AO, Miller KB, Hassoun PM. Pulmonary complications of bone marrow transplantation. Chest 1996;109:1066–77.

69. Peters SG, Afessa B. Acute lung injury after hematopoietic stem cell transplantation. Clin Chest Med 2005;26:561–9.

70. Capizzi SA, Kumar S, Huneke NE, et al. Periengraftment respiratory distress syndrome during autologous hematopoietic stem cell transplantation. Bone Marrow Transplant 2001;27:1299–303.

71. Panoskaltsis-Mortari A, Griese M, Madtes DK, et al. An official American Thoracic Society research statement: noninfectious lung injury after hematopoietic stem cell transplantation: idiopathic pneumonia syndrome. Am J Respir Crit Care Med 2011;183:1262–79.

72. Majhail NS, Parks K, Defor TE, et al. Diffuse alveolar hemorrhage and infection-associated alveolar hemorrhage following hematopoietic stem cell transplantation: related and high-risk clinical syndromes. Biol Blood Marrow Transplant 2006;12:1038–46.

73. Griese M, Rampf U, Hofmann D, et al. Pulmonary complications after bone marrow transplantation in children: twenty-four years of experience in a single pediatric center. Pediatr Pulmonol 2000;30: 393–401.

74. Solh M, Arat M, Cao Q, et al. Late-onset noninfectious pulmonary complications in adult allogeneic hematopoietic cell transplant recipients. Transplantation 2011;91:798–803.

75. Kim SH, Kee SY, Lee DG, et al. Infectious complications following allogeneic stem cell transplantation: reduced-intensity vs. myeloablative conditioning regimens. Transpl Infect Dis 2013;15:49–59.

76. Narreddy S, Mellon-Reppen S, Abidi MH, et al. Non-bacterial infections in allogeneic non-myeloablative stem cell transplant recipients. Transpl Infect Dis 2007;9:3–10.

77. Ziakas PD, Kourbeti IS, Mylonakis E. Systemic antifungal prophylaxis after hematopoietic stem cell transplantation: a meta-analysis. Clin Ther 2014; 36:292–306.

78. Wingard JR, Hsu J, Hiemenz JW. Hematopoietic stem cell transplantation: an overview of infection risks and epidemiology. Infect Dis Clin North Am 2010;24:257–72.

79. Shannon VR, Andersson BS, Lei X, et al. Utility of early versus late fiberoptic bronchoscopy in the evaluation of new pulmonary infiltrates following hematopoietic stem cell transplantation. Bone Marrow Transplant 2010;45:647–55.

80. Azoulay E, Mokart D, Rabbat A, et al. Diagnostic bronchoscopy in hematology and oncology

patients with acute respiratory failure: prospective multicenter data. Crit Care Med 2008;36:100–7.

81. Azoulay E, Mokart D, Lambert J, et al. Diagnostic strategy for hematology and oncology patients with acute respiratory failure: randomized controlled trial. Am J Respir Crit Care Med 2010; 182:1038–46.

82. Boersma WG, Erjavec Z, van der Werf TS, et al. Bronchoscopic diagnosis of pulmonary infiltrates in granulocytopenic patients with hematologic malignancies: BAL versus PSB and PBAL. Respir Med 2007;101:317–25.

83. Casal RF, Ost DE, Eapen GA. Flexible bronchoscopy. Clin Chest Med 2013;34:341–52.

84. Lamb K, Chang L, Wagner J, et al. Transbronchial and surgical lung biopsies in bone marrow transplant patients with pulmonary disease. Chest 2013;144:250A.

85. Feinstein MB, Mokhtari M, Ferreiro R, et al. Fiberoptic bronchoscopy in allogeneic bone marrow transplantation. Findings in the era of serum cytomegalovirus antigen surveillance. Chest 2001;120:1094–100.

86. Hofmeister CC, Czerlanis C, Forsythe S, et al. Retrospective utility of bronchoscopy after hematopoietic stem cell transplant. Bone Marrow Transplant 2006;38:693–8.

87. Hohenadel IA, Kiworr M, Genitsariotis R, et al. Role of bronchoalveolar lavage in immunocompromised patients with pneumonia treated with a broad spectrum antibiotic and antifungal regimen. Thorax 2001;56:115–20.

88. Patel NR, Lee PS, Kim JH, et al. The influence of diagnostic bronchoscopy on clinical outcomes comparing adult autologous and allogeneic bone marrow transplant patients. Chest 2005;127: 1388–96.

89. Starobin D, Fink G, Shitrit D, et al. The role of fiberoptic bronchoscopy evaluating transplant recipients with suspected pulmonary infections: analysis of 168 cases in a multi-organ transplantation center. Transplant Proc 2003;35:659–60.

90. Pfeiffer CD, Fine JP, Safdar N. Diagnosis of invasive Aspergillosis using a galactomannan assay: a meta-analysis. Clin Infect Dis 2006;42:1417–27.

91. D'Haese J, Theunissen K, Vereulen E, et al. Detection of galactomannan in bronchoalveolar lavage fluid samples of patients at risk for invasive pulmonary aspergillosis: analytical and clinical validity. J Clin Microbiol 2012;50:1258–63.

92. Pasqualotto AC, Xavier MO, Sanchez LB, et al. Diagnosis of invasive aspergillosis in lung transplant recipients by detection of galactomannan in the bronchoalveolar lavage fluid. Transplantation 2010;90:306–11.

93. Ernst A, Silvestri GA, Johnstone D. Interventional pulmonary procedures: guidelines from the American College of Chest Physicians. Chest 2003;123:1693–717.

94. Carr IM, Koefelenberg CF, von Groote-Bidlingmaier F, et al. Blood loss during flexible bronchoscopy: a prospective observational study. Respiration 2012;84:312–8.

95. Zihlif M, Khanchandani G, Ahmed HP, et al. Surgical lung biopsy in patients with hematological malignancy or hematopoietic stem cell transplantation and unexplained pulmonary infiltrates: improved outcome with specific diagnosis. Am J Hematol 2005;78:94–9.

96. Naiditch JA, Barsness KA, Rothstein DH. The utility of surgical lung biopsy in immunocompromised children. J Pediatr 2013;162:133–6.

97. Powell K, Davis JL, Morris AM, et al. Survival for patients with HIV admitted to the ICU continues to improve in the current era of combination antiretroviral therapy. Chest 2009;135:11–7.

98. Yoon C, Greene M, Weir D, et al. Have we plateaued? Outcomes of HIV-infected patients admitted to the intensive care unit in the combined antiretroviral therapy era. Presented at the American Thoracic Society (ATS) 2011 International Conference. Denver, CO, May 13-18, 2011.

99. Chiang HH, Hung CC, Lee CM, et al. Admission to intensive care unit of HIV-infected patients in the era of highly active antiretroviral therapy: etiology and prognostic factors. Crit Care 2011;15:R202.

100. Mendez-Tellez PA, Damluji A, Ammerman D, et al. Human immunodeficiency virus infection and hospital mortality in acute lung injury patients. Crit Care Med 2010;38:1530–5.

101. Turtle L, Vyakernam R, Menon-Johansson A, et al. Intensive care usage by HIV-positive patients in the HAART era. Interdiscip Perspect Infect Dis 2011;2011:847835.

102. Park DR, Sherbin VL, Goodman MS, et al. The etiology of community-acquired pneumonia at an urban public hospital: influence of human immunodeficiency virus infection and initial severity of illness. J Infect Dis 2001;184:268–77.

103. Barbier F, Coquet I, Legriel S, et al. Etiologies and outcome of acute respiratory failure in HIV-infected patients. Intensive Care Med 2009;35:1678–86.

104. Ganesan A, Masur H. Critical care of persons infected with the human immunodeficiency virus. Clin Chest Med 2013;34:307–23.

105. Vincent B, Timsit JF, Auburtin M, et al. Characteristics and outcomes of HIV-infected patients in the ICU: impact of the highly active antiretroviral treatment era. Intensive Care Med 2004;30:859–66.

106. Sarkar P, Rasheed HF. Clinical review: respiratory failure in HIV-infected patients–a changing picture. Crit Care 2013;17:228.

107. Klein MB, Yang H, DelBalso L, et al. Viral pathogens including human metapneumovirus are the

primary cause of febrile respiratory illness in HIV-infected adults receiving antiretroviral therapy. J Infect Dis 2010;201:297–301.

108. Ormsby CE, De la Rosa-Zamboni D, Vázquez-Pérez J, et al. Severe 2009 pandemic influenza A (H1N1) infection and increased mortality in patients with late and advanced HIV disease. AIDS 2011; 25:435–9.

109. Khater FJ, Moorman JP, Myers JW, et al. Bronchiolitis obliterans organizing pneumonia as a manifestation of AIDS: case report and literature review. J Infect 2004;49:159–64.

110. Angel-Moreno-Maroto A, Suárez-Castellano L, Hernández-Cabrera M, et al. Severe efavirenz-induced hypersensitivity syndrome (not-DRESS) with acute renal failure. J Infect 2006;52:e39–40.

111. Tobin-D'Angelo MJ, Hoteit MA, Brown KV, et al. Dapsone-induced hypersensitivity pneumonitis mimicking Pneumocystis carinii pneumonia in a patient with AIDS. Am J Med Sci 2004;327:163–5.

112. Yokogawa N, Alcid D. Acute fibrinous and organizing pneumonia as a rare presentation of abacavir hypersensitivity reaction. AIDS 2007;21:2116–7.

113. Jagannathan P, Davis E, Jacobson M, et al. Life-threatening immune reconstitution inflammatory syndrome after Pneumocystis pneumonia, a cautionary case series. AIDS 2009;23:1794–6.

114. Murdoch DM, Venter W, Feldman C, et al. Incidence and risk factors for the immune reconstitution inflammatory syndrome in HIV patients in South Africa, a prospective study. AIDS 2008;22:601–10.

115. Sungkanuparph S, Filler SG, Chetchotisakd P, et al. Cryptococcal immune reconstitution inflammatory syndrome after antiretroviral therapy in AIDS patients with cryptococcal meningitis: a prospective multicenter study. Clin Infect Dis 2009;49:931–4.

116. Pathak V, Rendon IS, Atrash S, et al. Comparing outcome of HIV versus non-HIV patients requiring mechanical ventilation. Clin Med Res 2012;10:57–64.

117. Nirappil F, Maheshwari A, Andrews J, et al. Characteristics and outcomes of HIV-1-infected patients with acute respiratory distress syndrome. Am J Respir Crit Care Med 2013;187:A4464.

118. Hirschtick RE, Glassroth J, Jordan MC, et al. Bacterial pneumonia in persons infected with the human immunodeficiency virus. Pulmonary Complications of HIV Infection Study Group. N Engl J Med 1995;333:845–51.

119. Stansell JD, Osmond DH, Charlebois E, et al. Predictors of Pneumocystis carinii pneumonia in HIV-infected persons. Pulmonary Complications of HIV Infection Study Group. Am J Respir Crit Care Med 1997;155:60–6.

120. Visnegarwala F, Graviss EA, Lacke CE, et al. Acute respiratory failure associated with cryptococcosis in patients with AIDS: analysis of predictive factors. Clin Infect Dis 1998;27:1231–7.

121. Huang L, Schnapp LM, Gruden JF, et al. Presentation of AIDS-related pulmonary Kaposi's sarcoma diagnosed by bronchoscopy. Am J Respir Crit Care Med 1996;153:1385–90.

122. Rabaud C, May T, Lucet JC, et al. Pulmonary toxoplasmosis in patients infected with human immunodeficiency virus: a French National Survey. Clin Infect Dis 1996;23:1249–54.

123. Tokman F, Huang L. Evaluation of respiratory disease. Clin Chest Med 2013;34:191–204.

124. Daher EF, Silva GB Jr, Barros FA, et al. Clinical and laboratory features of disseminated histoplasmosis in HIV patients from Brazil. Trop Med Int Health 2007;12:1108–15.

125. Baughman RP, Dohn MN, Frame PT. The continuing utility of bronchoalveolar lavage to diagnose opportunistic infection in AIDS patients. Am J Med 1994; 97:515–22.

126. Benito N, Rano A, Moreno A, et al. Pulmonary infiltrates in HIV-infected patients in the highly active antiretroviral therapy in Spain. J Acquir Immune Defic Syndr 2001;27:35–43.

127. Broaddus C, Dake MD, Stulbarg MS, et al. Bronchoalveolar lavage and transbronchial biopsy for the diagnosis of pulmonary infections in the acquired immunodeficiency syndrome. Ann Intern Med 1985;102:747–52.

128. Danés C, González-Martín J, Pumarola T, et al. Pulmonary infiltrates in immunosuppressed patients: analysis of a diagnostic protocol. J Clin Microbiol 2002;40:2134–40.

129. Velez L, Correa LT, Maya MA, et al. Diagnostic accuracy of bronchoalveolar lavage samples in immunosuppressed patients with suspected pneumonia: analysis of a protocol. Respir Med 2007;101:2160–7.

130. Salzman SH, Bernstein LE, Villamena PC, et al. Bronchoscopic lung biopsy improves the diagnostic yield of bronchoscopy in patients with known or suspected HIV. Journal of Bronchology 1996;3: 88–95.

131. Batungwanayo J, Taelman H, Lucas S, et al. Pulmonary disease associated with the human immunodeficiency virus in Kigali, Rwanda: a fiberoptic bronchoscopic study of 111 cases of undetermined etiology. Am J Respir Crit Care Med 1994; 149:1591–6.

132. Golden J, Hollander H, Stulbarg M, et al. Bronchoalveolar lavage as the exclusive diagnostic modality for Pneumocystis carinii pneumonia. A prospective study among patients with acquired immunodeficiency syndrome. Chest 1986;90:18–22.

133. Huang L, Hecht FM, Stansell JD, et al. Suspected Pneumocystis carinii pneumonia with a negative induced sputum examination. Is early bronchoscopy useful? Am J Respir Crit Care Med 1995; 151:1866–71.

134. Jules-Elysee KM, Stover DE, Zaman MB, et al. Aerosolized pentamidine: effect on diagnosis and presentation of *Pneumocystis carinii* pneumonia. Ann Intern Med 1990;112:750–7.

135. Baughman RP, Dohn MN, Shipley R, et al. Increased *Pneumocystis carinii* recovery from the upper lobes in *Pneumocystis* pneumonia: the effect of aerosol pentamidine prophylaxis. Chest 1993;103:426–32.

136. Yung RC, Weinacker AB, Steiger DJ, et al. Upper and middle lobe bronchoalveolar lavage to diagnose *Pneumocystis carinii* pneumonia. Am Rev Respir Dis 1993;148:1563–6.

137. Alvarez-Martinez MJ, Miro JM, Valls ME, et al. Sensitivity and specificity of nested and real-time PCR for the detection of *Pneumocystis jiroveci* in clinical specimens. Diagn Microbiol Infect Dis 2006;56:153–60.

138. Maillet M, Maubon D, Brion JP, et al. *Pneumocystis jirovecii* (Pj) quantitative PCR to differentiate Pj pneumonia from Pj colonization in immunocompromised patients. Eur J Clin Microbiol Infect Dis 2014;33:331–6.

139. Conde MB, Soares SL, Mello FC, et al. Comparison of sputum induction with fiberoptic bronchoscopy in the diagnosis of tuberculosis: experience at an acquired immune deficiency syndrome reference center in Rio de Janeiro, Brazil. Am J Respir Crit Care Med 2000;162:2238–40.

140. Joos L, Chhajed PN, Wallner J, et al. Pulmonary infections diagnosed by BAL: a 12-year experience in 1066 immunocompromised patients. Respir Med 2007;101:93–7.

141. Boehme CC, Nabeta P, Hillemann D, et al. Rapid molecular detection of tuberculosis and rifampin resistance. N Engl J Med 2010;363:1005–15.

142. Meyohas MC, Roux P, Bollens D, et al. Pulmonary cryptococcosis: localized and disseminated infections in 27 patients with AIDS. Clin Infect Dis 1995;21:628–33.

143. Salzman SH, Smith RL, Aranda CP. Histoplasmosis in patients at risk for the acquired immunodeficiency syndrome in a nonendemic setting. Chest 1988;93:916–21.

144. Martynowicz MA, Prakash UB. Pulmonary blastomycosis: an appraisal of diagnostic techniques. Chest 2002;121:768–73.

145. DiTomasso JP, Ampel NM, Sobonya RE, et al. Bronchoscopic diagnosis of pulmonary coccidioidomycosis: comparison of cytology, culture, and transbronchial biopsy. Diagn Microbiol Infect Dis 1994;18:83–7.

146. Wallace JM, Catanzaro A, Moser KM, et al. Flexible fiberoptic bronchoscopy for diagnosing pulmonary coccidioidomycosis. Am Rev Respir Dis 1981;123:286–90.

147. Lotholary O, Meyohas M, Dupont B, et al. Invasive aspergillosis in patients with acquired immunodeficiency syndrome: report of 33 cases. French Cooperative Study Group on Aspergillosis in AIDS. Am J Med 1993;95:177–87.

148. Bergeron A, Belle A, Sulahian A, et al. Contribution of galactomannan antigen detection in BAL to the diagnosis of invasive pulmonary aspergillosis in patients with hematologic malignancies. Chest 2010;137:410–5.

149. Buess M, Cathomas G, Halter J, et al. Aspergillus-PCR in bronchoalveolar lavage for detection of invasive pulmonary aspergillosis in immunocompromised patients. BMC Infect Dis 2012;12:237.

150. Miles PR, Baughman RP, Linnemann CC Jr. Cytomegalovirus in the bronchoalveolar lavage fluid of patients with AIDS. Chest 1990;97:1072–6.

151. Rodriguez-Barradas MC, Stool E, Musher DM, et al. Diagnosing and treating cytomegalovirus pneumonia in patients with AIDS. Clin Infect Dis 1996;23:76–81.

152. Waxman AB, Goldie SJ, Brett-Smith H, et al. Cytomegalovirus as a primary pulmonary pathogen in AIDS. Chest 1997;111:128–34.

153. Narayanswami G, Salzman SH. Bronchoscopy in the human immunodeficiency virus-infected patient. Semin Respir Infect 2003;18:80–6.

154. Feller-Kopman D, Ernst A. The role of bronchoalveolar lavage in the immunocompromised host. Semin Respir Infect 2003;18:87–94.

155. Griffiths MH, Kocjan G, Miller RF, et al. Diagnosis of pulmonary disease in human immunodeficiency virus infection: role of transbronchial biopsy and bronchoalveolar lavage. Thorax 1989;44:554–8.

156. Miller RF, Pugsley WB, Griffiths MH. Open lung biopsy for investigation of acute respiratory episodes in patients with HIV infection and AIDS. Genitourin Med 1995;71:280–5.

157. Pass HI, Potter D, Shelhammer J, et al. Indications for and diagnostic efficacy of open-lung biopsy in the patient with acquired immunodeficiency syndrome (AIDS). Ann Thorac Surg 1986;41:307–12.

Clinical Trial Design in Prevention and Treatment of Acute Respiratory Distress Syndrome

Gerard F. Curley, MSc, MB, PhD, FCARCSI[a],
Daniel F. McAuley, MB, MD, MRCP[b],*

KEYWORDS

- Acute respiratory distress syndrome • Clinical trial design • Prevention • Treatment

KEY POINTS

- Preclinical studies, involving in vitro and in vivo evidence of efficacy and mechanism of action, are an essential first step toward testing a hypothesis, and can usefully inform clinical trial design. However, in vitro models are limited in their complexity, although important genetic and immunologic differences between animals and humans, together with simplistic in vivo acute respiratory distress syndrome (ARDS) models, limit reliable extrapolation to clinical trials. More complex in vitro systems that mimic the alveolar-capillary interface, together with more clinically relevant animal models and human models of ARDS, could increase the reliability of preclinical investigation.
- Observational studies and systematic reviews and meta-analyses can support a potential clinical effect of an intervention, as well as providing important information for clinical trial design, including event rates and standard deviations in treatment or control groups, recruitment and withdrawal rates, and adverse events.
- Inadequate phase 2 trials provide suboptimal information for the decision to move to phase 3 and the design of the phase 3 trials. Larger phase 2 trials are probably indicated to reduce the risk of studying inactive drugs in phase 3 studies. Biomarkers, such as Ang-2 and surfactant proteins, are promising surrogates for phase 2 studies.
- Phase 3 trial design factors that need to be addressed in ARDS include (1) recruitment of insufficient numbers of patients to detect changes in mortality; (2) excessive heterogeneity; and (3) a lack of standardization of outcome measures.

INTRODUCTION

Over the past several decades, the medical community has strived toward the goal of being guided, to the best of our abilities, by evidence-based practice. There is potentially no other field in medicine in which this goal is more important than in critical care, in which there is a high degree of morbidity and mortality; the cost of care in the United States alone approaches 1% of the country's gross domestic product.[1] Few, if any, other specialties have experienced a more complicated history when it comes to applying clinical trial findings to everyday care.

Disclosures: none.
[a] Department of Anesthesia, Keenan Research Centre for Biomedical Science, Li Ka Shing Knowledge Institute, St Michael's Hospital, 30, Bond Street, Toronto, Ontario M5B 1W8, Canada; [b] School of Medicine, Dentistry and Biomedical Science, Centre for Infection and Immunity, Queen's University Belfast, Health Sciences Building, 97 Lisburn Road, Belfast, Northern Ireland BT9 7BL, UK
* Corresponding author.
E-mail address: d.f.mcauley@qub.ac.uk

Clin Chest Med 35 (2014) 713–727
http://dx.doi.org/10.1016/j.ccm.2014.08.009

Acute respiratory distress syndrome (ARDS) represents a recognizable common pattern of acute alveolar-capillary injury in critically ill patients. However, this pathway is triggered by a wide range of primary disease processes. Despite numerous randomized clinical trials aimed at regulating the lung inflammatory response during ARDS,[2] the only proven therapy to consistently reduce mortality is a protective ventilation strategy.[3] Over the last 4 decades since the first description of the syndrome, and despite new insights into disease pathophysiology and clinical trial design, numerous randomized controlled trials (RCTs) of therapies in ARDS have failed to show convincing benefit (eg, nitric oxide, surfactant, corticosteroids, β-agonists).[2]

In response, some have argued that more basic research is required, because there is not enough understanding of the underlying mechanisms of alveolar-capillary barrier dysfunction in ARDS.[4,5] Although this is no doubt true, others have also emphasized the need to better understand the data required to inform and improve the design of RCTs in ARDS.[6,7] The motive to improve study design is simple. Although studies have failed to show effect, lack of proof does not equal lack of effect. Given the ongoing high incidence and mortality of ARDS, and the high cost of developing potential new therapies, the concept that a therapy should fail to be approved simply because it was inadequately studied is an obvious concern. The development of therapeutic agents also has an ethical dimension, if many patients are exposed to a therapy that did not provide a possibility for clinical improvement.

In this article, the focus is on a stepwise approach (**Fig. 1**) to inform ARDS trial design: preclinical investigation, observational studies and meta-analysis, and phase 2 and 3 trial design, including patient recruitment, heterogeneity, and appropriate outcomes. The review concludes with a short discussion of how a stepwise approach to the evaluation of therapies in ARDS could reduce the likelihood of erroneously dismissing a potentially valuable therapy.

PRECLINICAL EVIDENCE TO INFORM A STUDY

Although much of the focus in ARDS research has been on clinical trial design, including validation of biomarkers and surrogate end points, many preclinical contributions have been made as well. The body of research required before undertaking a phase 3 trial has not been defined adequately.[7] It usually includes basic science discoveries, testing in animal models or human models of disease, as well as evidence from observational studies, phase 1 and 2 studies, and meta-analyses of previous trials. Before embarking on drug trials, pharmaceutical companies and independent investigators conduct extensive preclinical studies. In vitro and in vivo (animal experiments) studies examine preliminary efficacy, toxicity, and pharmacokinetics. Early in vivo testing specifically aims to show safety, which assists investigators to determine whether a candidate drug has

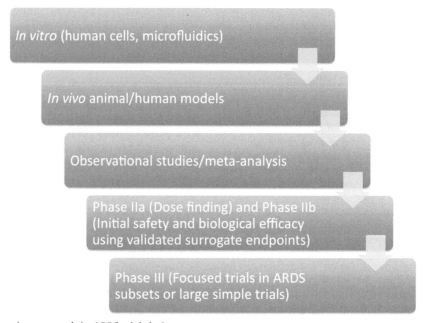

Fig. 1. A stepwise approach in ARDS trial design.

scientific merit to justify further development. Both the US Food and Drug Administration (FDA) and Health Canada require that animal tests be conducted before humans are exposed to a new molecular entity.[8,9]

In Vitro Studies as a First Step Toward Clinical Testing

Any intervention, be it therapeutic or supportive, requires biological plausibility before clinical testing. In vitro mechanistic studies allow researchers to strip away the complexity of systems to study individual biological steps or organs. For example, in 1974, Webb and Tierney[10] reported that high tidal volume ventilation induced pulmonary edema and diffuse alveolar damage histologically indistinguishable from ARDS in isolated rat lungs. Twenty-seven years later, a large multicenter randomized clinical trial confirmed the clinical benefit arising from lung-protective mechanical ventilation in patients with ARDS.[3] In vitro studies are not only an essential first step toward testing a hypothesis, but these studies also provide valuable insight that allows one to better tailor subsequent in vivo studies. For example, the in vitro observations that hypercapnic acidosis retards wound healing and the innate immune response have diminished enthusiasm for a clinical trial of therapeutic hypercapnia in ARDS.[11]

Toxicity and poor efficacy result in most clinical trials failures because it remains difficult to predict these factors with preclinical models.[12] This situation emphasizes the value of reliable, predictive in vitro model systems. However, one of the abiding weaknesses of in vitro experiments is that they fail to replicate the precise cellular conditions of an organism. Although considerable advances have been made in the development of cell culture models as surrogates of tissues and organs for these types of studies and the use of primary human cells,[13] cultured cells commonly fail to maintain differentiation and expression of tissue-specific functions. Improved tissue organization can be promoted by growing cells in three-dimensional extracellular matrix (ECM) gels[14]; however, these methods still fail to reconstitute structural and mechanical features of whole living organs, which are central to their function. In particular, existing model systems do not recreate the active tissue-tissue interface between the microvascular endothelium and neighboring parenchymal tissues, where critical transport of fluids, nutrients, immune cells, and other regulatory factors occur, nor do they permit application of dynamic mechanical forces (eg, breathing movements in lung, shear in blood vessels, peristalsis in gut, tension in skin), which are critical for the development and function of living organs.[15]

A potential solution to this problem is the development of human organs-on-chips, in which microscale engineering technologies are combined with cultured living human cells to create microfluidic devices that attempt to more accurately recapitulate the physiologic and mechanical microenvironment of whole living organs.[16,17] These organomimetic microdevices enable the study of complex human physiology in an organ-specific context, and more importantly, they offer the potential opportunity to develop specialized in vitro human disease models that could revolutionize drug development. The recently developed lung-on-a-chip that reconstituted the alveolar-capillary interface of the human lung and exposed it to physiologic mechanical deformation and flow is such an example. This versatile system enables direct visualization and quantitative analysis of diverse biological processes of the intact lung organ in ways that have not been possible in traditional cell culture or animal models and has shown promise as an initial efficacy test of potential therapies for alveolar-capillary barrier dysfunction.[18,19]

Animal Studies

Experimental discoveries are believed to begin at the bench with basic research, progress through preclinical animal studies, then show therapeutic efficacy in human clinical trials. Animal models provide a bridge between patients and the laboratory bench. Hypotheses generated in human studies can be tested directly in animal models, and the results of studies in more simple in vitro systems can be tested in animal models to assess their relevance in intact living systems. Animal models provide a means to test clinical hypotheses generated in patients using intact biological systems and to validate the importance of fundamental laboratory findings without going directly to human experimentation.

Until recently, there was no consensus in the scientific community as to what constitutes ARDS in an animal, in part because there is no single marker or parameter that has sufficient sensitivity and specificity to identify the occurrence of all forms and severities of lung injury. As a result, it was difficult for investigators to determine if lung injury had been achieved in an experimental model. For example, if an experimental drug decreases leukocyte migration into the lungs but has no effect on permeability changes, is this a potentially promising therapy for ARDS or not? In addition, a comparison of studies is difficult, because of the diversity of assays used by investigators to assess lung injury. In 2011, an American Thoracic Society report[20] concluded that the main features of experimental acute lung injury include histologic evidence of tissue injury, alteration of the alveolar-capillary barrier, presence of an inflammatory response, and evidence of physiologic dysfunction; they recommended that, to determine if ARDS has occurred, at least 3 of these 4 main features of ARDS should be present.

Notwithstanding these advances, extrapolation from animal to human in diseases such as ARDS remains problematic. Although animal models continue to play a role in the evaluation of efficacy and safety of new therapeutic interventions, genetic, molecular, and physiologic limitations often hinder their usefulness. Despite successful preclinical testing, 85% of early clinical trials for novel drugs fail; of those that survive through to phase 3, only half become approved for clinical use.[21] Almost 90% of the failures across all therapeutic areas were attributable to either lack of efficacy (66%) or safety issues (21%).[12] Although logistical and study design issues are often identified as the root cause of clinical trial failures, most futilities originate from molecular mechanisms of the drug(s) tested.[22]

There is a growing awareness of the limitations of animal research and its inability to make reliable predictions for human clinical trials.[23] Animal studies seem to overestimate by about 30% the likelihood that a treatment will be effective, because negative results are often unpublished.[24] Similarly, little more than a third of highly cited animal research is tested later in human trials.[25] Of the one-third that enter into clinical trials, as little as 8% of drugs pass phase 1 successfully.[26]

The major preclinical tools for new-agent screening before clinical testing are experimental models of ARDS in rodents. Although mice are most commonly used, they are poor models for most human diseases.[27] Crucial genetic, molecular, immunologic, and cellular differences between humans and mice prevent animal models from serving as effective and reliable surrogates of human ARDS. Among 4000+ genes in humans and mice, researchers[22] found that transcription factor binding sites differed between the species in 41% to 89% of cases. In many cases, mouse models serve to replicate specific processes or sets of processes within a disease but not the whole spectrum of physiologic changes that occur in humans in the disease setting.

A well-known example of a successful animal model that did not translate into clinical trials is the TGN1412 trial.[28] The drug TGN1412, developed by the company TeGenero, was described as an immunomodulatory humanized agonistic anti-CD28 monoclonal antibody developed for the treatment of immunologic diseases such as multiple sclerosis, rheumatoid arthritis, and certain cancers. Before conducting human trials, TGN1412 was tested on different animals, including mice, to ensure safety and efficacy in preclinical animal models.[29] These toxicity studies showed that doses 100 times higher than that administered to humans did not induce any toxic reactions. In the first human clinical trials of TGN1412, the drug caused catastrophic systemic organ failure in patients, despite being administered at a subclinical dose that was 500 times lower than the dose found safe in animal studies.[28]

The failure to translate from animals to humans is likely caused in part by poor methodology as well as failure of the models to accurately mimic the human disease condition. Unlike in human clinical trials,[30] no best-practice standards exist for animal testing. Several systematic reviews and meta-analyses[24,31] have identified a relationship between poor study quality and overestimation of treatment effect size in animal models of disease. It has been recommended that therapeutic agents should not only be evaluated in rodents but also in higher animal species and that randomization and outcomes assessor blinding should be performed. In addition, experiments should be designed in both genders and in different age groups of animals, and all data, both positive and negative, should be published.[21]

By paying due attention to experimental bias, to the breadth of physiologic variables known to influence ARDS outcome in patients, and by testing therapies in a range of model systems that might more faithfully reproduce the key facets of ARDS pathophysiology,[20] we are more likely to translate clear evidence of efficacy in animals to the more heterogeneous circumstances of human ARDS. Failure to adequately consider variables such as age, comorbidity, physiologic status, and timing of drug administration contribute to the disparity between the results of animal models and clinical trials.

Human Models of Acute Respiratory Distress Syndrome

Alternative translational approaches using humans have emerged that attempt to bridge the gap between in vitro and in vivo testing, and eliminate the uncertainty of animal testing. In the last decade, the FDA and the European Medicines Agency introduced guidelines for testing very small microdoses of drugs in humans.[32] These are concentrations less than one-hundredth of the therapeutic dose. Because the concentrations are so low, the drugs can be tested in a few patients without the level of safety data normally required before a phase 1 study. These early phase 0 studies collect human data quickly by showing how the drug is distributed and metabolized in the body, and whether it hits the right molecular target. Approximately one-quarter of the molecules entering clinical trials fail because of pharmacologic issues such as lack of absorption or penetration into the target organ.[32] With a direct test in humans, pharmaceuticals can determine earlier whether the drug is worth investing both time and money into clinical research. Phase 0 trials may be small in scope, but they require very sensitive tests to detect the minute quantities of the drug in the body and possibly its mechanism of action.

Patients undergoing 1-lung ventilation during esophagectomy,[33] lung lobectomy, or pneumonectomy[34] represent a cohort with a high risk of subsequent development of ARDS ($\leq$8% after lung resection, and 23.8% after esophagectomy) and an ideal population for the study of prophylactic or early disease-modifying therapy. ARDS after cardiopulmonary bypass is also common, occurring in 2% of patients, likely because of ischemic-reperfusion injury.[35] A recently published clinical trial evaluated the efficacy of hydroxymethylglutaryl–coenzyme A–reductase inhibitors (statins) to reduce postesophagectomy ARDS, using physiologic and biochemical end points to indicate efficacy.[36]

The development of a human model of endotoxemia using systemic administration of 4 ng/kg of reference endotoxin has been used to examine a wide range of inflammatory, hemostatic, cardiovascular, and respiratory responses characteristic of sepsis in humans.[37–39] Similarly, inhalation of lipopolysaccharide (LPS) results in a local alveolar inflammatory response with neutrophil recruitment and increased cytokine and chemokine production,[40,41] replicating many of the features of ARDS. This model has proved useful for preclinical testing using surrogate end points such as diminished inflammation[42] and enhanced epithelial repair[43] to provide proof of concept in humans before the initiation of clinical trials in established ARDS.[44,45]

Ex vivo human lung models of ARDS also offer an exciting clinically relevant alternative to animal studies. Ex vivo lung perfusion (EVLP) models of ARDS use consented donor organs that are unsuitable for transplantation based on International Society for Heart and Lung Transplant criteria. Organs are maintained in a viable state with established ventilation and perfusion systems and can be subjected to intrabronchial LPS or live bacteria, or further ischemia reperfusion injury.[46–48] EVLP models offer the potential to study detailed aspects of inflammation, repair, and alveolar-capillary dysfunction in the whole human lung. Sampling and subsequent cellular, molecular, proteomic, and genomic analyses can take place over time to generate a clear picture of the potential of a given therapeutic. For example, comprehensive characterization of the beneficial effects of mesenchymal stem cells in the isolated perfused human[46,47] lung complemented initial animal experiments[49,50] that had shown efficacy, leading to an early phase clinical trial of mesenchymal stem cells in ARDS (clinicaltrials.gov, NCT01775774).

OBSERVATIONAL STUDIES

Observational studies in the critically ill population can support a potential clinical effect of an intervention or an important pathophysiologic feature. An observational study that identifies an association between a specific intervention and improved clinical outcomes can support the need to test the hypothesis that an intervention may be effective. Observational studies are considered hypothesis generating only. For example, an observational cohort study[51] reported a reduced incidence of ARDS in critically ill patients taking chronic statin therapy. This protective effect was most notable in those with sepsis and the effect appeared to be potentiated by the coadministration of aspirin. This and other observations[52] have led to phase 2 randomized studies of statins in ARDS.[45]

Although RCTs are considered the gold standard for evaluating the efficacy and safety of a disease intervention, the carefully controlled environments required for RCTs to test the efficacy of a therapy do not include many practical treatment issues encountered by the clinician in practice. Observational studies may be an important addition by complementing RCT data with information on efficacy, safety, and patient compliance in a population of real-world patients.

Whereas RCTs allow one to determine whether a drug can bring about an intended effect, observational studies that use large databases allow one to assess the effectiveness of a drug to bring about the intended effect in the real world, by considering efficacy outcomes, safety, tolerability, and patient compliance in large patient populations and by using clinically relevant long-term outcomes. Large health care databases in Europe and the United States can provide useful information on a variety of medical conditions before, during, and after exposure to treatment interventions. Furthermore, health care providers can use data from observational studies to help identify clinically important differences between treatment options for a given medical condition.

Another limitation of RCTs is caused by shorter study durations and the use of restricted patient populations. Adverse events that might be seen in a larger patient population might not always be captured in RCTs. In addition, safety monitoring and reporting in RCTs can be incomplete. Ioannidis and Lau[53] evaluated 7 different medical areas, assessing different study designs and settings, and reported that severity of clinical adverse effects and laboratory-determined toxicity were inadequately defined in 61% and 71% of reports, respectively. The investigators called for improved and adequate safety reporting in randomized trials.

However, observational studies can result in spurious benefit that is not replicated in controlled trials. The treatment effect seen in observational studies often significantly overestimates the effect seen in prospective clinical trials, which should be considered when estimating the treatment effect for sample size calculations for subsequent clinical trials. The information gained from observational studies can also be generally limited if sample size is small, by indication bias, or by incomplete adjustment of confounding variables.

SYSTEMATIC REVIEWS AND META-ANALYSIS

Systematic reviews and meta-analysis of existing evidence are used to identify what is known about a particular area of research, and a systematic review, with or without a meta-analysis, should be undertaken to determine if the research question of interest has already been answered before a new trial begins. There is also an expectation that researchers applying for funding will use a systematic review to justify the need for a new trial. However, systematic reviews can also be used to aid planning and design of the trial. For example, a recent systematic review has been used to identify inconsistencies in outcome measures during trials of mechanically ventilated patients[54] and could be used to generate an agreed set of core outcomes in such clinical trials.[55] Systematic reviews can also be used to justify other important elements of trial design, such as event rate and standard deviation in treatment or control group, recruitment and withdrawal rate, duration of follow-up and adverse events.[56] Notwithstanding the information available to investigators from systematic reviews, previous research has shown that investigators of new randomized trials were often unaware of relevant reviews when designing trials. For example, Cooper and colleagues[57] found that 13 (55%) of 24 investigators of new published trials included in an updated Cochrane review were unaware of the review version available at the time of study

design, and 8 (33%) used the systematic review in study design. Goudie and colleagues[58] looked at how trials were designed and reported in the context of previous evidence in 2 journals (*Journal of the American Medical Association* and *Archives of Internal Medicine*) and reported that previous trial results were consulted during the design of 10 trials (37%). The CONSORT (Consolidated Standards of Reporting Trials) statement,[30] first published in 1996, required that data from a new trial should be interpreted "in the light of the totality of the available evidence." Researchers designing new trials should also begin by consulting previous evidence.[59]

PHASE 2 STUDIES

To develop effective therapies for ARDS, it is imperative to test them thoroughly in humans through well-designed and conducted clinical trials. These studies have traditionally been conducted in 3 separate phases (1, 2, and 3). Phase 1 treatment trials involve administering a new drug to a few healthy volunteers to assess initial safety and tolerability. However, in critical care, as in oncology, safety and dose-finding studies can be performed in patients with the disease of interest (referred to as phase 2a), particularly in the setting of concerns regarding toxicity of investigational therapies in healthy volunteers.

A major contributor to the high failure rate in phase 3 clinical trials is inadequate phase 2 programs, which provide suboptimal information for the decision to move to phase 3 and the design of the phase 3 trials. Deficient phase 2 programs are inadequately designed, do not contain the full complement of studies, incorporate end points that provide limited or misleading information regarding the efficacy of the test agent, or are improperly executed.

In recent times, several creative adaptations have been proposed that combine the different phases of drug development (eg, a seamless phase 2/3 adaptive design combines phases 2 and 3).[60] Pharmaceutical companies have started using these adaptations, which could save drug development costs and time. Among the future directions of ARDS research identified by the National Heart Lung and Blood Institute[61] was a call for improved trial design, conduct, and outcome assessment. As the number of experimental therapies undergoing clinical investigation in ARDS increases, there is an increasing need for more efficient statistical designs to (1) determine the optimal dose, (2) identify interventions with therapeutic potential, and (3) evaluate clinically relevant treatment effects.

Dose-Finding and Phase 2a Studies

The correct selection of the optimal dose, via a thorough understanding of the dose-toxicity and dose-efficacy relationships, is critical for establishing the efficacy of a potential therapeutic agent. Traditional rule-based dose-escalation designs,[62] such as the 3+3 design and its variations, have suboptimal statistical operating characteristics. The inefficiency in the 3+3 design is that it stems from the decision to escalate or de-escalate, a decision based solely on event data from the current dose, without considering event information available from neighboring doses. An alternative design, called the continual reassessment method,[63] is an adaptive dose-finding algorithm, wherein escalation or de-escalation through the dose region is determined by continuous re-estimation of the dose-toxicity curve, and each cohort of patients is treated at the dose currently believed to be the maximum tolerated dose. Although computationally more intensive than the 3+3 design, the continual reassessment method and its variations use all available toxicity data in the estimation of the maximum tolerated dose, and thus are statistically more efficient. Ethical considerations also favor the continual reassessment method, because it typically treats fewer patients at subtherapeutic doses.

Alternative Phase 2 Designs

Once the appropriate dose has been determined through a phase 1 trial, the next step is to evaluate efficacy potential in a phase 2 trial. The traditional concurrently controlled phase 2 design, intended to simultaneously estimate treatment effect and assess variability, is often criticized as an underpowered phase 3 comparative clinical trial. Proposed alternative designs, such as the selection design and the futility design, are instead intended to weed out ineffective or mediocre therapies.

The objective of the futility design, which has been successfully implemented in stroke,[64,65] is to discard treatments that do not show promise. Statistical hypotheses are stated such that the goal is to show that the intervention is futile. Failure to conclude futility would be considered evidence in favor of a need for a definitive phase 3 clinical trial. In the single-arm futility design,[66,67] the experimental treatment arm is compared with a target response rate, π_1, defined as the minimum proportion of successes in the treated group that would warrant further study. If the true success proportion π is less than π_1, the intervention is declared futile. Comparison of the experimental arm with a target response rate, which is fixed and has no variability, results in a smaller sample size than would be required for direct comparison with a concurrent control arm. The target response rate can be determined based on a clinically relevant treatment effect and historical control data.

Selection designs[67] can be used to prioritize candidate interventions, such that resources are allocated to the most promising of candidates. In a selection design, the objective is to select the best among K interventions (or K interventions and a control) for further testing. In the selection design, patients are randomized to one of the K interventions. The best intervention is defined as the intervention with the numerically, rather than statistically, highest response rate. The sample size is determined to ensure that, if the best treatment is superior by at least some margin D, then the best treatment is selected with high probability.

The selection design can be combined with a futility or superiority test in a sequential 2-stage design, such as in a trial of L-carnitine in septic shock.[68] At the conclusion of stage 1, a treatment would be selected, and the statistical hypothesis tested at the end of stage 2. Inclusion of stage 1 patients in the statistical hypothesis test has the advantage of using all available outcome data but introduces bias, which must be accounted for in the test statistical. If the stage 1 patients are excluded from the stage 2 hypothesis test, the parameter estimate is unbiased, but the overall sample size is increased.

Small phase 2 trials, like phase 3 trials stopped early for evidence of efficacy, are systematically susceptible to overestimating beneficial treatment effects.[69] In addition, phase 2 trials in ARDS have been hindered by the lack of a biomarker that the trial might be powered on and that correlates with clinically important outcome. The review of the data suggests that larger phase 2 trials are probably indicated to reduce the risk of studying inactive drugs in phase 3 studies. Large phase 2 trials ensure that there is adequate statistical power in calculating the effect size in a phase 3 clinical trial.

Outcomes in Phase 2 Trials

In phase 3 studies, the primary end point must incorporate a well-defined and generally accepted clinical benefit. In ARDS trials, this end point is typically mortality. In earlier development, one can use surrogate end points (usually pharmacodynamic parameters or disease progression criteria), which may not correspond directly to measurable clinical benefit but provide strong evidence of pharmacologic activity.

However, there are no end points for ARDS phase 2 studies that are well validated or that adequately predict subsequent differences in mortality or long-term clinically meaningful outcomes. For example, treatments that improve oxygenation in ARDS do not reliably result in a reduction in mortality.[3,70] This observation is consistent with other treatments in critical illness, in which organ failure reversal does not reliably correlate with mortality reduction.[71–73] Surrogate end points such as oxygenation and lung water measurements are valid only when they are causally related to a patient-centered outcome (ie, mortality), and there is no other link between the therapy for interest and the patient-centered outcomes.[74] Research in critical care is littered with numerous examples of therapies that improved surrogate outcomes but when studied in large trials were found to harm patients.[75] Although the process of validating phase 2 end points has been hindered by the relative paucity of phase 3 trials that report a treatment effect, recent landmark studies in ARDS (ARDSNet [Acute Respiratory Distress Syndrome Network] low tidal volume study,[3] PROSEVA [Proning Severe ARDS Patients] trial,[76] neuromuscular blockers in ARDS[77]) have reported differences between the control and intervention groups, representing an opportunity to explore potentially meaningful surrogate outcomes for phase 2 studies. The search for a reliable biomarker of ARDS is also ongoing, which would predict development of and outcome from ARDS, and which could be used as a reliable marker of potential treatment efficacy in a phase 2 study. The most encouraging data come from studies of Ang-2, but there are also compelling data for the interleukin 8, soluble intercellular adhesion molecule 1, the surfactant-associated proteins, and vascular endothelial growth factor.[78] However, no marker has supplanted clinical criteria in the diagnosis of ARDS and in phase 2 studies.

Current guidelines recommend surrogates of (1) 90-day mortality, (2) medium-term or long-term health-related quality of life, or (3) cost of treatment as primary end points for phase 2 trials.[79] Examples include hospital-free days to day 90, intensive care unit (ICU)-free days to day 28, or ventilator-free days to day 28. Interventions that increase mortality may reduce hospital length of stay, thereby creating a false impression that an intervention is having a beneficial effect. Thus, when using end points like hospital length of stay, it is preferable to report outcomes separately for both survivors and nonsurvivors. Free day end points may offer power advantages over mortality end points,[80] because they bring additional information from the ranking of outcomes among survivors: they are composite end points that combine the duration of support for survivors with mortality. Smaller sample sizes are therefore required for interventions that both reduce mortality and shorten the duration of support for survivors.

In addition, phase 2 trials should also report on several secondary end points relevant to a phase 3 trial, including 90-day mortality. Because sample size calculations are based solely on the primary outcome, secondary outcomes in phase 2 trials may be underpowered. When designing phase 2 trials, investigators should consider that the decision as to whether to progress to a phase 3 trial depends on the results of a range of end points measured in a phase 2 trial.

Phase 3 Studies

Despite 159 RCTs and 29 meta-analyses on ARDS treatment, only 3 specific interventions have been found to decrease ARDS mortality.[2] The available evidence seems to consistently support a reduction in overall mortality with low tidal volume ventilation and also with prone positioning and neuromuscular blockade in patients with severe ARDS. These 3 interventions may be the only ones that can be recommended for routine clinical use with rigorous support. The survival benefit of these specific interventions has been shown in only a single RCT for intervention,[3,76,77] without any further validation or confirmatory trial. There are several trial design factors that could explain the long list of negative RCTs in ARDS, including (1) recruitment of insufficient numbers of patients to detect changes in mortality; (2) excessive heterogeneity in study populations; and (3) a lack of standardization of outcome measures.

Patient Recruitment

Trial recruitment is challenging for medical researchers, who frequently overestimate the pool of qualified, willing participants.[81] A recent article in Nature[21] reported that at least 90% of trials are extended by at least 6 weeks because investigators fail to enroll patients on schedule. Recruitment challenges have been reported to be the cause of 45% of study delays, with delays often exceeding 6 months, whereas 17% of trials studied failed to reach even half their target recruitment.[82] Recruitment of a sufficient number of participants is a particular challenge for any clinical study that involves enrollment of participants receiving mechanical ventilatory support in the ICU. The desire to optimize the possibility of a positive finding leads most traditional RCTs to use strict study protocols and highly selected (in ARDS, high risk) patients, and to be conducted at the best medical centers. By necessity, traditional RCTs usually target a subgroup of individuals from the larger pool of potentially eligible patients by who is most likely to participate or respond to the therapy. This targeting further reduces the pool of eligible patients. Therefore, innovative strategies are needed to enhance recruitment.

To effectively validate phase 2 and single-center studies, we must cultivate nonindustry financial support and an infrastructure to perform multicenter comparative effectiveness studies. This approach has been exemplified by the ARDSnet, the Canadian Critical Care Trials Group, and the Australia and New Zealand Intensive Care Society Clinical Trials Group. For example, the ARDSnet low tidal volume study[3] clarified the conflicting results of previous smaller trials,[83,84] and its findings have since been incorporated into standard practice. If more such ICU-nets existed, the critical care community would have a vehicle by which carefully selected promising interventions could be validated using a multicenter approach. Ideally, by already having the network infrastructure in place, we may be able to reduce the time required to perform multicenter phase 3 trials. By expediting this process, ICU-nets could help to mitigate the recruitment delays created by the selective targeting of subsets of patients for ARDS research. Although the cost of such networks is substantial, they could prove to be a cost-effective approach if they prevent the needless expenditure of resources associated with delayed and incomplete trials.

One potential strategy to enhance recruitment and limit variability of the study population is to use a central clinical coordinating center to screen potential study participants. More protocol violations occur during initial patient enrollment in clinical trials in new centers, where a lack of full understanding of the patient population to be studied is evident. One role of the clinical coordinating center is to shorten or eliminate the duration of this learning curve for ARDS trials.[85] Center selection also constitutes an important aspect of patient recruitment. Should we use only centers for excellence that are familiar with the problems associated with clinical trials in ARDS and that see sufficiently large numbers of patients to maintain a high level of proficiency and interest in the study to ensure high-quality enrollment of patients? Perhaps phase 2 and even phase 3 trials should be conducted in level I ARDS clinical trial centers and study centers should be expanded to smaller ICUs in phase 4 trials. However, it is not clear that there are sufficient numbers of centers of excellence to generate the large number of patients in a reasonable period to complete large phase 3 trials. Furthermore, there is a question of external validity of the data if it is just performed in a few high-volume centers.

Heterogeneity in Phase 3 Studies of Acute Respiratory Distress Syndrome

Patient heterogeneity has been and continues to be a hallmark of populations with ARDS within clinical trials. This problem remains a major impediment to defining a responsive patient population for a specific intervention, and this issue remains a major unmet medical need in clinical trial design in ARDS studies (**Table 1**). Because the diagnosis of ARDS is based on a combination of clinical, oxygenation, hemodynamic, and radiographic criteria, most studies must include a highly heterogeneous group of patients. Even severe hypoxemia, the cardinal feature of ARDS, does not reliably delineate disease severity or predict the development and progression of the syndrome or response to treatment in any given patient. The Pao_2/Fio_2 ratio (arterial pressure of oxygen in arterial blood/fraction of inspired oxygen) is the hallmark for assessing hypoxemia in patients with ARDS. However, ARDS definitions do not mandate a standardized procedure for its measurement, despite our awareness that changes in positive end-expiratory pressure (PEEP) and Fio_2 alter Pao_2/Fio_2.[86,87] Most RCTs have enrolled patients with a wide range of lung injury, without acknowledging that some patients evolve with standard care to less severe forms of lung injury within 24 hours of diagnosis, whereas others evolve into more severe forms. This concern is highlighted in 2 recent observational reports in which Pao_2/Fio_2 at ARDS onset was incapable of separating patients into distinct categories of severity associated with significantly different mortalities.[88,89] However, persistently low Pao_2/Fio_2 is associated with a poor outcome and may be a marker of failure to respond to conventional therapy.[5,6] If patients in a trial with a low risk of death are not excluded or stratified, the trial will not show the efficacy of the intervention, regardless of the sample size. This limitation may explain why in the last 14 years since the publication of the ARDSnet trial, only 2 RCTs have had positive results.[76,77] In both trials, only patients with a Pao_2/Fio_2 threshold under a specific level of PEEP and Fio_2 that persisted 18 to 36 hours were enrolled. Thus, a standardized method for assessing lung injury severity must be mandatory to identify a homogeneous group of patients with ARDS.

Several strategies have been proposed to deal with the heterogeneity problem in ARDS trials. One approach is to conduct small, focused trials

Table 1
Recommendations to improve trial design

Trial Design Challenges	Recommendations to Improve Trial Design
In vitro models fail to recapitulate the precise microenvironment of the lung	Three-dimensional ECM gels, microfluidic devices and human organs-on-chips more accurately replicate the dynamics of the alveolar-capillary interface
Genetic, molecular, immunologic, and cellular differences between humans and mice prevent animal models from serving as effective and reliable surrogates of human ARDS	Microdose studies in humans, and human models of ARDS (1-lung ventilation during lobectomy/esophagectomy, inhaled LPS) and the ex vivo human lung model can provide proof of concept and complement initial animal studies
Poor preclinical in vivo study quality may overestimate potential treatment effects	Consider animal age, comorbidity, physiologic status, and timing of drug administration in the design of preclinical studies, as well as randomization and blinding
Event rate and standard deviation in treatment or control group are often overestimated in clinical trials, whereas recruitment and withdrawal rate are important unknowns	Observational studies and systematic reviews and meta-analysis can be used to inform trial design in these areas
Inadequate phase 2 trials provide suboptimal information for the decision to move to phase 3 and the design of the phase 3 trials	Larger phase 2 trials are probably indicated to reduce the risk of studying inactive drugs in phase 3 studies. Adaptive designs should be considered to increase statistical efficiency
End points for ARDS phase 2 studies do not adequately predict subsequent differences in mortality or long-term clinically meaningful outcomes in phase 3 trials	Phase 2 end points should include hospital-free days to day 90, ICU-free days to day 28, or ventilator-free days to day 28. Biomarkers, such as Ang-2 and surfactant proteins, are promising surrogates for phase 2 studies
Phase 3 trial design factors that could explain the long list of negative RCTs in ARDS include (1) recruitment of insufficient numbers of patients to detect changes in mortality; (2) excessive heterogeneity; and (3) a lack of standardization of outcome measures	The use of a network infrastructure to perform trials with a central coordinating center, focused trials with well-defined clinical subsets of ARDS, or very large simple studies increase the likelihood of detecting a treatment difference

with well-defined clinical subsets of ARDS (eg, severe community-acquired pneumonia, direct or indirect causes) or with the use of biomarkers to define more homogenous subsets. Biomarkers linked to the mechanism of action of the treatment may be used to either identify the subset or monitor response to therapy. For example, procollagen peptide III (PCP III), measured in bronchoalveolar lavage fluid, is a marker of fibroproliferation and has been shown to be increased in those patients with unresolving ARDS and to decrease with corticosteroid treatment.[90] Thus, targeting patients with unresolving ARDS who have increased PCP III levels could be 1 approach to identifying an antifibroproliferative therapy responsive subset. Other potential prognostic biomarkers include plasminogen activator inhibitor 1 (a marker of deranged coagulation)[91] and the receptor for advanced glycation end products (a marker of epithelial injury).[92] An alternative approach to focused trials to minimize heterogeneity is to conduct large, simple trial designs involving tens of thousands of patients to detect small but significant overall trends in large populations with ARDS. The major advantage of the large simple trial model, in which tens of thousands of patients are pooled together, is the greatly enhanced statistical power to find treatment benefits over current phase 3 trial sample size. The large sample size also provides face validity that similar benefits would accrue to the entire population of patients with ARDS should the drug be released. However, large simple trial designs in ARDS are difficult to perform and could lose discriminating power if only a subset of patients were benefited, whereas another subgroup of patients were worsened by the same treatment intervention. This issue would be difficult to decipher in a large trial in which extensive details such as microbiology and physiology of each individual patient are not collected.

Pathophysiologic mechanisms accounting for important differences in outcome within various patient subpopulations also would be obscured.

Outcomes in Phase 3 Studies

Mortality remains the most important outcome in phase 3 studies of ARDS.[61] As discussed in the section on phase 2 studies, free days (eg, ventilator-free days and ICU-free days) are increasingly used as end points in high-profile ARDS clinical trials[93–95] and offer power advantages over mortality end points.[80] However, these outcomes can be prone to bias, because the decision to discontinue mechanical ventilation is often subjective, unless driven by an explicit protocol.

Certain patient-centered or patient-important outcomes are also relevant: survival, cognitive function, pulmonary function, and quality of life are clearly important after ARDS, whereas substantial decreases in time on a ventilator, in the ICU, or in hospital may also have some, although likely less, importance. End points such as organ failure, if unaccompanied by changes in mortality or quality of life, are also likely to be of lesser importance from patients' perspectives.

Use of a primary composite end point as a strategy for reducing sample size may also be considered. However, each component should occur with equal frequency, and they should have similar risk reductions in response to effective interventions. Without these conditions, composite outcomes can be misleading. For example, a composite end point may be predominately determined by a component of lesser patient importance, such as time on mechanical ventilation, whereas a component of greater patient importance, such as mortality, shows no change or even potential harm.

EARLY TREATMENT AND PREVENTION TRIALS

Improving the time to diagnosis and intervention has been shown to have a significant impact on outcomes in acute myocardial infarction, stroke, and trauma. This finding was made possible through a better understanding of the early pathogenesis of these diseases, leading to more specific targeting for adjunctive therapies. Although the causes for previously failed ARDS trials are numerous, a prolonged and inconsistent time from disease onset to therapeutic intervention is a common feature. Clinical trials have largely targeted enrolling patients within 48 hours of meeting American-European Consensus Conference criteria while receiving mechanical ventilation, potentially delaying initiation of treatment until several days after onset of lung injury. Based on the successful paradigm of cardiovascular

trials and early goal-directed therapy for sepsis,[96] greater clinical benefit may derive from intervening earlier in the course of ARDS, before meeting current ARDS criteria or before the onset of respiratory failure and need for mechanical ventilation.

Levitt and colleagues[97] prospectively enrolled 100 patients with bilateral opacities on admission chest radiographs to identify risk factors associated with early ARDS. A supplemental oxygen of more than 2 L/min identified patients who progressed to ARDS with an area under the curve of 0.75 and with a sensitivity and specificity of 73% and 79%, respectively. Gajic and colleagues[98] have developed the Lung Injury Prediction Score to identify at-risk patients without current evidence of acute lung injury. These studies may result in useful clinical prediction tools to help identify target populations for enrollment in clinical trials of early treatment and prevention of ARDS.

SUMMARY

Progress in specific treatments for ARDS beyond lung-protective strategies of mechanical ventilation and conservative fluid management has not yet been realized. A stepwise approach incorporating preclinical in vitro and in vivo studies remains central to effective and safe clinical translation of potential therapies. However, important differences between murine and human immune systems highlight the need for improved model systems. Clinical trials for ARDS must incorporate the complex biology of this heterogeneous, and rapidly evolving clinical syndrome, which comprises an array of disparate diseases, different pathogens, and comorbid illnesses. Improved trial designs can incorporate the more intelligent use of point of care, rapid assays with biomarker panels to predictive responsiveness to specific therapies, and can increase the chance for success in the future. Another approach is to conduct trials in more defined target populations, such as those with community-acquired pneumonia or sepsis-induced ARDS. These diseases are more homogeneous, often occur in patients previously well with less comorbidity, and may be more reliably diagnosed. An emerging paradigm in ARDS is toward prevention and early treatment of at-risk populations. Observational studies and meta-analysis of interventions should also be used to inform clinical trial design. In this respect, standardization of outcome definitions in ARDS trials and core outcome sets allows comparison of effects across trials. A standardized format in ARDS trials for collecting data, including long-term quality of life and functional status outcomes, would facilitate patient-level meta-analyses from multiple trials. Given the increasing cost of drug development, it is important to design trials efficiently. By using a stepwise approach in conjunction with careful phase 2 trial design, it should be possible to subject fewer patients to ineffective therapies and increase the likelihood of detecting an important therapeutic effect.

REFERENCES

1. Halpern NA, Pastores SM. Critical care medicine in the United States 2000-2005: an analysis of bed numbers, occupancy rates, payer mix, and costs. Crit Care Med 2010;38(1):65–71.
2. Tonelli AR, Zein J, Adams J, et al. Effects of interventions on survival in acute respiratory distress syndrome: an umbrella review of 159 published randomized trials and 29 meta-analyses. Intensive Care Med 2014;40:769–87.
3. Ventilation with lower tidal volumes as compared with traditional tidal volumes for acute lung injury and the acute respiratory distress syndrome. The Acute Respiratory Distress Syndrome Network. N Engl J Med 2000;342(18):1301–8.
4. Kavanagh BP. Therapeutic hypercapnia: careful science, better trials. Am J Respir Crit Care Med 2005;171(2):96–7.
5. Marini JJ. Limitations of clinical trials in acute lung injury and acute respiratory distress syndrome. Curr Opin Crit Care 2006;12(1):25–31.
6. Donahoe M. Acute respiratory distress syndrome: a clinical review. Pulm Circ 2011;1(2):192–211.
7. McAuley DF, O'Kane C, Griffiths MJ. A stepwise approach to justify phase III randomized clinical trials and enhance the likelihood of a positive result. Crit Care Med 2010;38(10 Suppl):S523–527.
8. Junod SW. FDA and clinical drug trials: a short history. In: Kerimani F, Davies M, editors. A quick guide to clinical trials. Washington, DC: Bioplan; 2013. p. 25–55.
9. Guidance for industry: general considerations for clinical trials. Ottawa (Canada): Health Canada Publications; 1997.
10. Webb HH, Tierney DF. Experimental pulmonary edema due to intermittent positive pressure ventilation with high inflation pressures. Protection by positive end-expiratory pressure. Am Rev Respir Dis 1974;110(5):556–65.
11. Curley G, Contreras MM, Nichol AD, et al. Hypercapnia and acidosis in sepsis: a double-edged sword? Anesthesiology 2010;112(2):462–72.
12. Arrowsmith J. Trial watch: phase III and submission failures: 2007-2010. Nat Rev Drug Discov 2011; 10(2):87.
13. Davila JC, Rodriguez RJ, Melchert RB, et al. Predictive value of in vitro model systems in toxicology. Annu Rev Pharmacol Toxicol 1998;38:63–96.
14. Pampaloni F, Reynaud EG, Seltzer EH. The third dimension bridges the gap between cell culture and live tissue. Nat Rev Mol Cell Biol 2007;8(10):839–45.
15. Ingber DE. Cellular mechanotransduction: putting all the pieces together again. FASEB J 2006;20(7):811–27.
16. Huh D, Fujioka H, Tung YC, et al. Acoustically detectable cellular-level lung injury induced by fluid mechanical stresses in microfluidic airway systems. Proc Natl Acad Sci U S A 2007;104(48):18886–91.
17. Grosberg A, Alford PW, McCain ML, et al. Ensembles of engineered cardiac tissues for physiological and pharmacological study: heart on a chip. Lab Chip 2011;11(24):4165–73.
18. Huh D, Matthews BD, Mammoto A, et al. Reconstituting organ-level lung functions on a chip. Science 2010;328(5986):1662–8.
19. Huh D, Leslie DC, Matthews BD, et al. A human disease model of drug toxicity-induced pulmonary edema in a lung-on-a-chip micro device. Sci Transl Med 2012;4(159):159ra147.
20. Matute-Bello G, Downey G, Moore BB, et al. An official American Thoracic Society workshop report: features and measurements of experimental acute lung injury in animals. Am J Respir Cell Mol Biol 2011;44(5):725–38.
21. Ledford H. Translational research: 4 ways to fix the clinical trial. Nature 2011;477(7366):526–8.
22. Mak IW, Evaniew N, Ghert M. Lost in translation: animal models and clinical trials in cancer treatment. Am J Transl Res 2014;6(2):114–8.
23. Perel P, Roberts I, Sena E, et al. Comparison of treatment effects between animal experiments and clinical trials: systematic review. BMJ 2007; 334(7586):197.
24. Sena ES, van der Worp HB, Bath PM, et al. Publication bias in reports of animal stroke studies leads to major overstatement of efficacy. PLoS Biol 2010; 8(3):e1000344.
25. Hackam DG, Redelmeier DA. Translation of research evidence from animals to humans. JAMA 2006;296(14):1731–2.
26. Innovation or stagnation: challenge and opportunity on the critical path to new medical products. In: US Food and Drug Administration Critical Path Initiative; 2004. p. 1–30.
27. Seok J, Warren HS, Cuenca AG, et al. Genomic responses in mouse models poorly mimic human inflammatory diseases. Proc Natl Acad Sci U S A 2013;110(9):3507–12.
28. Suntharalingam G, Perry MR, Ward S, et al. Cytokine storm in a phase 1 trial of the anti-CD28 monoclonal antibody TGN1412. N Engl J Med 2006; 355(10):1018–28.
29. Attarwala H. TGN1412: from discovery to disaster. J Young Pharm 2010;2(3):332–6.

30. Begg C, Cho M, Eastwood S, et al. Improving the quality of reporting of randomized controlled trials. The CONSORT statement. JAMA 1996;276(8):637–9.

31. Dirnagl U, Lauritzen M. Fighting publication bias: introducing the Negative Results section. J Cereb Blood Flow Metab 2010;30(7):1263–4.

32. Marchetti S, Schellens JH. The impact of FDA and EMEA guidelines on drug development in relation to Phase 0 trials. Br J Cancer 2007;97(5):577–81.

33. Tandon S, Batchelor A, Bullock R, et al. Peri-operative risk factors for acute lung injury after elective oesophagectomy. Br J Anaesth 2001;86(5):633–8.

34. Dulu A, Pastores SM, Park B, et al. Prevalence and mortality of acute lung injury and ARDS after lung resection. Chest 2006;130(1):73–8.

35. Dodd-o JM, Welsh LE, Salazar JD, et al. Effect of bronchial artery blood flow on cardiopulmonary bypass-induced lung injury. Am J Physiol Heart Circ Physiol 2004;286(2):H693–700.

36. Shyamsundar M, McAuley DF, Shields MO, et al. Effect of simvastatin on physiological and biological outcomes in patients undergoing esophagectomy: a randomized placebo-controlled trial. Ann Surg 2014;259(1):26–31.

37. Hesse DG, Tracey KJ, Fong Y, et al. Cytokine appearance in human endotoxemia and primate bacteremia. Surg Gynecol Obstet 1988;166(2):147–53.

38. Michie HR, Manogue KR, Spriggs DR, et al. Detection of circulating tumor necrosis factor after endotoxin administration. N Engl J Med 1988;318(23):1481–6.

39. Suffredini AF, Fromm RE, Parker MM, et al. The cardiovascular response of normal humans to the administration of endotoxin. N Engl J Med 1989;321(5):280–7.

40. Sandstrom T, Bjermer L, Rylander R. Lipopolysaccharide (LPS) inhalation in healthy subjects causes bronchoalveolar neutrophilia, lymphocytosis, and fibronectin increase. Am J Ind Med 1994;25(1):103–4.

41. O'Grady NP, Preas HL, Pugin J, et al. Local inflammatory responses following bronchial endotoxin instillation in humans. Am J Respir Crit Care Med 2001;163(7):1591–8.

42. Shyamsundar M, McKeown ST, O'Kane CM, et al. Simvastatin decreases lipopolysaccharide-induced pulmonary inflammation in healthy volunteers. Am J Respir Crit Care Med 2009;179(12):1107–14.

43. Shyamsundar M, McAuley DF, Ingram RJ, et al. Keratinocyte growth-factor promotes epithelial survival and resolution in a human model of lung injury. Am J Respir Crit Care Med 2014;189:1520–9.

44. Cross LJ, O'Kane CM, McDowell C, et al. Keratinocyte growth factor in acute lung injury to reduce pulmonary dysfunction–a randomised placebo-controlled trial (KARE): study protocol. Trials 2013;14:51.

45. Craig TR, Duffy MJ, Shyamsundar M, et al. A randomized clinical trial of hydroxymethylglutaryl-coenzyme A reductase inhibition for acute lung injury (the HARP Study). Am J Respir Crit Care Med 2011;183(5):620–6.

46. Lee JW, Fang X, Gupta N, et al. Allogeneic human mesenchymal stem cells for treatment of *E. coli* endotoxin-induced acute lung injury in the ex vivo perfused human lung. Proc Natl Acad Sci U S A 2009;106(38):16357–62.

47. Lee JW, Krasnodembskaya A, McKenna DH, et al. Therapeutic effects of human mesenchymal stem cells in ex vivo human lungs injured with live bacteria. Am J Respir Crit Care Med 2013;187(7):751–60.

48. McAuley DF, Curley GF, Hamid UI, et al. Clinical grade allogeneic human mesenchymal stem cells restore alveolar fluid clearance in human lungs rejected for transplantation. Am J Physiol Lung Cell Mol Physiol 2014;306:L809–15.

49. Gupta N, Su X, Popov B, et al. Intrapulmonary delivery of bone marrow-derived mesenchymal stem cells improves survival and attenuates endotoxin-induced acute lung injury in mice. J Immunol 2007;179(3):1855–63.

50. Curley GF, Hayes M, Ansari B, et al. Mesenchymal stem cells enhance recovery and repair following ventilator-induced lung injury in the rat. Thorax 2012;67(6):496–501.

51. O'Neal HR Jr, Koyama T, Koehler EA, et al. Prehospital statin and aspirin use and the prevalence of severe sepsis and acute lung injury/acute respiratory distress syndrome. Crit Care Med 2011;39(6):1343–50.

52. Irish Critical Care Trials Group. Acute lung injury and the acute respiratory distress syndrome in Ireland: a prospective audit of epidemiology and management. Crit Care 2008;12(1):R30.

53. Ioannidis JP, Lau J. Completeness of safety reporting in randomized trials: an evaluation of 7 medical areas. JAMA 2001;285(4):437–43.

54. Blackwood B, Clarke M, McAuley DF, et al. How outcomes are defined in clinical trials of mechanically ventilated adults and children. Am J Respir Crit Care Med 2014;189(8):886–93.

55. Williamson PR, Altman DG, Blazeby JM, et al. Developing core outcome sets for clinical trials: issues to consider. Trials 2012;13:132.

56. Jones AP, Conroy E, Williamson PR, et al. The use of systematic reviews in the planning, design and conduct of randomised trials: a retrospective cohort of NIHR HTA funded trials. BMC Med Res Methodol 2013;13:50.

57. Cooper NJ, Jones DR, Sutton AJ. The use of systematic reviews when designing studies. Clin Trials 2005;2(3):260–4.

58. Goudie AC, Sutton AJ, Jones DR, et al. Empirical assessment suggests that existing evidence

could be used more fully in designing randomized controlled trials. J Clin Epidemiol 2010; 63(9):983–91.

59. Clarke M, Hopewell S, Chalmers I. Clinical trials should begin and end with systematic reviews of relevant evidence: 12 years and waiting. Lancet 2010;376(9734):20–1.

60. Thall PF. A review of phase 2-3 clinical trial designs. Lifetime Data Anal 2008;14(1):37–53.

61. Spragg RG, Bernard GR, Checkley W, et al. Beyond mortality: future clinical research in acute lung injury. Am J Respir Crit Care Med 2010;181(10):1121–7.

62. Storer BE. Design and analysis of phase I clinical trials. Biometrics 1989;45(3):925–37.

63. O'Quigley J, Pepe M, Fisher L. Continual reassessment method: a practical design for phase 1 clinical trials in cancer. Biometrics 1990;46(1):33–48.

64. IMS Study Investigators. Combined intravenous and intra-arterial recanalization for acute ischemic stroke: the Interventional Management of Stroke Study. Stroke 2004;35(4):904–11.

65. IMS II Trial Investigators. The Interventional Management of Stroke (IMS) II Study. Stroke 2007; 38(7):2127–35.

66. Palesch YY, Tilley BC, Sackett DL, et al. Applying a phase II futility study design to therapeutic stroke trials. Stroke 2005;36(11):2410–4.

67. Simon R, Thall PF, Ellenberg SS. New designs for the selection of treatments to be tested in randomized clinical trials. Stat Med 1994;13(5–7): 417–29.

68. Lewis RJ, Viele K, Broglio K, et al. An adaptive, phase II, dose-finding clinical trial design to evaluate L-carnitine in the treatment of septic shock based on efficacy and predictive probability of subsequent phase III success. Crit Care Med 2013;41(7):1674–8.

69. Bassler D, Briel M, Montori VM, et al. Stopping randomized trials early for benefit and estimation of treatment effects: systematic review and meta-regression analysis. JAMA 2010;303(12):1180–7.

70. Adhikari NK, Burns KE, Friedrich JO, et al. Effect of nitric oxide on oxygenation and mortality in acute lung injury: systematic review and meta-analysis. BMJ 2007;334(7597):779.

71. Bakker J, Grover R, McLuckie A, et al. Administration of the nitric oxide synthase inhibitor NG-methyl-L-arginine hydrochloride (546C88) by intravenous infusion for up to 72 hours can promote the resolution of shock in patients with severe sepsis: results of a randomized, double-blind, placebo-controlled multicenter study (study no. 144-002). Crit Care Med 2004;32(1):1–12.

72. Friedrich JO, Adhikari N, Herridge MS, et al. Meta-analysis: low-dose dopamine increases urine output but does not prevent renal dysfunction or death. Ann Intern Med 2005;142(7):510–24.

73. NICE-SUGAR Study Investigators, Finfer S, Chittock DR, et al. Intensive versus conventional glucose control in critically ill patients. N Engl J Med 2009;360(13):1283–97.

74. Fleming TR, DeMets DL. Surrogate end points in clinical trials: are we being misled? Ann Intern Med 1996;125(7):605–13.

75. Rubenfeld GD. Surrogate measures of patient-centered outcomes in critical care. In: Angus D, Carlet J, editors. Surviving intensive care. Berlin-Heidelberg: Springer; 2003. p. 169–80.

76. Guerin C, Reignier J, Richard JC, et al. Prone positioning in severe acute respiratory distress syndrome. N Engl J Med 2013;368(23):2159–68.

77. Papazian L, Forel JM, Gacouin A, et al. Neuromuscular blockers in early acute respiratory distress syndrome. N Engl J Med 2010;363(12):1107–16.

78. Binnie A, Tsang JL, dos Santos CC. Biomarkers in acute respiratory distress syndrome. Curr Opin Crit Care 2014;20(1):47–55. http://dx.doi.org/10.1097/MCC.0000000000000048.

79. Young P, Hodgson C, Dulhunty J, et al. End points for phase II trials in intensive care: recommendations from the Australian and New Zealand Clinical Trials Group consensus panel meeting. Crit Care Resusc 2012;14(3):211–5.

80. Schoenfeld DA, Bernard GR, Network A. Statistical evaluation of ventilator-free days as an efficacy measure in clinical trials of treatments for acute respiratory distress syndrome. Crit Care Med 2002; 30(8):1772–7.

81. Galbreath AD, Smith B, Wood P, et al. Cumulative recruitment experience in two large single-center randomized, controlled clinical trials. Contemp Clin Trials 2008;29(3):335–42.

82. Haidich AB, Ioannidis JP. Patterns of patient enrollment in randomized controlled trials. J Clin Epidemiol 2001;54(9):877–83.

83. Amato MB, Barbas CS, Medeiros DM, et al. Effect of a protective-ventilation strategy on mortality in the acute respiratory distress syndrome. N Engl J Med 1998;338(6):347–54.

84. Stewart TE, Meade MO, Cook DJ, et al. Evaluation of a ventilation strategy to prevent barotrauma in patients at high risk for acute respiratory distress syndrome. Pressure- and Volume-Limited Ventilation Strategy Group. N Engl J Med 1998;338(6):355–61.

85. Macias WL, Vallet B, Bernard GR, et al. Sources of variability on the estimate of treatment effect in the PROWESS trial: implications for the design and conduct of future studies in severe sepsis. Crit Care Med 2004;32(12):2385–91.

86. Villar J, Perez-Mendez L, Lopez J, et al. An early PEEP/FIO2 trial identifies different degrees of lung injury in patients with acute respiratory distress syndrome. Am J Respir Crit Care Med 2007; 176(8):795–804.

87. Villar J, Perez-Mendez L, Blanco J, et al. A universal definition of ARDS: the PaO2/FiO2 ratio under a standard ventilatory setting–a prospective, multicenter validation study. Intensive Care Med 2013;39(4):583–92.

88. Hernu R, Wallet F, Thiolliere F, et al. An attempt to validate the modification of the American-European consensus definition of acute lung injury/acute respiratory distress syndrome by the Berlin definition in a university hospital. Intensive Care Med 2013;39(12):2161–70.

89. Caser EB, Zandonade E, Pereira E, et al. Impact of distinct definitions of acute lung injury on its incidence and outcomes in Brazilian ICUs: prospective evaluation of 7,133 patients. Crit Care Med 2014;42(3):574–82.

90. Meduri GU, Tolley EA, Chinn A, et al. Procollagen types I and III aminoterminal propeptide levels during acute respiratory distress syndrome and in response to methylprednisolone treatment. Am J Respir Crit Care Med 1998;158(5 Pt 1):1432–41.

91. Ware LB, Matthay MA, Parsons PE, et al. Pathogenetic and prognostic significance of altered coagulation and fibrinolysis in acute lung injury/acute respiratory distress syndrome. Crit Care Med 2007;35(8):1821–8.

92. Calfee CS, Ware LB, Eisner MD, et al. Plasma receptor for advanced glycation end products and clinical outcomes in acute lung injury. Thorax 2008;63(12):1083–9.

93. Strom T, Martinussen T, Toft P. A protocol of no sedation for critically ill patients receiving mechanical ventilation: a randomised trial. Lancet 2010; 375(9713):475–80.

94. Ferrer M, Sellares J, Valencia M, et al. Non-invasive ventilation after extubation in hypercapnic patients with chronic respiratory disorders: randomised controlled trial. Lancet 2009;374(9695):1082–8.

95. Mercat A, Richard JC, Vielle B, et al. Positive end-expiratory pressure setting in adults with acute lung injury and acute respiratory distress syndrome: a randomized controlled trial. JAMA 2008; 299(6):646–55.

96. Rivers E, Nguyen B, Havstad S, et al. Early goal-directed therapy in the treatment of severe sepsis and septic shock. N Engl J Med 2001;345(19): 1368–77.

97. Levitt JE, Bedi H, Calfee CS, et al. Identification of early acute lung injury at initial evaluation in an acute care setting prior to the onset of respiratory failure. Chest 2009;135(4):936–43.

98. Gajic O, Dabbagh O, Park PK, et al. Early identification of patients at risk of acute lung injury: evaluation of lung injury prediction score in a multicenter cohort study. Am J Respir Crit Care Med 2011; 183(4):462–70.

Beyond Low Tidal Volumes
Ventilating the Patient with Acute Respiratory Distress Syndrome

 CrossMark

Ray Guo, MD, Eddy Fan, MD, PhD*

KEYWORDS

- Acute respiratory distress syndrome • Mechanical ventilation • Lung protective ventilation
- Positive end expiratory pressure

KEY POINTS

- The goal of mechanical ventilation in patients with acute respiratory distress syndrome (ARDS) is minimizing ventilator-induced lung inujury (ie, alveolar overdistension and cyclical recruitment/derecruitment) while providing adequate oxygenation and ventilation.
- An effective conventional mechanical ventilation strategy in patients with ARDS uses low tidal volumes and an open lung strategy employing increased positive end-expiratory pressure (PEEP).
- The optimal level of PEEP in patients with ARDS is unclear, but higher levels may be warranted in patients with moderate/severe ARDS.
- Bedside monitoring techniques (eg, esophageal pressure monitoring and electrical impedance tomography) may help clinicians to individualize the delivery of mechanical ventilation, as well as detect complications.

INTRODUCTION

Since first described by Ashbaugh and colleagues[1] in 1967 as the acute onset of respiratory distress, cyanosis refractory to oxygenation therapy, decreased lung compliance and diffuse pulmonary infiltrates on chest radiography, acute respiratory distress syndrome (ARDS) has been recognized as a life-threatening syndrome associated with significant morbidity[2,3] and mortality[4] that affects many patients admitted to critical care units.

Although several ARDS definitions have been developed and used over time, the most recent was proposed in 2012 by the ARDS Definition Task Force.[5] The Berlin Definition of ARDS requires the development of bilateral opacities on chest imaging within 1 week of a known clinical insult and respiratory failure not fully explained by cardiac failure or fluid overload.[6] The severity of hypoxemia is determined by Pao_2/Fio_2 ratios measured on at least a positive-end expiratory pressure (PEEP) of 5 cm H_2O, resulting in 3 mutually exclusive categories: mild (Pao_2/Fio_2 300–201), moderate (Pao_2/Fio_2 200–101), and severe ($Pao_2/Fio_2 \leq 100$).

Despite the marked derangements in gas exchange, death from refractory hypoxemia is rare and accounts for approximately 13% of deaths in patients with ARDS; sepsis with resulting multiorgan failure remains the leading cause of death.[7] Therefore, although mechanical ventilation

No relevant disclosures.
Interdepartmental Division of Critical Care Medicine, University of Toronto, Toronto, Ontario, Canada
* Corresponding author. Toronto General Hospital, 585 University Avenue, PMB 11-123, Toronto, Ontario M5G 2N2, Canada.
E-mail address: eddy.fan@uhn.ca

Clin Chest Med 35 (2014) 729–741
http://dx.doi.org/10.1016/j.ccm.2014.08.010
0272-5231/14/$ – see front matter © 2014 Elsevier Inc. All rights reserved.

remains the cornerstone of ARDS management, increased recognition of the potential for injury from mechanical ventilation itself has shifted the focus from restoring normal physiology to mitigating ventilator-induced lung injury (VILI) in ARDS. Ashbaugh and colleagues' observation that ARDS does "not respond to usual and ordinary methods of respiratory therapy" remains relevant and insightful almost 50 years later.

VENTILATOR-INDUCED LUNG INJURY

Classically, the components of VILI include: barotrauma, volutrauma, and atelectrauma. Alveolar overdistention coupled with cyclical recruitment and atelectasis are the primary causes of VILI.[8] Barotrauma is generally recognized as pneumothoraces, pneumomediastinum, and subcutaneous emphysema. The concept of volutrauma originated after animal experiments showed that lung stretch through volume rather than purely high airway pressures was the primary determinant of lung injury.[9] Atelectrauma is thought to result from ventilation at low lung volumes, causing repetitive opening and closing of lung units, altered surfactant function, and regional hypoxia.[8] Collectively, these physical forces can disrupt the epithelial barrier[10] and wound plasma membranes of alveolar cells,[11] leading to increased alveolar–capillary permeability. The resulting increase in the production of inflammatory mediators induces biotrauma at both the local tissue and systemic levels.[12]

Chiumello and colleagues[13] have been influential in framing the understanding of these physiologic descriptions of VILI from a biomechanical perspective. The forces that develop in the lung tissue that react to the transpulmonary pressure (alveolar pressure, pleural pressure) are defined as stress, while the resulting lung deformation is termed strain.[14] Because stress varies in a linear fashion with strain, the relationship of "stress = k × strain" can be translated with clinical variables to be:

$$Transpulmonary\ Pressure\ (Stress) =$$

$$Specific\ Lung\ Elastance \times \frac{\Delta Volume}{FRC\ (strain)}$$

Using this relationship and animal data, it has been conjectured that a strain of greater than 2 is harmful and thus provides clinicians with alternate monitoring parameters to avoid VILI.[15]

The evaluation of ventilatory strategies in ARDS has been directly influenced by the understanding of VILI, with the goal of minimizing VILI as much as possible. Although there are several potential

adjunctive therapies to mechanical ventilation, such as proning,[16] neuromuscular blockade,[17] and extracorporeal life support,[18] these will be discussed elsewhere in this series.

TARGETING VOLUTRAUMA—LOWERING TIDAL VOLUMES

Both pathologic evidence[19] and radiographic evidence[20] exist demonstrating the heterogeneous distribution of lung injury in patients with ARDS, with relatively more nonaerated lung in gravitationally dependent regions. The remaining aerated nondependent lung regions can be relatively small; quantitative assessment of computed tomography (CT) images measured this aerated portion to be in the order of 200–500 g in severe ARDS, the amount normally found in a healthy 5- or 6–year-old child, the so-called baby lung concept.[21] This baby lung concept, coupled with animal studies demonstrating harm after receiving mechanical ventilation with high tidal volumes,[22] helped inform the design of a number of human clinical trials that tried to reproduce this finding but led to conflicting results. In 2000, the landmark randomized controlled trial (RCT) by the ARDS Network (ARDSNet) was published, demonstrating a nearly 9% absolute risk reduction in short-term mortality with a tidal volume and plateau pressure limited (6 mL/kg predicted body weight [PBW] and 30 cm H_2O) strategy.[23] Interestingly, in addition to more patients breathing without assistance and number of ventilator-free days by day 28, a statistically significant decrease in days without nonpulmonary organ failure (15 vs 12, $P = .006$) was observed.

Subsequently, a meta-analysis including 6 RCTs (1297 patients) comparing ventilation strategies targeting a tidal volume of 7 mL/kg or less and plateau pressures of 30 cmH_2O or less versus ventilation with tidal volumes between 10 and 15 mL/kg has confirmed a significant mortality benefit at 28 days (pooled relative risk [RR] 0.74; 95% confidence interval [CI] 0.51–0.88).[24]

Despite pressure- and volume-limited ventilation becoming the standard of care, the optimal tidal volume and plateau pressure limitations are still unclear, and even strict adherence to the ARDSNet strategy may induce VILI in some patients.[25] For instance, in 30 patients ventilated with the ARDSNet strategy, quantitative CT imaging revealed that a third of these patients still underwent tidal hyperinflation of the aerated nondependent baby lung.[26] Correspondingly, bronchoalveolar lavage concentrations of inflammatory mediators were also significantly elevated in the patients who experienced tidal hyperinflation. In addition to hyperinflation, CT imaging evidence continues to demonstrate cyclic recruitment–derecruitment even at tidal volumes of 6 mL/kg PBW.[27]

In response, studies have aimed to investigate the feasibility and potential efficacy of lowering tidal volume and plateau pressure further,[25,28] with ultralung protective strategies. A pilot physiologic study using conventional mechanical ventilation in 10 patients demonstrated the ability to ventilate patients at 4 mL/kg PBW without severe respiratory acidosis or hypercapnia.[29] Extracorporeal CO_2 removal ($ECCO_2R$) strategies coupled with ultralung protective strategies have been explored but have yet to demonstrate a mortality benefit.[30,31] Therefore, despite conventionally accepted tidal volume and plateau pressure limitations, absence of VILI may not be achieved in certain groups of patients given the heterogeneity of lung parenchyma affected in ARDS.

Spontaneous Breathing

The role of spontaneous breathing efforts during ARDS is controversial, with conflicting data regarding the potential risks and benefits of spontaneous breathing (**Table 1**).[32] Although several experimental studies support the notion that spontaneous breathing in ARDS results in decreased lung injury and inflammation, others have suggested the potential for increased lung damage during spontaneous breathing.[33] Indeed, spontaneous breathing in patients with severe ARDS may induce patient–ventilator asynchrony and

rapid–shallow breathing, further potentiating atelectrauma.[34] Several experimental observations also suggest that the type of spontaneous breathing (supported vs unsupported) and the amount of inspiratory effort plays an important role in the development of VILI, particularly in patients with severe ARDS. Finally, a recent study demonstrated that local changes in transpulmonary pressure generated by diaphragmatic contraction during spontaneous breathing are not uniformly transmitted through the injured lung, but concentrated in the dependent lung.[35] This results in a pendelluft phenomenon (movement of air within the lung from nondependent to dependent regions without a change in tidal volume), which can result in hidden, local overstretch injury to the dependent lung and increased VILI.

Perhaps the most striking evidence against the potential use of early (ie, within first 48 hours) spontaneous breathing in patients with ARDS is the recent RCT demonstrating a reduction in the incidence of barotrauma (ie, pneumothorax), an increase in the number of ventilator- and intensive care unit (ICU)-free days, and a reduction in 90-day mortality with cisatracurium in patients with severe ARDS ($Pao_2/Fio_2 <120$ mm Hg) (Papazian,[17] 2010). Importantly, the benefit was observed despite the control group receiving low tidal volume ventilation with the volume/assist-control mode, with the only major difference being the ability of the patient to trigger the ventilator in the control group. These results are particularly salient given that approximately 25% of patients may be ventilated with modes that allow spontaneous

Table 1	
Potential risks and benefits of spontaneous breathing in acute respiratory distress syndrome	
Benefits	**Risks**
Increased lung aeration/recruitment	Lack of control on delivered tidal volumes
Redistribution of ventilation leading to improved ventilation–perfusion matching	Patient–ventilator dyssynchrony
Redistribution of perfusion leading to improved ventilation–perfusion matching	Spread of inflammatory mediator-laden secretions from affected lung units to unaffected lung units
Improved gas exchange	Regional (dependent lung) overdistension due to pendelluft
Prevention of ventilator-induced diaphragmatic dysfunction	Increased mortality in early, severe ARDS
Improvement in hemodynamics and organ perfusion	Adverse effects of heavy sedation/analgesia required to suppress spontaneous breathing efforts
Avoid the adverse effects of heavy sedation/analgesia required to suppress spontaneous breathing efforts	
Decreased lung damage and inflammation	*Increased lung damage and inflammation*

breathing during the first 28 hours of lung injury.[36,37] Although the mechanism by which neuromuscular blockade leads to improved outcomes is unclear, important facets may include a reduction in VILI through reduced patient–ventilator asynchrony (minimizing barotrauma and volutrauma), abrogating reverse triggering[38] and pendelluft, better control of end-expiratory pressure by preventing active expiration (decreased atelectrauma), reduced minute ventilation, and reduced cardiac output and pulmonary blood flow due to reduced oxygen consumption.[39] However, the results of this clinical trial should be interpreted cautiously, as both groups were deeply sedated; additionally, there were no significant differences in plateau pressure between groups (to help explain the difference in pneumothoraces), and there was the possibility of a direct anti-inflammatory effect of cisatracurium.

TARGETING ATELECTRAUMA AND LUNG RECRUITMENT – HIGHER VERSUS LOWER POSITIVE END-EXPIRATORY PRESSURE

Although the focus of reduced tidal volumes has been to minimize volutrauma, PEEP has been used to prevent end-expiratory collapse of unstable lung units, resulting in cyclic (tidal) recruitment–derecruitment. However, the optimal strategy for setting PEEP remains unclear.

There have been 5 RCTs examining the use of higher PEEP in patients with ARDS. Unfortunately the 2 RCTs demonstrated a significant reduction in mortality using higher PEEP also utilized higher tidal volumes (9–12 mL/kg PBW) in their control group[40,41] making it difficult to make inferences regarding the relative benefit of higher PEEP alone. Details of the other 3 RCTs, Assessment of Low Tidal Volume and Elevated End-Expiratory Lung Volume to Obviate Lung Injury (ALVEOLI),[42] Lung Open Ventilation (LOV),[43] and Expiratory Pressure (ExPress),[44] which compare different levels of PEEP, are summarized in **Table 2**.

ALVEOLI[42] was stopped early for futility after randomizing 549 patients. Even after adjustment for baseline imbalances, there was no significant difference in in-hospital mortality, or many secondary outcomes. Subsequently, 2 additional large multicenter randomized trials, ExPress[44] and LOV,[43] also did not find a survival advantage with higher PEEP. However, in all 3 studies, oxygenation (as measured by Pao_2/Fio_2 ratios) was improved in the higher PEEP group. In the ExPress and LOV trials, this translated into a decreased need for rescue therapies such as proning, inhaled nitric oxide, almitrine bismesylate, high-frequency ventilation, and extracorporeal

membrane oxygenation in the higher PEEP group (ExPress: 35 vs 19%, $P<.001$ and LOV: 12% vs 8%, $P = .05$).

Several study-level[45,46] and individual patient data meta-analyses[47] have further evaluated the association between higher PEEP strategies and mortality. Although all included ALVEOLI, ExPress, and LOV, 1 meta-analysis[45] included a fourth study that used esophageal pressure measurements to ensure a positive end-expiratory transpulmonary pressure in the experimental group.[48] Despite the differences between these meta-analyses, overall findings were relatively consistent, with nonsignificant reductions in short-term mortality with higher PEEP (RR 0.90, 95% CI 0.79–1.02),[45] (adjusted RR 0.94, 95% CI 0.86–1.04),[47] and (RR 0.90, 95% CI 0.81–1.01).[46] Among patients with greater baseline severity of ARDS (Pao_2/Fio_2 ratios $\leq$ 200), the use of higher PEEP was associated with a significant reduction in in-hospital mortality (adjusted RR 0.90, 95% CI 0.81–1.00).[47]

Together, these experiments showcase that although the unselected application of higher PEEP in ARDS may have a mortality benefit, especially in those in the moderate-to-severe category, future efforts should help delineate the individual patients who may benefit most. From physiologic principles, it stands to reason that patients with recruitable lungs may benefit more from higher PEEP, while those with nonrecruitable lungs can only experience overdistension of their baby lung.

HIGH-FREQUENCY OSCILLATORY VENTILATION

Theoretically, high-frequency oscillatory ventilation (HFOV) should be an ideal lung protective mode of ventilation. Tidal overdistension is avoided through the delivery of very small tidal volumes (1–4 mL/kg PBW),[49] while atelectrauma is avoided by maintaining relatively high mean airway pressures. As the delivered tidal volumes may be less than the anatomic dead space, the traditional concepts regarding gas exchange and alveolar ventilation may not be primarily applicable in HFOV.[50] This ability to provide minute volumes on the descending limb of the pressure–volume curve while avoiding the zones of overdistension and atelectasis makes HFOV an attractive option.

HFOV is supported by a large body of experimental animal data[51] demonstrating its effectiveness at providing adequate oxygenation and ventilation while reducing evidence of inflammation,[52] improving respiratory compliance,[53] and reducing oxidative injury.[54] Several small randomized trials using HFOV have been done in people

Table 2
Comparison of key studies investigating the effects of low and high positive end-expiratory pressure in acute respiratory distress syndrome

Study	Groups	N	Ventilation Strategy	Target Tidal Volume (mL/kg PBW)	Primary Mortality Outcome	
ALVEOLI Brower et al,[42] 2004	High	276	Higher PEEP/FiO2 ladder	6	Hospital mortality	28% vs 25%, P = .48
	Control	273	Conventional PEEP/FiO2 adder, plateau pressures $\leq$ 30 cm H_2O, no recruitment maneuvers	6		
LOV Meade et al,[43] 2008	Experimental	475	Higher PEEP/FiO2 ladder, plateau pressures $\leq$ 40 cm H_2O, recruitment maneuvers	6	Hospital mortality	36% vs 40%, P = .19
	Control	508	Conventional PEEP/FiO2 adder, plateau pressures $\leq$ 30 cm H_2O, no recruitment maneuvers	6		
ExPress Mercat et al,[44] 2008	Experimental	385	PEEP as high as possible while keeping plateau pressures <28–30 cm H_2O	6	28-d mortality	28% vs 31%, P = .31
	Control	382	Conventional PEEP to meet oxygenation goals	6		
Villar et al,[40] 2006	Experimental	50	PEEP 2 cm H_2O above Pflex or 15 cm H_2O if no Pflex,	5–8	ICU mortality	32% vs 53%, P = .04
	Control	45	PEEP >5 cm H_2O	9–11		
Amato et al,[41] 1998	Experimental	29	PEEP 2 cm H_2O above Pflex or 16 cm H_2O if no Pflex, driving pressures <20 cm H_2O, recruitment maneuvers	6	28-d mortality	38% vs 71%, P<.001
	Control	24	PEEP to optimize FiO2 <0.6 with adequate systemic oxygen delivery	12		

Abbreviation: Pflex, lower inflection point.

with conflicting results. A systematic review and meta-analysis including 6 trials (365 patients) revealed a significant reduction in short-term mortality in favor of HFOV (pooled RR 0.77, 95% CI 0.61–0.98).[52] HFOV also improved oxygenation (Pao_2/Fio_2 ratio); however, because of a concurrent rise in mean airway pressures by 22% to 33%, the oxygenation index was not significantly different. Although these results were encouraging, there was significant variability in terms of patient populations included (6 adult and 2 pediatric ICUs), duration of treatment with HFOV (patients were treated <24 hours in 2 trials), and lack of lung-protective ventilation in the conventional group (279 patients were enrolled in trials without target tidal volumes of <8 mL/kg PBW). Based upon the favorable preclinical studies and these early clinical trials, a strong rationale existed for the design and conduct of the Oscillation for Acute Respiratory Distress Syndrome Treated Early (OSCILLATE)[55] and Oscillation in ARDS (OSCAR)[56] trials (**Table 3**).

OSCILLATE was a multicenter RCT comparing HFOV and conventional ventilation in patients with moderate/severe ARDS. The HFOV protocol was based upon the results of a pilot study[57] and expert roundtable discussion.[58] Of note, the conventional ventilation protocol used a strategy adapted from the LOV trial, with PEEP values between the previous control and open lung treatment groups. Both groups underwent a recruitment maneuver after enrollment. The trial was stopped early after randomizing 548 patients. In-hospital mortality (47 vs 35%, RR 1.33, 95% CI 1.09–1.64), in-ICU mortality (RR 1.45, 95% CI 1.17–1.81), and 28-day mortality (RR 1.41, 95% CI 1.12–1.79) were all increased in the HFOV group.

The OSCAR trial was a pragmatic multicenter RCT including 795 patients in 29 hospitals in the United Kingdom comparing and usual ventilatory care in patients with moderate/severe ARDS. In contrast to OSCILLATE, the control group in OSCAR was ventilated according to local practices and while use of pressure- and volume-limited ventilation was strongly encouraged, it was not mandated nor protocolized. There was no difference in 30-day mortality between the HFOV and control groups (42 vs 41%, $P = .85$). Similarly no differences were observed for in-hospital mortality (50 vs 48%, $P = .62$) and in-ICU mortality (44% vs 42%, $P = .57$).

Several differences exist between these 2 trials. First, sicker patients were enrolled in OSCILLATE (mean APACHE II scores of 29 vs 22). Second, ventilation strategies were different both in terms of HFOV (different machines, higher mean airway pressures in OSCILLATE to target an open lung, and different experience using HFOV at baseline) and conventional ventilation (strict protocol with low tidal volumes and open lung ventilation in OSCILLATE vs usual practice in OSCAR). Several possible explanations have been proposed for the increased mortality seen in the OSCILLATE study. As suggested by the OSCILLATE authors, hemodynamic compromise from multiple causes may have been the root cause. The high mean airway pressures are known to decrease right ventricle preload[59] and cause right ventricular dysfunction.[60] Compounding this was the increased use of neuromuscular blockade and doses of vasodilating sedation/analgesia among patients in the HFOV group. Common responses to hemodynamic insults are fluid administration and use of vasopressors. Indeed, the HFOV group had a higher 24-hour fluid balance, most noticeably on Day 1 (2897 mL vs 2400 mL, $P = .06$). Although the proportion of patients requiring vasopressors was similar prior to protocol initiation (66% vs 61%), more patients randomized to the HFOV group required vasopressors on Day 0 (73% vs 62%) and Day 1 (78% vs 58%).[55] In contrast, there were no significant differences with respect to inotropic or vasopressor use between groups in the OSCAR trial.

Despite the physiologic elegance of HFOV, the current evidence cannot support the early application of HFOV in adults with moderate/severe ARDS over a conventional ventilatory strategy using low tidal volumes and high PEEP, and allowing HFOV as rescue therapy for refractory hypoxemia. As a result, clinicians could consider HFOV in select patients with severe ARDS and refractory hypoxemia with close monitoring, if there is little response in oxygenation and/or a significant deterioration in hemodynamics, HFOV should be abandoned and patients returned to conventional ventilation. Whether HFOV still has a place in the armamentarium for ARDS remains to be seen, with future studies focused on identifying patients who may have a favorable response to HFOV, and an optimized strategy for setting mean airway pressure.[61]

OPTIMIZING MECHANICAL VENTILATION – MONITORING AT THE BEDSIDE

Although guiding principles have been established for the safe and effective ventilation of patients with ARDS, it is important to note the heterogeneity of the syndrome and the variable response individual patients have to the same interventions. Since the Respiratory Management in Acute Lung Injury ARDS (ARMA) trial, there have been accumulating data suggesting that 1 size does not fit all.[62,63] Indeed, an important advance in the management of patients with ARDS may

Table 3
High frequency oscillatory ventilation for early acute respiratory distress syndrome - Comparison of Oscillation Treated Early (OSCILLATE) and Oscillation in ARDS (OSCAR) trials

Study	OSCILLATE		OSCAR	
Groups	Conventional	HFOV	Conventional	HFOV
Patients	273	275	397	398
Ventilation strategy	6 mL/kg PBW tidal volume, high PEEP, plateau pressure ≤35 cm H$_2$O	Mean airway pressure as per Fio$_2$/ mean airway pressure ladder, highest possible frequency with pH >7.25	Local practice	Mean airway pressure and Fio$_2$ according to algorithm, highest, highest possible frequency with pH >7.25
Duration of mechanical ventilation before randomization (days)	1.9 ± 2.3	2.5 ± 3.3	2.1 ± 2.1	2.2 ± 2.3
APACHE II	29 ± 7	29 ± 8	22 ± 6	22 ± 6
Pao$_2$:Fio$_2$ ratio (mm Hg)	114 ± 38	121 ± 46	113 ± 38	113 ± 37
Day 1 tidal volume (mL/kg PBW)	6.1 ± 1.3		8.3 ± 2.9	
Day 1 plateau pressure (conventional) or mean airway pressures (HFOV)	32 ± 6	31 ± 3	31 ± 11	27 ± 6
Short-term mortality (conventional vs HFOV)	29% vs 40%, P = .004		41% vs 42%, P = .85	

All values are mean (±standard deviation) unless otherwise specified.
Abbreviation: APACHE, Acute Physiology and Chronic Health Evaluation.

include approaches to individualize mechanical ventilation strategies in recognition of the heterogeneous ARDS phenotype.

Lung Mechanics

Lung mechanical measurements, such as the pressure–volume (PV) curve, may help guide PEEP titration. In patients with ARDS, the PV curve exhibits sigmoid inspiratory and expiratory limbs separated by hysteresis.[64] On the inspiratory limb, the lower inflection point is felt to represent opening pressure of the collapsed lung and therefore the interface between lung recruitment and derecruitment.[65] The upper inflection point is felt to represent airway pressures at which overdistension occurs. Logically, it follows that 1 strategy would be to set PEEP above the lower inflection point while limiting plateau pressures below the upper infection point.[66] Unfortunately, the construction of PV curves using either traditional (eg, supersyringe) or contemporary ventilator-automated techniques (eg, pressure ramping) requires deep sedation and often paralysis.[67] Even after obtaining a PV curve, there is considerable inter- and intraobserver variability in the determination of key values such as the lower inflection point.[68] Attempts to compare the idealized PV curve (ie, with identifiable upper and lower inflection points) with CT imaging have shown that in a heterogeneously affected lung such as that seen in ARDS, the constructed PV curves only reflect the residual healthy zones of lung.[69] As well, given that PEEP by definition is a pressure at end-expiration used to prevent alveolar derecruitment, it does not necessarily interact with the lower inflection point of the inspiratory arm of a PV curve.[70] Consequently, alveolar derecruitment associated with PEEP decrements can be seen across a wide range of pressures rather than focused at the lower inflection point.[71] In the heterogeneously injured lung, the closing pressures will differ across the spectrum of alveoli, from the most severely injured and densely consolidated alveolus in the dependent lung zones, to the relatively spared and aerated alveolus close to the sternum. Despite a meta-analysis[72] showing a marked improvement in overall survival (odds ratio [OR] 2.7, 95% CI 1.5–4.9), when using PV curves to guide PEEP titration, this conclusion is limited by the lack of any RCTs using PV curve-guided PEEP titrations with low tidal volume ventilation in both treatment and control groups. The true utility of PV curves may be in quantifying alveolar recruitment through plotting multiple PV curves at different PEEP levels for each individual together and assessing the volume shift between different PEEP levels for the same airway pressure.[73]

Esophageal Pressure Monitoring and Transpulmonary Pressure

An alternative approach has centered on titration of PEEP guided by transpulmonary pressures (P_L). Defined as the pressure at the airway opening (P_{aw}) minus the pleural pressure (P_{pl}), esophageal pressure (P_{es}) monitoring has been used as a surrogate for the more difficult to measure pleural pressure. Unfortunately, the validity of this relationship has been questioned because of controversy regarding the underlying assumptions. Under ideal circumstances, P_{es} can serve as an estimate of pleural pressure at midlung height (where the catheter is positioned), as there is a cranial–caudal gradient of P_{pl} (as a function of gravity).[74] Absolute values of P_{es} can be affected by many factors such as the weight of the mediastinal structures, the abdomen, tension across the esophageal smooth muscle wall, and asymmetry of lung disease.[75] P_{es} monitoring in patients with ARDS demonstrated marked variability across patients.[76] Interestingly, although P_{es} was not correlated with body mass index (BMI), there was a weak correlation with chest wall stiffness at end inflation (R2 = 0.43, $P<.0001$) as well as gastric pressures (R2 = 0.354, $P<.0001$). These results confirm that P_L can be affected by chest wall compliance and intra-abdominal pressures, and the strength of these correlations necessitates actual measurements of P_{es}.

Although the use of esophageal pressures as a surrogate of pleural pressures may be inaccurate in supine mechanically ventilated patients with injured lungs,[77] artifacts introduced may not be large enough to negate the usefulness of the measurement. To that end, Talmor and colleagues[48] designed a small single-center pilot RCT comparing esophageal balloon-guided versus conventional mechanical ventilation in patients with ARDS. Importantly, in approximately one-third of patients, the esophageal balloon could not be successfully inserted into the stomach, and esophageal placement was confirmed by noting pressure changes in response to tidal ventilation and cardiac artifact. Within the esophageal pressure group, PEEP was set to maintain a positive transpulmonary pressure of 0 to 10 cm H_2O at end expiration. Although tidal volumes were limited to keep P_L at less than 25 H_2O at end inspiration, the initial setting of 6 mL/kg PBW never had to be reduced for this rule. The control group was ventilated according to the low tidal volume strategy used in ARMA. The study was stopped after enrolling 61 patients after an interim analysis met prespecified stopping criteria. Patients randomized to the esophageal pressure group had significantly higher PEEP (17 vs 10, $P<.001$), higher Pao_2/Fio_2 ratios (280 vs 191, $P = .002$), and better respiratory system compliance (45 vs 35, $P = .005$) at 72 hours. Interestingly, although patients in the esophageal pressure group had higher set PEEP overall, changes to PEEP on Day 1 based upon measured P_{es} resulted in a greater range of adjustments than following the ARDSNet protocol. As a pilot study not powered to detect clinical outcomes, none reached statistical significance; however, there was a trend toward 28-day mortality benefit (17 vs 39%, $P = .055$) and 180 day mortality benefit (27 vs 45%, $P = .13$) favoring the esophageal pressure group. No differences were observed for length of ICU stay, ICU-free days at 28 days, ventilator-free days at 28 days, and days of ventilation among survivors. Building on these encouraging results, the multicenter phase 2 EPVent2 study (Esophageal-Pressure Guided Mechanical Ventilation) is currently underway (ClinicalTrials.gov NCT01681225).

Imaging—Computed Tomography and Electrical Impedance Tomography

Imaging has been linked to the diagnosis of ARDS since the initial description by Ashbaugh. CT has greatly improved the understanding of the morphologic features and distribution of parenchymal changes in ARDS.[78,79] Moreover, through comparison of tissue densities representing derecruited dense lung zones, recruited aerated lung zones, and hypodense areas of hyperinflation under different airway pressures, CT has now shown promise in determining the potential for lung recruitment and titration of PEEP[80] and to monitor VILI through quantification of repeated recruitment/derecruitment as well as hyperinflation.[81] Concerns regarding the cumulative risk of radiation exposure with serial CT scans to guide mechanical ventilation have prompted research demonstrating that even low-dose CT (70% reduction in effective dose) can provide accurate quantitative results.[82] However, the practical limitations of moving critically ill patients to obtain serial CT scans makes newer, bedside imaging modalities increasingly attractive.

Electrical impedance tomography (EIT) is a noninvasive, radiation-free method to monitor regional ventilation on a breath-to-breath basis at the bedside. Measured through electrode pairs applied around the thorax, impedance changes are related to tidal volume through complex mathematical algorithms relying on the principle that gas is an electrical insulator when compared to blood and lung tissue.[83] Small studies with EIT have demonstrated value in monitoring recruitment during slow inflation maneuvers,[84] measuring potentially recruitable lung volume,[85] and assessing regional lung recruitment/derecruitment during incremental and decremental PEEP trials.[86] The use of EIT during spontaneous efforts in mechanically ventilated patients has also allowed investigators to detect VILI, with the observation of occult pendelluft that was not easily detected by other readily available means by the clinician.[35] Although EIT represents a promising noninvasive imaging modality that can aid in the tailoring of mechanical ventilation at the individual level, no experimentally validated approach has been indentified thus far. Several small clinical trials ranging from feasibility studies (NCT01272882) to pilot interventional trials (NCT02056977, NCT01326208) are currently underway, and their results will be useful for the evaluation of this technology.

Novel work by Gattinoni's group investigated the relationship between different bedside PEEP titration strategies and their relationship to lung recruitability as assessed by CT imaging and severity of ARDS.[87] From current understanding, an optimal strategy should provide lower PEEP targets to patients with low recruitability to prevent overdistention and higher PEEP targets to patients with high recruitability to prevent atelectrauma. Multiple PEEP titration strategies based upon lung mechanics (ExPress and Stress Index), esophageal pressure, and oxygenation (LOV) were included. Surprisingly, only the expert-opinion derived $PEEP/Fio_2$ table from the LOV study weakly correlated target PEEP with lung recruitability ($r^2 = 0.29$, $P<.0001$); the more physiologically derived strategies arrived at similar PEEP targets across the spectrum of lung recruitability and severity of ARDS. Interpretation of these findings needs to be tempered with the reminder that although there is a weak correlation between the LOV strategy and lung recruitability, this does not necessarily result in any significant effects on clinically important outcomes such as mortality. Whether this is a reflection on the relative value of using recruitability to guide PEEP titrations remains unclear. RCTs, possibly incorporating other methods of bedside monitoring such as EIT, may improve understanding of the role of lung recruitability in managing ARDS.

SUMMARY

Contemporary use of mechanical ventilation in patients with ARDS has evolved steadily since its original description by Ashbaugh and colleagues in 1967. More recently, the desire to move ventilatory support in these patients beyond low tidal volumes has sparked many promising approaches.

Unfortunately, despite sound physiologic rationale and encouraging preclinical evidence, many interventions have not translated into the improvements in patient-important outcome that were envisioned. Therefore until further evidence arises, a ventilatory strategy focused on minimizing VILI, with low tidal volumes and an open lung strategy employing increased PEEP, while targeting modest physiologic goals should represent the standard of care in the ventilatory management of ARDS.

REFERENCES

1. Ashbaugh DG, Bigelow DB, Petty TL, et al. Acute respiratory distress in adults. Lancet 1967;ii:319–23.
2. Herridge MS, Tansey CM, Matte A, et al. Functional disability 5 years after acute respiratory distress syndrome. N Engl J Med 2011;364:1293–304.
3. Fan E, Dowdy DW, Colantuoni E, et al. Physical complications in acute lung injury survivor: a 2-year longitudinal prospective study. Crit Care Med 2013;42(4):849–59.
4. Phua J, Badia JR, Adhikari NK, et al. Has mortality from acute respiratory distress syndrome decreased over time?: a systematic review. Am J Respir Crit Care Med 2009;179:220–7.
5. The ARDS definition task force. Acute respiratory distress syndrome. JAMA 2012;307:3526–33.
6. Ferguson ND, Fan E, Camporota L, et al. The Berlin definition of ARDS: an expanded rationale, justification, and supplementary material. Intensive Care Med 2012;38:1573–82.
7. Stapleton RD, Wang BM, Hudson JD, et al. Causes and timing of death in patients with ARDS. Chest 2005;128:525–32.
8. Slutsky AS, Ranieri VM. Ventilator-induced lung injury. N Engl J Med 2013;369:2126–36.
9. Dreyfuss D, Soler P, Basset G, et al. High inflation pressure pulmonary edema: respective effects of high airway pressure, high tidal volume, and positive end-expiratory pressure. Am Rev Respir Dis 1988;137:1159–64.
10. Cavanaugh KJ Jr, Margulies SS. Measurement of stretch-induced loss of alveolar epithelial barrier integrity with a novel in vitro method. Am J Physiol Cell Physiol 2002;283:C1801–8.
11. Vlahakis NE, Hubmayr RD. Cellular stress failure in ventilator-injured lungs. Am J Respir Crit Care Med 2005;171:1328–42.
12. Tremblay LN, Slutsky AS. Ventilator-induced injury: from barotrauma to biotrauma. Proc Assoc Am Physicians 1998;110:482–8.
13. Chiumello D, Carlesso E, Cadringher P, et al. Lung stress and strain during mechanical ventilation for acute respiratory distress syndrome. Am J Respir Crit Care Med 2008;178:346–55.
14. Gattinoni L, Protti A, Caironi P, et al. Ventilator-induced lung injury: the anatomical and physiological framework. Crit Care Med 2010;38(10 Suppl): S539–48.
15. Protti A, Cressoni M, Santini A, et al. Lung stress and strain during mechanical ventilation: any safe threshold? Am J Respir Crit Care Med 2011;183: 1354–62.
16. Guerin C, Reignier J, Richard JC, et al. Prone positioning in severe acute respiratory distress syndrome. N Engl J Med 2013;368:2159–68.
17. Papazian L, Forel JM, Gacouin A, et al. Neuromuscular blockers in early acute respiratory distress syndrome. N Engl J Med 2010;363:1107–16.
18. Sorbo LD, Cypel M, Fan E. Extracorporeal life support for acute respiratory failure. Lancet Respir Med 2014;2:154–64.
19. Thille AW, Esteban A, Fernandez-Segoviano P, et al. Chronology of histological lesions in acute respiratory distress syndrome with diffuse alveolar damage: a prospective cohort study of clinical autopsies. Lancet Respir Med 2013;1:395–401.
20. Maunder RJ, Shuman WP, McHugh JW, et al. Preservation of normal lung regions in the adult respiratory distress syndrome. Analysis by computed tomography. JAMA 1986;255:2463–5.
21. Gattinoni L, Pesenti A. The concept of the "baby lung". Intensive Care Med 2005;31:776–84.
22. Kolobow T, Moretti MP, Fumagalli R, et al. Severe impairment in lung function induced by high peak airway pressure during mechanical ventilation. An experimental study. Am Rev Respir Dis 1987;135: 312–5.
23. The acute respiratory distress syndrome network. Ventilation with lower tidal volumes as compared with traditional tidal volumes for acute lung injury and the acute respiratory distress syndrome. N Engl J Med 2000;342:1301–8.
24. Petrucci N, De Feo C. Lung protective ventilation strategy for the acute respiratory distress syndrome. Cochrane Database Syst Rev 2013;(2):CD003844.
25. Hager DN, Krishnan JA, Hayden DL, et al. Tidal volume reduction in patients with acute lung injury when plateau pressures are not high. Am J Respir Crit Care Med 2005;172:1241–5.
26. Terragni PP, Rosboch G, Tealdi A, et al. Tidal hyperinflation during low tidal volume ventilation in acute respiratory distress syndrome. Am J Respir Crit Care Med 2007;175:160–6.
27. Bruhn A, Bugedo D, Riquelme F, et al. Tidal volume is a major determinant of cyclic recruitment-derecruitment in acute respiratory distress syndrome. Minerva Anestesiol 2011;4:418–26.
28. Needham DM, Colantuoni E, Mendez-Tellez PA, et al. Lung protective mechanical ventilation and two year survival in patients with acute lung injury: prospective cohort study. BMJ 2012;344:e2124.

29. Retamal J, Libuy J, Jimenez M, et al. Preliminary study of ventilation with 4 mL/kg tidal volume in acute respiratory distress syndrome: feasibility and effects on cyclic recruitment–derecruitment and hyperinflation. Crit Care 2013;17:R16.

30. Terragni PP, Del Sorbo L, Mascia L, et al. Tidal volume lower than 6 mL/kg enhances lung protection. Anesthesiology 2009;111:826–35.

31. Bein T, Weber-Carstens W, Goldmann A, et al. Lower tidal volume strategy (3 mL/kg) combined with extracorporeal CO_2 removal versus 'conventional' protective ventilation (6 mL/kg) in severe ARDS. Intensive Care Med 2013;39:847–56.

32. Gama de Abreu M, Guldner A, Pelosi P. Spontaneous breathing activity in acute lung injury and acute respiratory distress syndrome. Curr Opin Anaesthesiol 2012;25:148–55.

33. Henzler D, Hochhausen N, Bensberg R, et al. Effects of preserved spontaneous breathing activity during mechanical ventilation in experimental intra-abdominal hypertension. Intensive Care Med 2010;36:1427–35.

34. Thille AW, Rodriguez P, Cabello B, et al. Patient-ventilator asynchrony during assisted mechanical ventilation. Intensive Care Med 2006;32:1515–22.

35. Yoshida T, Torsani V, Gomes S, et al. Spontaneous effort causes occult pendelluft during mechanical ventilation. Am J Respir Crit Care Med 2013;188:1420–7.

36. Esteban A, Ferguson ND, Meade MO, et al. Evolution of mechanical ventilation in response to clinical research. Am J Respir Crit Care Med 2008;177:170–7.

37. Esteban A, Frutos-Vivar F, Muriel A, et al. Evolution of mortality over time in patients receiving mechanical ventilation. Am J Respir Crit Care Med 2013;188:220–30.

38. Akoumianaki E, Lyazidi A, Rey N, et al. Mechanical ventilation-induced reverse-triggered breaths: a frequently unrecognized form of neuromechanical coupling. Chest 2013;143:927–38.

39. Slutsky AS. Neuromuscular blocking agents in ARDS. N Engl J Med 2010;363:1176–80.

40. Villar J, Kacmarek RM, Perez-Mendez L, et al. A high positive end-expiratory pressure, low tidal volume ventilatory strategy improves outcomes in persistent acute respiratory distress syndrome: a randomized, controlled trial. Crit Care Med 2006;34:1311–8.

41. Amato MB, Barbas CS, Medeiros DM, et al. Effect of a protective-ventilation strategy on mortality in the acute respiratory distress syndrome. N Engl J Med 1998;338:347–54.

42. Brower RG, Lanken PN, MacIntyre N, et al. Higher versus lower positive end-expiratory pressures in patients with the acute respiratory distress syndrome. N Engl J Med 2004;351:327–36.

43. Meade MO, Cook DJ, Guyatt GH, et al. Ventilation strategy using low tidal volumes, recruitment maneuvers, and high positive end-expiratory pressure for acute lung injury and acute respiratory distress syndrome: a randomized controlled trial. JAMA 2008;299:637–45.

44. Mercat A, Richard JC, Vielle B, et al. Positive end-expiratory pressure setting in adults with acute lung injury and acute respiratory distress syndrome: a randomized controlled trial. JAMA 2008;299:646–55.

45. Dasenbrook EC, Needham DM, Brower RG, et al. Higher PEEP in patients with acute lung injury: a systematic review and meta-analysis. Respir Care 2011;56:568–75.

46. Cruz RS, Rojas JI, Nervi R, et al. High versus low positive end-expiratory pressure (PEEP) levels for mechanically ventilated adult patients with acute lung injury and acute respiratory distress syndrome. Cochrane Database Syst Rev 2013;(6):CD009098.

47. Briel M, Meade M, Mercat A, et al. Higher vs lower positive end-expiratory pressure in patients with acute lung injury and acute respiratory distress syndrome: systematic review and meta-analysis. JAMA 2010;303:865–73.

48. Talmor D, Sarge T, Malhotra A, et al. Mechanical ventilation guided by esophageal pressure in acute lung injury. N Engl J Med 2008;359:2095–104.

49. Hager DN, Fessler HE, Kaczka DW, et al. Tidal volume delivery during high-frequency oscillatory ventilation in adults with acute respiratory distress syndrome. Crit Care Med 2007;35:1522–0.

50. Slutsky AS, Drazen JM. Ventilation with small tidal volumes. N Engl J Med 2002;347:630–1.

51. Ferguson ND, Villar J, Slutsky AS. Understanding high-frequency oscillation: lessons from the animal kingdom. Intensive Care Med 2007;33:1316–8.

52. Muellenbach RM, Kredel M, Said HM, et al. High-frequency oscillatory ventilation reduces lung inflammation: a large -animal 24-h model of respiratory distress. Intensive Care Med 2007;33:1423–33.

53. Imai Y, Nakagawa S, Ito Y, et al. Comparison of lung protection strategies using conventional and high-frequency oscillatory ventilation. J Appl Physiol (1985) 2001;91:1836–44.

54. Rotta AT, Gunnarsson B, Fuhrman BP, et al. Comparison of lung protective ventilation strategies in a rabbit model of acute lung injury. Crit Care Med 2001;29:2176–84.

55. Ferguson ND, Cook DJ, Guyatt GH, et al. High-frequency oscillation in early acute respiratory distress syndrome. N Engl J Med 2013;368:795–805.

56. Young DM, Lamb SE, Shah S, et al. High-frequency oscillation for acute respiratory distress syndrome. N Engl J Med 2013;368:806–13.

57. Ferguson ND, Chiche JD, Kacmarek RM, et al. Combining high-frequency oscillatory ventilation and recruitment maneuvers in adults with early acute respiratory distress syndrome: the Treatment with Oscillation and an Open Lung Strategy (TOOLS) Trial pilot study. Crit Care Med 2005;33: 479–86.

58. Fessler HE, Derdak S, Ferguson ND, et al. A protocol for high-frequency oscillatory ventilation in adults: results from a roundtable discussion. Crit Care Med 2007;35:1649–54.

59. Fougeres E, Teboul JL, Richard C, et al. Hemodynamic impact of a positive end-expiratory pressure setting in acute respiratory distress syndrome: importance of the volume status. Crit Care Med 2010;38:802–7.

60. Guervilly C, Forel JM, Hraiech S, et al. Right ventricular function during high-frequency oscillatory ventilation in adults with acute respiratory distress syndrome. Crit Care Med 2012;40:1539–45.

61. Malhotra A, Drazen JM. High-frequency oscillatory ventilation on shaky ground. N Engl J Med 2013; 368:863–5.

62. Dean KJ, Minneci P, Cui X, et al. Mechanical ventilation in ARDS: one size does not fit all. Crit Care Med 2005;33:1141–3.

63. Brower R, Thompson BT. Tidal volumes in acute respiratory distress syndrome—one size does not fit all. Crit Care Med 2006;34:263–4.

64. Hata JS, Simmons JS, Kuma AB, et al. The acute effectiveness and safety of the constant-flow, pressure-volume curve to improve hypoxemia in acute lung injury. J Intensive Care Med 2012;27: 119–27.

65. Brochard L. Respiratory pressure-volume curves. In: Tobin MJ, editor. Principles and practice of intensive care monitoring. New York: McGraw-Hill; 1998. p. 579–616.

66. Artigas A, Bernard GB, Carlet J, et al. The American–European Consensus Conference on ARDS, part 2. Ventilatory, pharmacologic, supportive therapy, study design strategies, and issues related to recovery and remodeling. Am J Respir Crit Care Med 1998;157:1332–47.

67. Piacentini E, Wysocki M, Blanch L. A new automated method versus continuous positive airway pressure method for measuring pressure-volume curves in patients with acute lung injury. Intensive Care Med 2009;35:565–70.

68. Harris RS, Hess DR, Venegas JG. An objective analysis of the pressure-volume curve in the acute respiratory distress syndrome. Am J Respir Crit Care Med 2000;161:432–9.

69. Gattinoni L, Pesenti A, Avalli L, et al. Pressure-volume curve of total respiratory system in acute respiratory failure. Computed tomographic scan study. Am Rev Respir Dis 1987;136:730–6.

70. Maggiore SM, Richard JC, Brochard L. What has been learnt from P/V curves in patients with acute lung injury/acute respiratory distress syndrome. Eur Respir J 2003;22:22s–6s.

71. Maggiore S, Jonson B, Richard JC, et al. Alveolar derecruitment at decremental positive end-expiratory pressure levels in acute lung injury. Comparison with the lower inflection point, oxygenation, and compliance. Am J Respir Crit Care Med 2001;164:795–801.

72. Hata JS, Togashi K, Kumar AB, et al. The effect of the pressure-volume curve for positive end-expiratory pressure titration on clinical outcomes in acute respiratory distress syndrome: a systematic review. J Intensive Care Med 2013. [Epub ahead of print].

73. Ranieri VM, Eissa NT, Corbeil C, et al. Effects of positive end-expiratory pressure on alveolar recruitment and gas exchange in patients with the adult respiratory distress syndrome. Am Rev Respir Dis 1991;144:544–51.

74. Pelosi P, Goldner M, McKibben A, et al. Recruitment and derecruitment during acute respiratory failure: an experimental study. Am J Respir Crit Care Med 2001;164:122–30.

75. Akoumianaki E, Maggiore SM, Valenza F, et al. The application of esophageal pressure measurement in patients with respiratory failure. Am J Respir Crit Care Med 2014;185:520–31.

76. Talmor D, Sarge T, O'Donnell CR, et al. Esophageal and transpulmonary pressures in acute respiratory failure. Crit Care Med 2006;34:1389–94.

77. de Chazal I, Hubmayr RD. Novel aspects of pulmonary mechanics in intensive care. Br J Anaesth 2004;91:81–91.

78. Gattinoni L, Bombino M, Pelosi P, et al. Lung structure and function in different stages of severe adult respiratory distress syndrome. JAMA 1994;271: 1772–9.

79. Goodman LR, Fumagalli R, Tagliabue P, et al. Adult respiratory distress syndrome due to pulmonary and extra pulmonary causes: CT, clinical, and functional correlations. Radiology 1999;213:545–52.

80. Gattinoni L, Caironi P, Cressoni M, et al. Lung recruitment in patients with the acute respiratory distress syndrome. N Engl J Med 2006;354: 1775–86.

81. David M, Karmrodt J, Bletz C, et al. Analysis of atelectasis, ventilated, and hyperinflated lung during mechanical ventilation by dynamic CT. Chest 2005;128:3757–70.

82. Vecchi V, Langer T, Bellomi M, et al. Low-dose CT for quantitative analysis in acute respiratory distress syndrome. Crit Care 2013;17:R183.

83. Muders T, Leupschen M, Putensen C. Impedance tomography as a new monitoring technique. Curr Opin Crit Care 2010;16:269–75.

84. Wrigge H, Zinserling J, Muders T, et al. Electrical impedance tomography compared with thoracic computed tomography during a slow inflation maneuver in experimental models of lung injury. Crit Care Med 2008;36:903–9.

85. Lowhagen K, Lindgren S, Odenstedt H, et al. A new non-radiological method to assess potential lung recruitability: a pilot study in ALI patients. Acta Anaesthesiol Scand 2011;55:165–74.

86. Meier T, Luepschen H, Karsten J, et al. Assessment of regional lung recruitment and derecruitment during a PEEP trial based on electrical impedance tomography. Intensive Care Med 2008;34:543–50.

87. Chiumello D, Cressoni M, Carlesso E, et al. Bedside selection of positive end-expiratory pressure in mild, moderate, and severe acute respiratory distress syndrome. Crit Care Med 2014;42: 252–64.

Prone Positioning for Acute Respiratory Distress Syndrome

 CrossMark

Alexander B. Benson, MD[a,b], Richard K. Albert, MD[a,b],*

KEYWORDS

- Prone position • Acute respiratory distress syndrome • Ventilator-induced lung injury • Hypoxemia

KEY POINTS

- Prone positioning can be applied safely to most patients with acute respiratory distress syndrome (ARDS).
- Prone positioning when applied early for an appropriate duration improves mortality in ARDS and should be used in most patients with moderate/severe ARDS.
- The mechanism by which prone ventilation reduces mortality in ARDS is likely a reduction in ventilator-induced lung injury.
- Prone positioning in patients with ARDS also improves oxygenation when compared with supine positioning.
- A protocolized approach to application of prone ventilation in ARDS reduces potential complications and maximizes benefit.

HISTORY

The benefits of prone positioning were first theorized in 1974 from studies on the effects of sedation and paralysis on the diaphragm.[1] However, the deleterious effects of supine ventilation were noted as early as the 1940s.[2,3] In 1976, Piehl and Brown[4] described marked improvement in oxygenation in 5 patients with hypoxemic respiratory failure, and a year later, Douglas and Finlayson,[5] reported similar findings in 6 individuals and also found that oxygenation worsened after turning patients back to the supine position in most instances. Despite these promising reports, no additional clinical or mechanistic studies on prone positioning were published for the next decade. In 1987, Albert and colleagues[6] used a model of acute lung injury (ALI), replicated the improvement in gas exchange that had been seen in humans, measured shunt using the multiple inert gas technique, and showed that it decreased from a mean of 23% supine to 8% prone and that the improvement occurred without changes in cardiac output, pulmonary vascular pressure, regional perfusion distribution, end-expiratory lung volume, or regional diaphragmatic movement (**Fig. 1**).

Since these initial clinical and physiologic findings, multiple animal and human studies have shown that prone positioning improves oxygenation and reduces ventilator-induced lung injury (VILI) in the setting of ALI or acute respiratory distress syndrome (ARDS). In this article, the physiologic changes explaining the improvement in oxygenation are reviewed, how prone positioning

Funding Sources: National Institutes of Health K23 HL108991 (Dr A.B. Benson); NHLBI 1 U10 HL074409-01; NHLBI-HR-06-07 (Dr R.K. Albert).
Conflict of Interest: None.
[a] University of Colorado, 12605 E, 16th avenue, Aurora, CO 80045, USA; [b] Department of Medicine, Denver Health, 777 Bannock, MC 4000, Denver, CO 80204-4507, USA
* Corresponding author. Department of Medicine, Denver Health, 777 Bannock, MC 4000, Denver, CO 80204-4507.
E-mail address: ralbert@dhha.org

Clin Chest Med 35 (2014) 743–752
http://dx.doi.org/10.1016/j.ccm.2014.08.011
0272-5231/14/$ – see front matter © 2014 Elsevier Inc. All rights reserved.

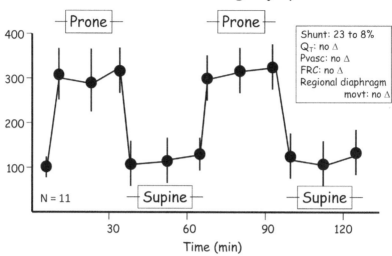

Fig. 1. Changes in oxygenation and pulmonary physiology between prone and supine positions in dogs with oleic acid induced lung injury. FRC, functional residual capacity; Movt, movement; Pvasc, pulmonary artery pressures; Qt, pulmonary blood flow. (*Data from* Albert RK, Leasa D, Sanderson M, et al. The prone position improves arterial oxygenation and reduces shunt in oleic-acid-induced acute lung injury. Am Rev Respir Dis 1987;135(3):628–33.)

reduces VILI is described, randomized controlled trials of prone ventilation in patients with ARDS are evaluated, the complications associated with prone ventilation are summarized, suggestions are made as to how these might be reduced or avoided, and when prone ventilation should start and stop and for what duration it should be used are discussed.

PHYSIOLOGIC RATIONALE

Multiple anatomic and physiologic changes take place when changing from supine to prone. These changes affect both normal and diseased lungs, but the consequences are more pronounced in the setting of atelectasis or conditions that predispose to atelectasis (eg, anesthesia, obesity, sedation, paralysis, abdominal distension).

Mechanism Behind Improvements in Oxygenation

Both observational studies and randomized trials have shown that oxygenation improves in 66% to 75% of patients with ARDS who are turned from supine to prone.[7]

Regional changes in perfusion
Computed tomography (CT) imaging and autopsy studies indicate that atelectasis preferentially develops and is more extensive in the dorsal caudal portions of the lung when normal individuals and patients with ALI/ARDS are supine. To the extent that these regions receive perfusion (Q) low ventilation-to-perfusion areas or shunt result. It was initially hypothesized that the mechanism of improved oxygenation on turning prone was the redistribution of Q to the better ventilated ventral lung in response to the change in the directional effect of gravity. However, Wiener and colleagues[8] reported that the increasing Q gradient from ventral to dorsal lungs changed little on turning from supine to prone (ie, dorsal lung regions continued to receive the greatest fraction of the perfusion, regardless of whether the animals were supine or prone). This finding has been confirmed by many others, resulting in revisions in the zonal perfusion distribution theory, which was previously used to explain regional Q variations.[9] In addition, Weiner and colleagues[8] also found that regional edema resulting from lung injury was uniformly distributed throughout the lung, regardless of position.

Regional changes in ventilation/recruitment
If shunt decreases but regional perfusion remains unchanged on turning from supine to prone, then, the regional distribution of ventilation must be changing. Measurements of regional pleural pressure (Ppl) in animals and estimates in normal individuals indicate that Ppl is more negative in nondependent regions and less negative (or even positive) in dependent regions, with a gravitational Ppl gradient in normal lungs of approximately

0.5 cm H_2O/cm distance.[10–13] This gradient is the same in the upright, supine, and right and left lateral decubitus positions. However, in the prone position, the gradient is almost zero, because of the reduction in lung distortion that occurs on turning prone.[10–14] This factor translates to less atelectasis in dorsal regions, and because most of the perfusion continues to be distributed to these regions even when they are in the nondependent position, shunt decreases, and regions of low V/Q ratios are reduced.

Positional differences in distortion result from several factors, including the generally triangular shape of the lung in the ventral-dorsal plane (**Fig. 2**), the heart mass and mediastinal mass that compress the dorsal lung in the supine position, but not when prone, and differences in the shapes of the ventral and dorsal portions of the diaphragm in the 2 positions (with large portions of the dorsal lung being compressed by abdominal contents when supine, but not when prone, and only small portions of ventral lung being affected by abdominal pressure when turning prone).

In the occasional patient (perhaps 1 in 15 or 20), turning prone results in immediate and copious drainage of airspace liquid. This factor may also contribute to the improvement in gas exchange and occurs as a result of the reversal to a downward angle of the central airways and of airways serving the dorsal lung when turning prone, favoring drainage of the liquid by gravity.

Effect on Ventilator-Induced Lung Injury

VILI is attributed to 1 of 2 mechanisms that are not mutually exclusive: alveolar overdistension and cyclical airspace opening and closing. Overdistension can result from very negative Ppls, which can occur in ventral lung regions in response to high end-inspiratory lung volumes or to gravitational stresses resulting from the weight of more dorsal regions, or throughout the lung in any region because of heterogeneity in alveolar distension that occurs as a result of heterogeneous atelectasis.[15] Low tidal volume ventilation reduces overdistension occurring from any of these mechanisms. Overdistension from either of these problems cannot be reliably excluded by global measurements of pulmonary mechanics, but both problems are reduced by prone positioning, the former resulting from the decrease in Ppl that occurs in nondependent lung regions (ie, Ppl becoming less negative) and the latter because of the reduction in dorsal lung atelectasis as Ppl in this region becomes less positive.[11]

The second proposed mechanism of VILI is cyclical airspace opening and closing, resulting in intra-airway shear forces that injure airway epithelial cells.[16] Much has been written about the concept of opening the lung and keeping it open after the idea was first coined by Berkhard Lachman in 1992.[17] If all airways could remain open at end exhalation, this mechanism of VILI would be eliminated. There is substantial heterogeneity with respect to airway opening and closing pressures to the extent that very large levels of positive end-expiratory pressure (PEEP) are needed to ensure that all airways are open at end exhalation.[16,18] In addition, low tidal volume ventilation administered with the idea of reducing overdistension, to the extent that hysteresis contributes to lung mechanics, limits the ability to open collapsed airways. Continuous low tidal volume ventilation can also limit surfactant release from type 2 pneumocytes and thereby increase airway closure. However, prone positioning reduces some of the forces contributing to airway closure and partially accomplishes the objective of maintaining airway patency without additional PEEP.

A

Triangular Shape of the Lung

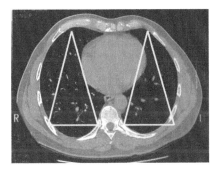

B

Effect of Lung Weight on Regional Lung Distension

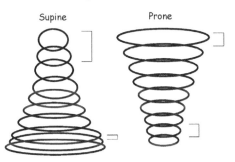

Fig. 2. (*A*) Triangular shape of the lung in the transverse plane. (*B*) The triangular shape of the lung represented by springs. Prone positioning leads to more homogenous end-expiratory lung volume.

Studies in several species show less VILI when animals are ventilated in the prone position.[19–21] Although there is no way to document the mechanism by which prone ventilation decreases mortality in humans, studies do indicate that the improved survival seen in patients with ARDS who are ventilated prone is not related to changes in Pao_2, the P/F ratio or the $Paco_2$, the Fio_2, or the level of PEEP.[22]

CLINICAL STUDIES

Most human clinical trials have reported that prone ventilation improves oxygenation in most (but not all) patients with ARDS (ie, 60%–70%). These benefits can, on occasion, be maintained after returning the patient to the supine position after a few hours but are more frequently lost on turning supine, requiring that prone ventilation be continued longer.

The first 4 randomized trials found that, despite improvements in oxygenation, prone ventilation had no effect on mortality. However, each of these trials was limited by problems with study design, sample size, or methods of analysis.

The first study published by Gattinoni and colleagues[23] enrolled patients with ALI or ARDS (ie, P/F <300). Problems with this study include the fact that prone ventilation was performed for only ~7 hours each day, and only for 10 days, and many of the patients were studied late in the course of their ARDS/ALI (ie, 25% had decubiti at the time of enrollment). This factor would likely bias the study against finding a significant mortality difference, in that prone positioning is less likely to reverse lung distortions in patients in the fibrotic versus the exudative phase of ARDS. In addition, no ventilator or weaning protocols were used, and the levels of PEEP and Fio_2 were kept constant, despite improvements in Pao_2, which would negate any possible effect of PEEP or Fio_2 on mortality (although subsequent studies indicate that changes in these variables are not related to improved survival).[24]

Surprisingly, given that the study was published in the New England Journal of Medicine, the methods section of the article included no sample size estimate or power analysis. A total of 308 patients were enrolled, and other studies using mortality reduction in ARDS as the primary end point that were conducted at about this same time estimated that approximately 800 patients would be needed to accurately assess mortality as an end point, indicating that the Gattinoni study was markedly underpowered. Enrollment was curtailed because of bias toward prone ventilation, to the extent that investigators were no longer willing to enroll subjects in the control (ie, supine) arm.

In this study, mortality in the supine arm was 25% and in the prone arm, 16%, but this difference did not reach statistical significance. However, a post hoc analysis found that patients in the lowest quartile of Pao_2/Fio_2 ratio on enrollment had a significant reduction in 10-day mortality. This difference did not translate into a reduction in intensive care unit (ICU) mortality. This post hoc analysis has influenced the design and interpretation of several subsequent studies (see later discussion).

The second study reporting improvements in oxygenation with prone ventilation, but no difference in mortality, was published by Guerin and colleagues.[22] These investigators enrolled 810 patients who had a P/F less than 300, but only 413 (51%) had ARDS or ALI, and using the investigators' own assumptions for their sample size estimate, 713 patients with ARDS were needed. Prone ventilation was used only 8 h/d, and 21% of the patients who were randomized to the supine arm crossed over to the prone arm and 41% crossed from the prone to the supine arm. Ventilator modes and settings were left up to the individual treating physician, although the levels of PEEP and Fio_2 were titrated to maintain an Sao_2 greater than 90%.

The third study enrolled patients within 48 hours of intubation, sought to apply prone ventilation for 20 h/d and achieved 17 h/d. Evidence-based ventilation and weaning protocols were used.[25] Because of financial incentives paid to investigators to enroll patients in pharmaceutical company–sponsored studies, enrollment in the prone ventilation study (which came with no financial incentives) decreased to the point that it had to be stopped early. The primary outcome was ICU mortality, which was 59% (34/58) in those ventilated in supine and 44% (33/75) in those ventilated prone. This 15% absolute and 25% relative reduction was not statistically significant (P = .12), but became significant when adjusted for severity of illness (P = .02) with less severely ill patients doing better, the opposite of what was found by Gattinoni and colleagues in their post hoc analysis noted earlier. Despite an appropriate study design based on our current understanding of prone ventilation and VILI, enrollment targets were not met and the mortality difference from this study was not significant unless adjusted, and therefore the results were inconclusive.

The fourth study enrolled patients within 72 hours of diagnosis, attempted to use prone ventilation 20 h/d, achieving 18 h/d, and used predefined ventilation and weaning protocols.[26]

Because of the post hoc analysis described earlier, patients were stratified into 2 subgroups: those with severe and less severe oxygenation based on P/F ratio. Prone ventilation had no effect on mortality in either subgroup, although oxygenation improved in both. Problems with this study include the following: first, of the 169 patients randomized to receive prone ventilation, 34 (20%) did not receive it on 51% of the patient days. The investigators attributed this failure to the patients being too clinically unstable to undertake turning (mostly because of hypotension when supine, a problem not noted in any of the previous studies).

Second, the rate of complications (eg, airway obstruction, arrhythmias and need for vasopressors, loss of venous access, displacement of endotracheal tubes) in the group receiving prone ventilation was considerably higher than any previously published study of prone ventilation. A possible explanation for this increase in complications was a "need for increased sedation/muscle relaxants" in 81% of the patients randomized to the prone ventilation, but in only 66.7% of those randomized to the supine arm. This need was not further described nor is it apparent to us from our experience caring for numerous patients ventilated prone. Importantly, 20 of the 25 centers participating in the study used the Rotoprone bed to facilitate proning, the only study of the ones summarized in this review that did so. This bed provides continuous rotational therapy in addition to prone positioning, and others have reported[27] that continuous rotational therapy alone performed without prone positioning requires increased sedation. We theorize that patients randomized to the prone arm of this study had increased complications, particularly hypotension, which precluded turning many of them prone, and that this hypotension resulted indirectly from use of Rotoprone beds, because the continuous rotational therapy resulted in the need for additional administration of sedatives and muscle relaxants.

Several meta-analyses of these 4 studies and several smaller ones have come to the conclusion that prone ventilation reduced mortality, but only for patients with severe hypoxia (ie, a P/F ratio <150).[28] The validity of meta-analyses that group results of studies that enroll patients with a variety of diagnoses, at various points in the course of their ARDS, and apply prone ventilation for varying durations each day and for a varying number of days is highly questionable at best.

The final study to be considered was recently published by Guerin and colleagues.[29] Again, from the post hoc analysis, the inclusion criteria limited enrollment to patients with severe hypoxia (ie, P/F $\leq$ 150 when the Fio_2 was $\geq$ 0.6 and the level of PEEP was $\geq$5 cm H_2O). This study enrolled an appropriate number of patients (n = 466) within 48 hours of their diagnosis and after a 24-hour stabilization period, administered prone ventilation for approximately 17 h/d and used standardized ventilation and weaning protocols. Protocol violation and complications were rare. Those randomized to supine ventilation had a 32% ICU mortality (consistent with the ICU mortality of patients with ARDS reported in other studies) compared with 16% mortality for those in the prone ventilation arm (hazard ratio = 0.39; 95% confidence interval, 0.25–0.63, P<.001).

Meta-analyses including the results of this last study with the others previously summarized have already started to appear. However, we suggest that aggregating the results of a well-designed, well-conducted trial with those of studies with clear flaws in study design or conduct that used prone ventilation for shorter periods of time makes little sense.

COMPLICATIONS

Although several potential complications related to prone positioning have been described, the only 3 that occur with any frequency are facial edema, skin breakdown, and transient desaturation, which occurs during, and for a short period after, the turning process.

Facial edema is common and occurs as a result of the high compliance of facial tissues that allows edema to accumulate when the face is dependent. It can be minimized by placing patients in slight Trendelenberg position while prone (ie, approximately 20°). Family members should be cautioned about facial edema before visiting their loved ones, because it can be pronounced and disconcerting, but they can also be told that it resolves rapidly when patients no longer require prone positioning.

Pressure necrosis can lead to skin breakdown. Some studies suggest that skin breakdown occurs more frequently when patients are prone; others suggest that the incidence of skin breakdown is the same in patients ventilated supine or prone, but that the areas affected are different. Areas of concern when prone include the chin, perioral region and forehead, the humeral and iliac tuberosities, and the patellar surfaces of the knees. Aside from the face, we use protective coverings on these areas of concern.

As with any movement in patients with profound hypoxemia from shunt, the Spo_2 frequently decreases during, and shortly after, the turning process, but the change is almost always extremely transient (ie, 15–60 seconds) and needs no specific intervention.

Box 1
Checklist for the application of prone ventilation

1. Preparing for prone ventilation before assembly of team for turning procedure
   - Check for contraindications (see above).
   - Consider possible adverse effects of prone positioning on chest tube drainage if tube thoracostomy present.
   - Stop tube feeding, check residuals, evacuate stomach, and cap or clamp the feeding and gastric tubes.
   - Explain risks/benefits of maneuver to the patient or their family.
   - Confirm from a recent chest roentgenogram that the tip of the endotracheal tube is located 2 to 4 cm above the main carina.
   - Secure endotracheal tube and all central and peripheral vascular access devices.

2. Preparing to turn the patient with team (3–5 ICU staff members)
   - Consider how the patient's head, neck, and shoulder girdle will be supported after they are turned prone.
   - Assemble pillows, foam pads, or other types of support devices.
   - Prepare endotracheal suctioning equipment, and review what the process will be if copious airway secretions abruptly interfere with ventilation.
   - Decide whether the turn will be rightward or leftward.
   - Prepare all intravenous tubing and other catheters and tubing for connection when the patient is prone.
     - Ensure sufficient tubing length. Relocate all drainage bags on the opposite side of the bed.
     - Move chest tube drains between the legs.
     - Reposition intravenous tubing toward the patient's head, on the opposite side of the bed.

3. The turning procedure with team (3–5 ICU staff members)
   - Place 1 (or more) people on both sides of the bed (to be responsible for the turning processes) and another at the head of the bed (to ensure the central lines and the endotracheal tube do not become dislodged or kinked).
   - Increase the Fio_2 to 1.0 and note the mode of ventilation, the tidal volume, the minute ventilation, and the peak and plateau airway pressures.
   - Pull the patient to the edge of the bed furthest from whichever lateral decubitus position will be used while turning.
   - Place a new draw sheet on the side of the bed that the patient will face when in this lateral decubitus position. Leave most of the sheet hanging.
   - Turn the patient to the lateral decubitus position, with the dependent arm tucked slightly under the thorax. As the turning progresses, the nondependent arm can be raised in a cocked position over the patient's head. Alternatively, the turn can progress using a log-rolling procedure.
   - Remove electrocardiographic (ECG) leads and patches. Suction the airway, mouth, and nasal passages if necessary.
   - Continue turning to the prone position.
   - Reposition in the center of the bed using the new draw sheet.
   - If the patient is on a standard hospital bed, turn their face toward the ventilator. Ensure that the airway is not kinked and has not migrated during the turning process. Suction the airway if necessary.
   - Support the face and shoulders appropriately, avoiding any contact of the supporting padding with the orbits or the eyes.
   - Position the arms for patient comfort. If the patient cannot communicate, avoid any type of arm extension that might result in a brachial plexus injury.

4. Postturning assessment and maintenance

- Auscultate the chest to check for right mainstem intubation. Reassess the tidal volume and minute ventilation.
- Adjust all tubing and reassess connections and functions.
- Reattach ECG patches and leads to the back.
- Tilt the patient into 20° Trendelenberg position. Slight, intermittent lateral repositioning (20°–30°) should also be used, changing sides at least every 2 hours.
- Document a thorough skin assessment every shift, specifically inspecting weight bearing

There is a risk of dislodging central or peripheral intravascular catheters, Foley catheters, chest tubes, or endotracheal tubes when turning patients prone, or returning them supine. When we prone patients in our unit, we station 1 health care provider at the head of the bed and give them the sole responsibility of watching the endotracheal tube during the turn, protecting against its movement.

Positioning the head, neck, and upper thorax requires special attention. Our preference is to place pillows under the upper chest to raise that portion of the thorax off the bed, thereby allowing the neck and head to move more freely, have less contact with the bed, and it is hoped reduce skin breakdown from pressure necrosis. We use additional pillows to support the head after turning so that the endotracheal tube hangs freely and is subjected to minimal tension. In doing so, our primary objectives are to minimize pressure to the face and avoid endotracheal tube kinking. Anesthesiologists use circular facial pillows when positioning patients prone in the operating room. Our experience with these is poor, because they seem to result in more facial skin breakdown than is seen using pillows. As with any patient in the ICU, positions should be changed slightly every 2 to 3 hours (alternating between 15° and 20° left and right semiprone with straight prone).

On rare occasions, immediately after turning to the prone position, copious secretions can drain from the lung and completely fill the endotracheal tube. If not suctioned immediately, these secretions can obstruct ventilation and precipitate life-threatening hypoxia and hypercarbia. Accordingly, suctioning equipment should be prepared, checked for proper functioning before turning, and ready for use immediately if needed. All complications of proning cannot be avoided, but if caregivers are aware of the concerns and are prepared to deal with them, adverse effects from these complications can be avoided.

There are numerous issues to consider when turning patients prone, but our experience is that if a checklist is used and care is taken before turning, complications are minor and uncommon (**Box 1**).[30]

A meta-analysis of several clinical trials found that the only complications seen more commonly in patients ventilated prone were pressure ulcers and endotracheal tube obstruction.[31] The former can be minimized, but not eliminated, by applying barrier protections, and the latter should not occur if the turning process is orchestrated properly and includes a person whose sole responsibility is to ensure patency and maintenance of the endotracheal tube.

One study found that ventilator-associated pneumonia occurred less frequently in patients ventilated prone.[32] The reduction in dorsal lung atelectasis that occurs on turning prone could result in a reduction in pneumonia, and certainly reduces dorsal lung atelectasis on both chest radiographs and CT scans. Depending on how ventilator-associated pneumonias are defined, this reduction could account for this observation, as could improved removal of airway secretions.

CONTRAINDICATIONS

There are no absolute contraindications to prone ventilation, but several relative contraindications should be considered. Serious burns or open wounds on the face or ventral body surface could put patients at higher risk of infection when they are prone. Spinal instability requires extreme care in the turning process, possibly to include the support of a back board. In patients with rheumatoid arthritis or cervical spine trauma, it is not possible to turn the head to the left or right and facial positioning has to take this into account (patients can be positioned with their heads on tables at the top of the bed, cushioned with pillows, leaving the endotracheal tube free to dangle dorsally between the table and the head of the bed). Facial, pelvic, or other fractures may be destabilized by turning patients. Intracranial pressure could increase on marked turning of the head to 1 side or the other, or simply by turning prone, but both can be minimized by applying reverse Trendelenberg position.

Providers should be prepared to rapidly return patients supine if there are concerns for cardiac arrhythmias that might require cardiopulmonary resuscitation or defibrillation.

PREVENTION OF ACUTE RESPIRATORY DISTRESS SYNDROME

Recently, one of us hypothesized that most instances of ARDS might be iatrogenic.[33] In this scenario, patients without ARDS develop atelectasis as a result of sedation, anesthesia, or supine positioning, or from ventilator-induced changes in surfactant that increase surface tension in the airspace and precipitate atelectasis. Once atelectasis develops, cyclical airspace opening and closing occur (during spontaneous or mechanical ventilation), resulting in VILI, which can progress to ARDS. Albert[33] summarized an extensive literature documenting that (1) ventilation with a fixed tidal volume (large or small) reduces surfactant secretion from type 2 alveolar epithelial cells and increases surface tension, which predispose to atelectasis, (2) ventilation with large compared with small tidal volumes reduces surfactant function more rapidly (providing what might be a more likely explanation for the benefit of low tidal volume ventilation than its effect on reducing overdistension), (3) qualitative and quantitative changes in surfactant occur before the onset of ARDS, (4) supine positioning of normal individuals causes dorsal lung atelectasis, (5) sedation and anesthesia result in atelectasis in normal individuals, and (6) ventilation of normal lungs can produce ARDS. If this hypothesis is correct, prone positioning might have an important role in preventing ARDS by reducing the amount of dorsal lung atelectasis that occurs as a result of being supine and undergoing constant tidal volume ventilation.

WHEN SHOULD PRONE VENTILATION BE STARTED?

There are 3 ways to answer this question.

If one aims to practice evidence-based medicine, the only study documenting that prone ventilation reduces mortality limited enrollment to patients with severe ARDS (ie, a P/F ratio <150 while being ventilated with an Fio_2 >0.6 and a PEEP $\geq$5 cm H_2O). Accordingly, if the decision to institute prone ventilation is based on literature, only those with severe ARDS would be turned prone.

If the decision to institute prone ventilation is based on physiology, specifically, how and why prone positioning reduces VILI, it makes little sense to withhold this intervention until sufficient

VILI has occurred to produce the degree of hypoxia outlined earlier. In this scenario, everyone with ARDS, regardless of their P/F ratio, should be ventilated prone. As reviewed in the earlier comments, the idea that prone ventilation is effective only in patients with severe hypoxemia originated from a post hoc analysis of a study that had numerous design flaws, and the reduction in mortality observed at 10 days in this analysis did not extend to ICU mortality. One study with prespecified stratification of patients into severe and less severe hypoxemia found similar mortality in both groups, and another study found a reduced mortality in patients with the least severe ARDS.[25,26,34] The beneficial effects of prone ventilation on mortality are not related to either basal gas exchange or the improvement in gas exchange that occurs on turning prone.[35] Accordingly, the evidence indicating that prone ventilation is effective only in patients with severe ARDS is limited at best, and the physiologic changes resulting from prone positioning reduce cyclical airspace opening and closing as well as overdistension regardless of the P/F ratio.

If the hypothesis reviewed earlier is correct (ie, that ARDS is largely iatrogenic), an argument can be made for instituting prone positioning whenever mechanical ventilation is needed, irrespective of whether the patient has ARDS, because supine positioning and sedation increase atelectasis, and whenever there is atelectasis, cyclical airspace opening and closing occur. Prone positioning of all patients limits these effects.

WHEN SHOULD PRONE VENTILATION BE DISCONTINUED?

The same considerations as noted earlier apply. If the decision is based on published literature, prone ventilation should continue until the P/F ratio when supine exceeds 150 on 60% O_2 and 6 or more of PEEP as defined by Guerin and colleagues.[29] If prone ventilation is initiated primarily to minimize VILI, patients should be maintained prone until they are sufficiently improved to be extubated.

WHAT PORTION OF THE DAY SHOULD PATIENTS BE KEPT PRONE?

This question assumes that the normal position for hospitalized patients is supine. Although this position is the standard practice, only a few normal individuals sleep on their backs; given a choice, most sleep prone or semiprone. Many studies in both humans and animals indicate that the supine position is the worst possible position for the lung, because it results in more distortion. The beneficial physiologic effects of prone positioning are partially or completely reversed immediately on returning supine. It follows, therefore, that patients should be kept prone as much of the day as possible to reduce the contribution that atelectasis occurring from supine positioning makes to VILI.

REFERENCES

1. Froese AB, Bryan AC. Effects of anesthesia and paralysis on diaphragmatic mechanics in man. Anesthesiology 1974;41(3):242–55.

2. Drinker CK, Hardenbergh E. The effects of the supine position upon the ventilation of the lungs of dogs. Surgery 1948;24(1):113–8.

3. Dock W. The evil sequelae of complete bed rest. JAMA 1944;94:1371–3.

4. Piehl MA, Brown RS. Use of extreme position changes in acute respiratory failure. Crit Care Med 1976;4(1):13–4.

5. Douglas FG, Finlayson DC. Effect of positive end-expiratory pressure on lung mechanics during anaesthesia in dogs. Can Anaesth Soc J 1977; 24(4):425–32.

6. Albert RK, Leasa D, Sanderson M, et al. The prone position improves arterial oxygenation and reduces shunt in oleic-acid-induced acute lung injury. Am Rev Respir Dis 1987;135(3):628–33.

7. Pelosi P, Brazzi L, Gattinoni L. Prone position in acute respiratory distress syndrome. Eur Respir J 2002;20(4).1017–28.

8. Wiener CM, Kirk W, Albert RK. Prone position reverses gravitational distribution of perfusion in dog lungs with oleic acid-induced injury. J Appl Physiol (1985) 1990;68(4):1386–92.

9. Glenny RW, Lamm WJ, Albert RK, et al. Gravity is a minor determinant of pulmonary blood flow distribution. J Appl Physiol (1985) 1991;71(2):620–9.

10. Wiener-Kronish JP, Gropper MA, Lai-Fook SJ. Pleural liquid pressure in dogs measured using a rib capsule. J Appl Physiol (1985) 1985;59(2): 597–602.

11. Mutoh T, Guest RJ, Lamm WJ, et al. Prone position alters the effect of volume overload on regional pleural pressures and improves hypoxemia in pigs in vivo. Am Rev Respir Dis 1992;146(2):300–6. http://dx.doi.org/10.1164/ajrccm/146.2.300.

12. Lai-Fook SJ, Rodarte JR. Pleural pressure distribution and its relationship to lung volume and interstitial pressure. J Appl Physiol (1985) 1991;70(3): 967–78.

13. Margulies SS, Rodarte JR. Shape of the chest wall in the prone and supine anesthetized dog. J Appl Physiol (1985) 1990;68(5):1970–8.

14. Bar-Yishay E, Hyatt RE, Rodarte JR. Effect of heart weight on distribution of lung surface pressures in vertical dogs. J Appl Physiol (1985) 1986;61(2): 712–8.

15. Mead J, Takishima T, Leith D. Stress distribution in lungs: a model of pulmonary elasticity. J Appl Physiol 1970;28(5):596–608.

16. Gattinoni L, Taccone P, Carlesso E, et al. Prone position in acute respiratory distress syndrome. Rationale, indications, and limits. Am J Respir Crit Care Med 2013;188(11):1286–93. http://dx.doi.org/10.1164/rccm.201308-1532CI.

17. Lachmann B. Open up the lung and keep the lung open. Intensive Care Med 1992;18(6):319–21.

18. Pelosi P, Goldner M, McKibben A, et al. Recruitment and derecruitment during acute respiratory failure: an experimental study. Am J Respir Crit Care Med 2001; 164(1):122–30. http://dx.doi.org/10.1164/ajrccm.164.1.2007010.

19. Valenza F, Guglielmi M, Maffioletti M, et al. Prone position delays the progression of ventilator-induced lung injury in rats: does lung strain distribution play a role? Crit Care Med 2005;33(2):361–7.

20. Nishimura M, Honda O, Tomiyama N, et al. Body position does not influence the location of ventilator-induced lung injury. Intensive Care Med 2000; 26(11):1664–9.

21. Broccard A, Shapiro RS, Schmitz LL, et al. Prone positioning attenuates and redistributes ventilator-induced lung injury in dogs. Crit Care Med 2000; 28(2):295–303.

22. Guérin C, Gaillard S, Lemasson S, et al. Effects of systematic prone positioning in hypoxemic acute respiratory failure. JAMA 2004;292(19):2379. http://dx.doi.org/10.1001/jama.292.19.2379.

23. Gattinoni L, Tognoni G, Pesenti A, et al. Effect of prone positioning on the survival of patients with acute respiratory failure. N Engl J Med 2001;345(8):568–73. http://dx.doi.org/10.1056/NEJMoa010043.

24. Gattinoni L, Carlesso E, Brazzi L, et al. Positive end-expiratory pressure. Curr Opin Crit Care 2010;16(1):39–44. http://dx.doi.org/10.1097/MCC.0b013e3283354723.

25. Mancebo J, Fernández R, Blanch L, et al. A multicenter trial of prolonged prone ventilation in severe acute respiratory distress syndrome. Am J Respir Crit Care Med 2006;173(11):1233–9. http://dx.doi.org/10.1164/rccm.200503-353OC.

26. Taccone P, Pesenti A, Latini R, et al. Prone positioning in patients with moderate and severe acute respiratory distress syndrome. JAMA 2009;302(18): 1977. http://dx.doi.org/10.1001/jama.2009.1614.

27. Goldhill DR, Badacsonyi A, Goldhill AA, et al. A prospective observational study of ICU patient position and frequency of turning. Anaesthesia 2008; 63(5):509–15. http://dx.doi.org/10.1111/j.1365-2044.2007.05431.x.

28. Sud S, Friedrich JO, Taccone P, et al. Prone ventilation reduces mortality in patients with acute respiratory

failure and severe hypoxemia: systematic review and meta-analysis. Intensive Care Med 2010;36(4):585–99. http://dx.doi.org/10.1007/s00134-009-1748-1.

29. Guérin C, Reignier J, Richard JC, et al. Prone positioning in severe acute respiratory distress syndrome. N Engl J Med 2013;368(23):2159–68. http://dx.doi.org/10.1056/NEJMoa1214103.

30. Messerole E, Peine P, Wittkopp S, et al. The pragmatics of prone positioning. Am J Respir Crit Care Med 2002;165(10):1359–63. http://dx.doi.org/10.1164/rccm.2107005.

31. Sud S, Sud M, Friedrich JO, et al. Effect of mechanical ventilation in the prone position on clinical outcomes in patients with acute hypoxemic respiratory failure: a systematic review and meta-analysis. CMAJ 2008;178(9):1153–61. http://dx.doi.org/10.1503/cmaj.071802.

32. Voggenreiter G, Aufmkolk M, Stiletto RJ, et al. Prone positioning improves oxygenation in post-traumatic lung injury–a prospective randomized trial. J Trauma 2005;59(2):333–41 [discussion: 341–3].

33. Albert RK. The role of ventilation-induced surfactant dysfunction and atelectasis in causing acute respiratory distress syndrome. Am J Respir Crit Care Med 2012;185(7):702–8. http://dx.doi.org/10.1164/rccm.201109-1667PP.

34. Gattinoni L. Effect of prone positioning on the survival of patients with acute respiratory failure. N Engl J Med 2001;345:568–73.

35. Albert RK, Keniston A, Baboi L, et al. Prone position-induced improvement in gas exchange is not associated with survival in the acute respiratory distress syndrome. Am J Respir Crit Care Med 2014;189: 494–6.

The Use of Paralytics in Patients with Acute Respiratory Distress Syndrome

Sami Hraiech, MD[a,b], Stéphanie Dizier, MD[a],
Laurent Papazian, MD, PhD[a,b],*

KEYWORDS

- Acute respiratory distress syndrome • Mechanical ventilation • Neuromuscular blocking agents
- Protective ventilation • Spontaneous ventilation • Transpulmonary pressure
- ICU-acquired weakness

KEY POINTS

- Neuromuscular blocking agents (NMBAs), largely used in the treatment of acute respiratory distress syndrome (ARDS), have been shown to improve the oxygenation and decrease the mortality of the most hypoxemic patients.
- NMBAs most likely decrease ventilator-induced lung injury by facilitating the adaptation to protective ventilation and prevention of high levels of transpulmonary pressures, and by limiting barotrauma and biotrauma. NMBAs also limit the derecruitment induced by active expiration.
- The use of NMBAs should be considered in the most severe ARDS patients at the early phase of the injury and for a limited period. In the less hypoxemic forms and/or after the improvement of oxygenation, spontaneous ventilator efforts should be maintained.

INTRODUCTION

Almost 50 years after its first description,[1] acute respiratory distress syndrome (ARDS) remains a hot topic, and its definition and treatment are still debated. The mortality of ARDS patients remains high (40%–50% of patients) despite medical advances.[2] The recent definition of the European Society of Intensive Care Medicine (ESICM) task force[3] has identified 3 levels of severity that are associated with significantly different prognoses and management strategies. For the last 15 years, only 3 therapeutic strategies have been shown to increase the survival of ARDS patients in randomized controlled trials (RCTs). A reduction in the tidal volume[4] has now entered the current standard of care.[5] Two other recent studies have unsettled the management of more severe ARDS patients[6,7]: the administration of neuromuscular blocking agents (NMBAs) for a 2-day period in the early phase of ARDS and the use of prone positioning (PP). These 2 recent advances are frequently associated, and call into question the ventilatory strategy in early ARDS. Consequently, exploration of the role of NMBAs in the care of such patients must define the respective role of entirely controlled ventilation versus ventilation allowing a part of spontaneous breathing (SB). The purpose of this review is to recall both older and more recent literature with a focus on NMBAs in ARDS, thereby to propose a pathophysiologic explanation for the actions of NMBAs and to

Disclosures: None.
[a] Assistance Publique - Hôpitaux de Marseille, Medical Intensive Care Unit APHM, CHU Nord, Marseille 13015, France; [b] Faculté de Médecine, University of Aix-Marseilles, URMITE UMR CNRS 7278, Marseille 13005, France
* Corresponding author. Assistance Publique - Hôpitaux de Marseille, Medical Intensive Care Unit APHM, CHU Nord, Chemin des Bourrely, Marseille 13015, France.
E-mail address: laurent.papazian@ap-hm.fr

Clin Chest Med 35 (2014) 753–763
http://dx.doi.org/10.1016/j.ccm.2014.08.012
0272-5231/14/$ – see front matter © 2014 Elsevier Inc. All rights reserved.

attempt to define their place in the ventilation strategy for the treatment of patients with ARDS.

FROM CASE REPORTS TO RANDOMIZED CONTROLLED TRIALS: THE SAGA OF NEUROMUSCULAR BLOCKING AGENTS IN ACUTE RESPIRATORY DISTRESS SYNDROME
Clinical Practice

NMBAs are frequently used by intensivists, especially for the management of ARDS; in a recent large survey[8,9] 25% to 55% of ARDS patients were involved. Indeed, the adaptation of the patients to the ventilator, the control of patient/ventilator asynchrony, the use of low tidal volumes, the use of permissive hypercapnia, and the use of PP or high-frequency oscillatory (HFO) ventilation is cited to justify this large use.[9,10] Moreover, several RCTs studying the effects of tidal volume, positive end-expiratory pressure (PEEP), or HFO report the frequent use of NMBAs.[4,11–13]

Historical Context

Despite their frequent use, the guidelines concerning the use of NMBAs have not been revised since 2002[14] and have included paralytics for facilitating mechanical ventilation (MV) when sedation alone is inadequate, most notably in patients with severe gas-exchange impairment. Regarding the recent data in the literature, these guidelines appear to be restrictive and outdated. The first publications concerning NMBAs were case reports and small nonrandomized studies that reported controversial results concerning the improvement in oxygenation.[15–18] Physiologic studies on ventilator mechanics in healthy subjects found that sedation induced a reduction in pulmonary compliance, whereas NMBAs induced an increase in thoracic compliance[19] and improved the mechanical viscoelastic properties of the chest wall.[20] The absence of strong data showing a benefit to the prognosis or potential adverse events, especially intensive care unit (ICU)-acquired neuromyopathy,[21] were often responsible for a distrust of paralytics. Larger studies focusing on the clinical effects of paralytics in ARDS patients began with Lagneau and colleagues,[22] who demonstrated that the continuous infusion of NMBAs for 2 hours improved the partial pressure of arterial oxygen (Pao_2)/fraction of inspired oxygen (Fio_2) ratio in a prospective randomized control trial (PRCT) including 102 patients presenting moderate to severe ARDS (**Table 1**).

The Era of Randomized Controlled Trials

Recent randomized studies have helped to clarify positions. In the first multicenter PRCT conducted by Gainnier and colleagues,[23] there was a significant improvement in the Pao_2/Fio_2 ratio in the group of patients with ARDS receiving neuromuscular blockade continuously for 48 hours. The beneficial effects were observed as early as the 48th hour and persisted throughout the study

Table 1
Main characteristics and results of clinical studies investigating the effect of NMBAs on oxygenation in ARDS patients

Authors,[Ref.] Year	No. of Patients	Study Design	Setting	Type of Lung Failure	Drug Infused	Duration of Infusion	Effect on Oxygenation
Bishop,[16] 1984	9	NRCT	ICU	4 ALI/5 ARDS	Pancuronium	Single bolus	No effect
Coggeshall et al,[17] 1985	1	Case	ICU	1 ARDS	Pancuronium	Repeated boluses	Improvement
Conti et al,[18] 1985	13	PNRCT	ICU	9 ALI/4 ARDS	Pancuronium	Single bolus	No effect
Lagneau et al,[22] 2002	102	PRCT	ICU	102 ARF with Pao_2/Fio_2 <200	Cisatracurium	2 h	Improvement
Gainnier et al,[23] 2004	56	PRCT	ICU	56 ARDS (Pao_2/Fio_2 <150)	Cisatracurium	48 h	Improvement
Forel et al,[24] 2006	36	PRCT	ICU	36 ARDS (Pao_2/Fio_2 <200)	Cisatracurium	48 h	Improvement
Papazian et al,[6] 2010	339	PRCT	ICU	339 ARDS (Pao_2/Fio_2 <150)	Cisatracurium	48 h	Improvement

Abbreviations: ALI, acute lung injury; ARDS, acute respiratory distress syndrome; ARF, acute respiratory failure; Fio_2, fraction of inspired oxygen; ICU, intensive care unit; NRCT, nonrandomized controlled trial; Pao_2, partial pressure of arterial oxygen; PNRCT, prospective nonrandomized controlled trial; PRCT, prospective randomized controlled trial.

period (120 hours after randomization). Curiously the investigators reported a strong tendency toward a lower mortality rate in the group of patients receiving the NMBAs. In a second study,[24] the same group analyzed the effects of muscle paralysis on inflammation in ARDS. The results were in accordance with the previous work, confirming the beneficial effects of the NMBAs on oxygenation. Decreases in the plateau pressure, Fio_2, and PEEP were also observed during the study period of 120 hours in the NMBA group. In this second study there was a trend toward decreased mortality in patients receiving the NMBAs. This decrease was the rationale for the design of the ACURASYS study conducted by Papazian and colleagues,[6] the only PRCT to date that has investigated the impact of neuromuscular blockade on the survival of patients with ARDS. In this multicenter, double-blind trial (with equal levels of deep sedation in both groups), 339 patients who had exhibited severe ARDS for less than 48 hours (ie, with a Pao_2/Fio_2 ratio <150 mm Hg and PEEP $\geq$5 cm H_2O) were randomized into 2 groups, a group receiving a continuous infusion of cisatracurium besylate (177 patients) and a placebo group (162 patients). Either the placebo or the NMBA was administered over a 48-hour period. The group of patients treated with cisatracurium showed an improvement in the adjusted 90-day survival rate compared with the placebo group. After adjusting for the baseline Pao_2/Fio_2 ratio, the plateau pressure and the Simplified Acute Physiology Score II, the hazard ratio for death at 90 days in the cisatracurium group compared with the placebo group was 0.68 (95% confidence interval [CI] 0.48–0.98; $P = .04$). Furthermore, the mortality at 28 days was 23.7% with cisatracurium and 33.3% with the placebo ($P = .05$). The beneficial effects of cisatracurium on the mortality of the most severe patients included a Pao_2/Fio_2 ratio of less than 120. Among these patients, the 90-day mortality was 30.8% in the cisatracurium group and 44.6% in the control group ($P = .04$). The cisatracurium group had significantly more ventilator-free days than the placebo group during the first 28 and 90 days and more days free of organ failure (other than the lung) during the first 28 days. The investigators also found that significantly more days were spent outside of the ICU between day 1 and day 90 in the cisatracurium group. The NMBAs also had a protective effect against the adverse effects of MV, as demonstrated by the larger proportion of pneumothoraces in the placebo group in comparison with the cisatracurium group (11.7%, vs 4.0%; $P = .01$).[6]

Importantly the ventilatory strategy in the ACURASYS study associated a 48-hour period of NMBA use with protective ventilation, and used a quick transition toward ventilator modes allowing SB, such as pressure support ventilation (PSV), as soon as possible, typically from the third day.

Summary of the Evidence-Based Data

Two recent meta-analyses based on PRCTs have investigated the role of NMBA use in ARDS. In the meta-analysis of Alhazzani and colleagues,[25] there was a reduction in the 28-day mortality rate among patients receiving NMBAs in the early phase of ARDS. The investigators concluded that 9 patients needed to be treated for every life saved, given the in-hospital mortality rate (**Fig. 1**). There was also a reduced risk of barotrauma and an increase in the number of days without MV during the first 28 days in the patients receiving the NMBAs. NMBAs also improved the Pao_2/Fio_2 ratio at 24, 48, and 72 hours of randomization.

The meta-analysis conducted by Neto and colleagues[26] substantially confirmed all of these results, and stated that the use of NMBAs was associated with a decrease in the PEEP and the plateau pressure over time in a group of paralyzed patients, reflecting improved ventilation.

The main criticism that can be levied is that both studies were based on only 3 randomized controlled studies conducted by the same group, which may have introduced bias into the conclusions. However, as noted by Neto and colleagues, the main study on which these meta-analyses were based consisted of 20 different ICUs, which reduces the risk of bias.

RCTs evaluating NMBAs in ARDS patients have some limitations as well. First, the benefits observed may not apply to all NMBAs, considering that cisatracurium besylate has been used in all RCTs. Second, more data are necessary with which to assess precisely the Pao_2/Fio_2 cutoff for use of NMBAs and duration of infusion. Twenty-four hours of paralysis may indeed be sufficient in some cases. Future studies evaluating NMBA use in patients with late ARDS may also be of important interest. Moreover, monitoring transpulmonary pressures concomitantly with the administration of NMBAs may provide precious data to aid in understanding the pathophysiologic mechanisms of action of paralyzing agents.

In summary, the data from RCTs provide a strong argument in favor of using a 48-hour infusion of cisatracurium in patients with most hypoxemic ARDS (especially with a Pao_2/Fio_2 ratio <120 mm Hg), with a direct benefit on survival. In these studies, the use of time-limited NMBAs

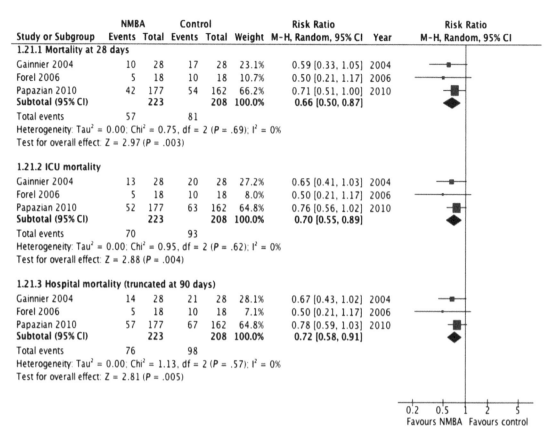

Fig. 1. Risk ratios for mortality at 28 days, intensive care unit (ICU) mortality, and hospital mortality at 90 days observed in the 3 randomized controlled trials evaluating the effects of NMBAs during ARDS. (*From* Alhazzani W, Alshahrani M, Jaeschke R, et al. Neuromuscular blocking agents in acute respiratory distress syndrome: a systematic review and meta-analysis of randomized controlled trials. Crit Care 2013;17(2):R43.)

was not associated with an increased incidence of ICU-acquired neuromyopathy. However, considering the reduced number of RCTs that were all conducted by the same group, confirmatory studies are needed. Of note, in a recent large retrospective study Steingrub and colleagues[27] investigated the outcomes of mechanically ventilated patients with severe sepsis who had received NMBAs within the 2 days following their admission into the ICU. Twenty-three percent of the patients had NMBAs at the early phase of the treatment, and the mean duration of treatment was 1.5 days. The unadjusted in-hospital mortality rate of those patients initially treated with NMBAs was 31.9%, compared with 38.3% among those who did not receive NMBAs (*P*<.001). Using a propensity-matched analysis, the investigators showed that the risk ratio of in-hospital mortality was 0.88 (95% CI 0.80–0.96) in favor of the treated group. Even if all the patients included were not ARDS patients and were most likely less severe than in the ACURASYS study, these results are in line with those of Papazian and colleagues.[6]

PROPOSED PATHOPHYSIOLOGIC EFFECTS OF NEUROMUSCULAR BLOCKING AGENTS DURING ACUTE RESPIRATORY DISTRESS SYNDROME

If the beneficial effects of NMBAs in the early phase of ARDS now seem strongly supported, the pathophysiology underlying their action remains unclear. Several mechanisms may be involved and are most likely interrelated (**Table 2**).

Neuromuscular blockade causes an increase in thoracopulmonary compliance with an improved adaptation to the ventilator and the inhibition of expiratory muscle activity. These changes are accompanied by an increase in the functional residual capacity and a decrease in the intrapulmonary shunt. Finally, changes in the ventilation-perfusion ratios may be related to a more uniform distribution of pulmonary perfusion owing to the application of lower pulmonary pressures, favoring the perfusion of ventilated areas and a decreasing intrapulmonary shunt.[28] Another hypothesis could be a better regional distribution of the tidal volume,

Table 2
Potential physiopathologic effects explaining the benefits of NMBAs on the survival of most hypoxemic ARDS patients

Neuromuscular Blockers	
Increase	Decrease
Thoracopulmonary compliance	Pulmonary shunt
Functional residual capacity	Muscular O_2 consumption
Perfusion of ventilated areas	Overdistension of high-compliance territories
Recruitment of areas with small compliance	End-expiratory collapse and derecruitment
	Patient-ventilator asynchrony
	VILI (barotrauma, volutrauma, atelectrauma, biotrauma)

Abbreviation: VILI, ventilator-induced lung injury.

avoiding or limiting the overdistension of high-compliance territories and favoring the recruitment of areas with smaller compliance. NMBAs could prevent patient-ventilator asynchrony and limit the occurrence of high transpulmonary pressures during inspiratory efforts, in addition to expiratory collapse, by inhibiting active expiration, limiting derecruitment and allowing the maintenance of PEEP.[29] In recently published experimental studies, Yoshida and colleagues[30] demonstrated that important ventilatory efforts added to controlled ventilation resulted in an increased transpulmonary pressure and significantly more ventilator-induced lung injury (VILI), even if the plateau pressures had been maintained below 30 cm H_2O.

The use of NMBAs may also have a protective role against VILI (ie, atelectrauma, barotrauma, volutrauma, and biotrauma), as shown by the decrease in the incidence of barotrauma and pneumothoraces in the ACURASYS study and the decreased production of proinflammatory cytokines in both the lung and blood observed by Forel and colleagues.[24] In this latter study, the investigators evaluated the pulmonary and systemic inflammation in 36 ARDS patients receiving a 48-hour continuous infusion of cisatracurium besylate or a placebo at the early phase. Inflammation markers were dosed in bronchoalveolar lavage and serum. Forty-eight hours after randomization, the lung concentrations of interleukin (IL)-1β, IL-6, and IL-8, in addition to the serum concentrations of IL-1β and IL-6, were lower in the cisatracurium group than in the control group. These results are consistent with the decrease in the number of organ failures in patients in the cisatracurium group noted in the ACURASYS study, possibly related to the reduction of biotrauma. However, the direct anti-inflammatory role of muscle relaxants remains uncertain and warrants confirmation.

NEUROMUSCULAR BLOCKING AGENTS AND INTENSIVE CARE UNIT–ACQUIRED WEAKNESS

In a recent review,[31] the incidence of ICU-acquired weakness (ICUAW) was 34% to 60% in patients with ARDS. ICUAW is responsible for severe and durable morbidity and, since it was first described in the early 1980s, has become a major concern.[32] Risk factors have been discussed widely in the literature, and independent risk factors such as female sex, multiple organ dysfunctions (≥2), duration of MV, and administration of corticosteroids[33] have been identified. Duration of vasopressor support, duration of ICU stay, hyperglycemia, low serum albumin, and neurologic failure have also identified as risk factors.[34–36]

NMBAs have been dispraised because of a supposed association with ICUAW. However, Sharshar and colleagues[37] found that NMBAs were not associated with muscular weakness. In a prospective observational study performed in 40 ICUs, Weber-Carstens and colleagues[38] showed that NMBA use was not a significant risk factor for the development of impaired muscle membrane excitability. However, Griffiths and Hall[39] reported that simultaneous use of NMBAs and corticosteroids may be associated with muscle weakness. Moreover, the use of steroid NMBAs and duration of infusion exceeding 48 hours seem to further favor the occurrence of myopathies.[40,41] Confirming these data, in the ACURASYS study, in which patients received a short course of nonsteroid NMBAs,[6] the incidence of ICU-acquired paresis (evaluated based on the Medical Research Council[33] score on day 28 or at the time of ICU discharge) was not higher in paralyzed patients than in the control group. Furthermore, in the meta-analysis by Alhazzani and colleagues,[25] the use of NMBAs was not associated with an increased risk of ICUAW. The occurrence of neuromyopathy was evaluated by clinical assessment of quadriparesis in 2 studies[23,24] and by using the Medical Research Council score at day 28 or ICU discharge in the ACURASYS study.[6] To summarize, there is actually no evidence that nonsteroid NMBAs, when used for a short duration and without the simultaneous administration of corticosteroids, increase the risk of ICUAW.

NEUROMUSCULAR BLOCKING AGENTS IN ACUTE RESPIRATORY DISTRESS SYNDROME VENTILATOR STRATEGY: SPONTANEOUS BREATHING OR CONTROLLED VENTILATION?

Discussing the role of NMBAs in the care of ARDS patients raises the question of the ventilation strategy to adopt with these patients. In this field, the debate is ongoing. This section summarizes what can be concluded from the recent literature.

Spontaneous Breathing During Acute Respiratory Distress Syndrome: From Theory to Practice

If the preservation of SB in patients during MV is considered to be potentially beneficial, the role of SB during ARDS remains in doubt. The preservation of SB efforts seems to be a seductive alternative to controlled ventilation with respect to its potential physiologic benefits.

First, avoiding sedation (hypnotics and opioids) is essential to promoting SB. Several studies[42,43] assessing a daily interruption of sedation showed positive impacts on the prognosis of ICU patients, the duration of MV, and the incidence of ventilator-acquired pneumonia. Lowering the doses of sedatives also decreased the hemodynamic side effects, as was observed in studies comparing airway pressure release ventilation (APRV) with pressure-controlled ventilation.[44]

However, it is important that in these studies most patients did not fulfill the ARDS criteria. Thus, even if a ventilatory strategy favoring SB to reduce sedation as soon as possible is most likely associated with an improved prognosis for some patients, this cannot be generalized to all patients, especially those with acute-phase ARDS.

One of the supposed main positive effects of SB preservation during ARDS is the reduction of diaphragmatic dysfunction and the consequent improvement of recruitment in dependent lung areas. Levine and colleagues[45] demonstrated the presence of a diaphragmatic impairment in 14 ventilated patients in brain death compared with patients ventilated a few hours after surgical lung reduction. Jaber and colleagues[46] confirmed a decrease in the contractile force of the diaphragm and the onset of muscle atrophy by showing a correlation with the duration of MV. Thus, spontaneous ventilation preservation helps in the recruitment of vertebrobasilar diaphragmatic lung areas ("dependent areas") that are often the most affected during ARDS.

Spontaneous ventilation could ensure a redistribution of ventilation to the vertebrobasilar diaphragmatic areas and improve alveolar recruitment.[47,48]

Regarding studies evaluating the benefits of SB during ARDS, the clinical data are scarce. The majority compare partial ventilatory support modalities such as APRV, bilevel positive airway pressure (BIPAP), or PSV with controlled ventilation. APRV is a singular mode that permits the superposition of SB onto pressure-controlled ventilation with no possibility of release (no inspiratory trigger). Thus, it prevents from the risks of high tidal volumes, plateau pressure, or important levels of transpulmonary pressure (TPP). APRV has been compared with synchronized intermittent MV in moderate ARDS patients, with comparable results concerning the Pao_2/Fio_2 ratio, number of ventilator-free days, and mortality.[49] APRV has also been evaluated during PP, and appeared to be feasible in the treatment of patients with acute lung injury. APRV after 24 hours appears to enhance the improvements in oxygenation in response to PP.[50] The main clinical data evaluating APRV during ARDS are limited and arise primarily from Putensen and colleagues.[47,48] In a first study,[47] 24 ARDS patients (most of whom had moderate ARDS and a mean Pao_2/Fio_2 ratio of 140 mm Hg) were ventilated in APRV with or without SB or PSV. The results were in favor of APRV with SB, with a decrease in the intrapulmonary shunt, improved arterial oxygenation, venous oxygen saturation, and an increase in the cardiac index and end-diastolic right ventricle volume. Another study by the same group[48] comparing 30 patients with mild ARDS who were ventilated with APRV + SB or PSV found improved oxygenation in the APRV group, a lower proportion of patients developing severe ARDS, and a shorter duration of ventilation (APRV = 15 vs PSV = 21 days) and hospitalization in the ICU (APRV = 23 vs PSV = 30 days).

If the results of this work are encouraging and seem to argue for maintaining partial SB during ARDS, although it should be noted that the number of patients included was limited and that most of them had mild or moderate but not severe ARDS. In addition, the timing of these studies was at least 1 week after the development of ARDS, and their results cannot be extrapolated to the initial phase of lung injury. Finally, APRV has potential disadvantages, such as the increase of work of breathing associated with important respiratory efforts that may increase the transcapillary pressure gradient, thus enhancing pulmonary edema formation or the increase in tidal volumes with potential increase in VILI.[51]

The results of the BiRDS study (NCT01862016), which compares a strategy using a short period of controlled ventilation with rapid transition to APRV with a strategy using prolonged controlled ventilation, will certainly introduce new results to the debate concerning SB in ARDS.

By separating ARDS according to severity based on the Pa_{O_2}/Fi_{O_2} ratio, the new Berlin Definition[3] highlights the differences related to the prognosis of each of the ARDS subgroups. To summarize, it is not certain that what has been demonstrated in patients with mild ARDS can be generalized to all ARDS patients. Instead, at the initial phase of ARDS and for most hypoxemic patients, RCTs[6,7,21,22] have provided strong evidence supporting controlled and protective ventilation, NMBAs for a short period, and PP.

Deleterious Effects of Spontaneous Breathing at the Acute Phase of Acute Respiratory Distress Syndrome

The beneficial effect of the paralysis of most hypoxemic patients at the initial phase of ARDS is, in itself, a strong argument against the use of spontaneous ventilation during this period. This idea is reinforced by some experimental studies suggesting a deleterious role of ventilatory efforts during ARDS. In a model of ARDS in rabbits, Yoshida and colleagues[30] studied the impact of ventilatory efforts added to controlled ventilation on oxygenation, ventilatory mechanics, and lung histology. Two groups of animals were ventilated with either low (6 mL/kg) or moderate (7–9 mL/kg) tidal volumes. Within each of these groups, the inspiratory efforts were either highly preserved or, by increasing sedation, diminished. The TPPs in each group were evaluated by measuring the esophageal pressure. The investigators found no improvement in the Pa_{O_2}/Fi_{O_2} ratio at the fourth hour in the group of animals receiving ventilation with moderate volumes and important ventilatory efforts. By contrast, in this group of animals they observed a significant decrease in the dynamic compliance associated with increased TPP that was, on average, greater than 33 cm H_2O throughout the observation period, whereas it remained below 30 cm H_2O in the other groups. This increase in TPP was observed although the plateau pressure remained below 30 cm H_2O. In this same group of animals, the analysis of bronchoalveolar lavage revealed significantly more inflammatory markers than in other groups. Lung histologic lesions were also more prominent, and a morphologic analysis of the lungs showed the largest areas of atelectasis and overdistension damage. These results support the idea that SB during ARDS can potentially generate a high TPP, increasing the risk of VILI, and that measuring only plateau pressure does not ensure protective ventilation. Important ventilatory efforts (triggering) in patients with ARDS may be the cause of an uncontrolled increase in the TPP, despite plateau

pressures maintained below values that are considered safe; this could be particularly true in patients with the most severe forms of ARDS, as suggested by the recent experimental work of Yoshida and colleagues.[52] In a model of ARDS in rabbits, the preservation of ventilatory efforts lacked the same effects on oxygenation, pulmonary ventilation, and lung injury, depending on the severity of ARDS (mild or severe). The preservation of SB induced an improvement in the pulmonary ventilation and oxygenation for mild ARDS but resulted in increased TPP and VILI in the group of animals with severe ARDS (**Fig. 2**A, B). This deterioration of ventilatory and histologic parameters was prevented by abolishing SB via administration of NMBAs to the severe ARDS group.

In summary, and contrary to what happens to patients with mild to moderate ARDS, in the initial phase of severe ARDS the prevention of VILI and optimization of alveolar recruitment seem to be based on controlled protective ventilation and the use of NMBAs and, consequently, the abolition of spontaneous ventilatory efforts.

SYNTHESIS

Whatever the mode of MV in ARDS, the protection of the lung parenchyma must be constantly kept in mind, especially in the initial acute phase of the pulmonary complications. For this reason, it is necessary to strictly limit the current volume (approximately 6 mL/kg of predicted weight), to maintain the plateau pressures below 30 cm H_2O and to titrate the PEEP.

During the initial phase of ARDS (first 48 hours, but sometimes longer), the complete abolition of spontaneous ventilation by deep muscle relaxation for a period of 48 hours improves survival. This paralysis in the early phase of ARDS is not incompatible with the rapid use of spontaneous ventilation when the ventilatory parameters improve. Indeed, in the ACURASYS study,[6] after the initial 48-hour period the NMBAs were discontinued, sedatives were diminished, and PSV was introduced in all patients with an Fi_{O_2} less than or equal to 0.6. This short duration of use may explain the low incidence of neuromyopathy observed in this study. This concept is also present in the PROSEVA study. Guerin and colleagues[7] reported the use of NMBAs in 85.4% of the included patients. The average duration of NMBA use was 5.6 ± 5.0 days, the average duration of each session of PP was 17 ± 3 hours, and the average number of PP sessions was 4 ± 4 per patient. However, when the Pa_{O_2}/Fi_{O_2} ratio was 150 mm Hg or higher, PEEP 10 cm H_2O or less, and Fi_{O_2} 60% or less, the

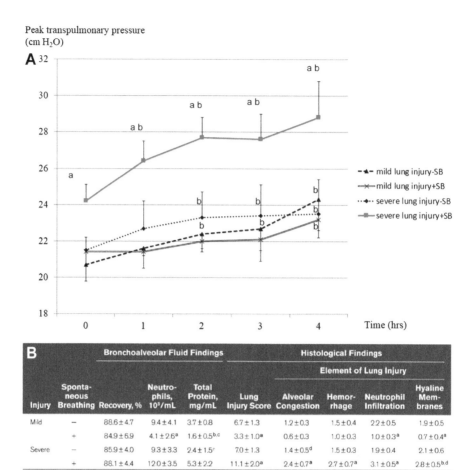

Fig. 2. Peak transpulmonary pressure, bronchoalveolar fluids, and pulmonary histology in 4 groups of rabbits with mild or severe lung injury and with preserved or abolished (by the use of NMBAs) spontaneous breathing (SB). (A) The changes in peak transpulmonary pressure during a 4-hour experiment in all groups. The severe lung injury + SB group showed the highest peak transpulmonary pressure throughout the study period. [a] $P<.05$ compared with other groups; [b] $P<.05$ compared with 0 (at the start of the protocol) within groups. (B) Bronchoalveolar fluids and histologic findings in all groups. [a] $P<.05$ compared with other groups. [b] $P<.05$ compared with mild lung injury minus SB. [c] $P<.05$ compared with severe lung injury plus SB. [d] $P<.05$ compared with mild lung injury plus SB. (*From* Yoshida T, Uchiyama A, Matsuura N, et al. The comparison of spontaneous breathing and muscle paralysis in two different severities of experimental lung injury. Crit Care Med 2013;41(2):536–45; with permission.)

PP sessions, sedation, and paralysis were stopped to allow spontaneous efforts.

The recommended duration of SB abolition (deep sedation ± paralysis) remains unclear. A period of 24 hours in patients with rapid favorable developments could be considered. On the contrary, in the most severe cases a longer period may be required (72–96 hours), particularly for patients requiring several days of PP (as in the PROSEVA study[7]) or in patients requiring extracorporeal life support. Indeed, in the PROSEVA study,[7] the acute phase of ARDS before improvement marked by a Pao_2/Fio_2 ratio of at least 150 mm Hg with a PEEP 10 cm H_2O or less is approximately 5 to 6 days.

The improved survival of ARDS patients reported by the ACURASYS[6] and PROSEVA[7] studies clearly indicates that protective ventilatory strategies in the most acute phase of lung injury are the cornerstone of ARDS treatment. The early and limited use of NMBAs, in addition to PP requiring deep sedation and often paralysis, have in common the limitation of spontaneous ventilation during the peak of the lung parenchyma complications. The ARMA study[4] and many other experimental studies[53] have clearly demonstrated the great interest in a strategy to protect the lung parenchyma during MV in ARDS. The abolition of spontaneous ventilation in the initial acute phase, dominated by inflammatory processes and biotrauma, seems to have a positive impact on survival in most hypoxemic patients. By contrast, the literature in favor of the preservation of SB

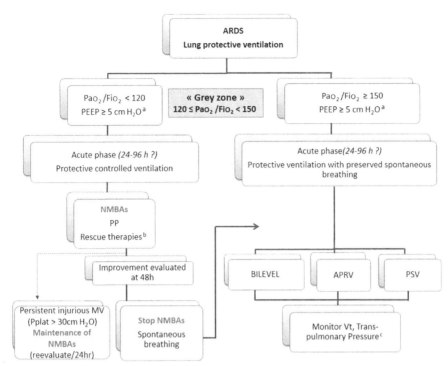

Fig. 3. The role of neuromuscular blocking agents in the ventilatory strategy of ARDS patients. [a] Thresholds of Pao_2/Fio_2 ratio and PEEP have been arbitrarily determined and correspond to those used in the ACURASYS[6] and PROSEVA[7] studies. [b] Rescue therapies: extracorporeal membrane oxygenation, high-frequency oscillatory ventilation, inhaled nitric oxide. [c] Monitoring of transpulmonary pressure can be proposed during the acute phase of ARDS. APRV, airway pressure release ventilation; ARDS, acute respiratory distress syndrome; MV, mechanical ventilation; NMBAs, neuromuscular blocking agents; PEEP, positive end-expiratory pressure; PP, prone positioning; Pplat, plateau pressure; PSV, pressure support ventilation; Vt, tidal volume.

relates essentially to mild (formerly acute lung injury) or moderate ARDS, when lung injury is not severe. Similarly, the extensive literature on the use of titrated sedation or the reevaluation of sedation and, consequently, the preservation of SB, support this idea. However, the most severe ARDS patients were not included in these studies, particularly those in the most hypoxemic acute phase.[42,43]

Taking into account the new definition of ARDS,[3] the use of NMBAs with protective controlled ventilation and the abolition of SB at the early phase of severe ARDS should be promoted. In mild or moderate ARDS or when severe patients improve, NMBAs should be interrupted and sedation decreased to allow SB and to enhance lung recruitment and oxygenation. The Pao_2/Fio_2 ratio and PEEP thresholds to determine the best ventilatory strategy remain unclear. A threshold for the use of SB of a Pao_2/Fio_2 ratio of at least 150 mm Hg may be proposed, pending new data, but an area of uncertainty persists for patients with a Pao_2/Fio_2 ratio between 120 and 150 mm Hg. The optimal level of SB (percentage of spontaneous

cycles, percentage of SB in minute ventilation) and its modalities (APRV, PSV, and so forth) also remain to be determined. Taking into account the most recent data and pending new evidence, an algorithm of clinical decision can be proposed (**Fig. 3**).

SUMMARY

The use of NMBAs during ARDS has been controversial for a long time despite their frequent use in clinical practice. The recent RCTs have demonstrated their benefit in the care of severe ARDS patients at the acute phase. NMBAs can be integrated into protective ventilation. Even if their precise mechanism of action remains unknown, the prevention of VILI and the improvement of lung recruitment are most likely strongly implicated in the increased survival of the most hypoxemic patients. This positive effect has been demonstrated in severe ARDS, in which SB can be deleterious. The use of NMBAs should be restricted to those patients with acute-phase ARDS. For mild and moderate patients and after improvement in the more severe cases, SB breathing should be encouraged. Short-term use of NMBAs is most likely not associated with an increase in the occurrence ICU-acquired neuromyopathy. Controlled ventilation with NMBAs and protective ventilation with SB should not be opposed, but rather should be considered in the continuum of care for ARDS patients.

REFERENCES

1. Ashbaugh DG, Bigelow DB, Petty TL, et al. Acute respiratory distress in adults. Lancet 1967; 2(7511):319–23.
2. Phua J, Badia JR, Adhikari NK, et al. Has mortality from acute respiratory distress syndrome decreased over time?: a systematic review. Am J Respir Crit Care Med 2009;179(3):220–7.
3. Ranieri VM, Rubenfeld GD, Thompson BT, et al. Acute respiratory distress syndrome: the Berlin definition. JAMA 2012;307(23):2526–33.
4. Ventilation with lower tidal volumes as compared with traditional tidal volumes for acute lung injury and the acute respiratory distress syndrome. The Acute Respiratory Distress Syndrome Network. N Engl J Med 2000;342(18):1301–8.
5. Esteban A, Frutos-Vivar F, Muriel A, et al. Evolution of mortality over time in patients receiving mechanical ventilation. Am J Respir Crit Care Med 2013; 188(2):220–30.
6. Papazian L, Forel JM, Gacouin A, et al. Neuromuscular blockers in early acute respiratory distress syndrome. N Engl J Med 2010;363(12):1107–16.
7. Guerin C, Reignier J, Richard JC, et al. Prone positioning in severe acute respiratory distress syndrome. N Engl J Med 2013;368(23):2159–68.
8. Raoof S, Goulet K, Esan A, et al. Severe hypoxemic respiratory failure: part 2–nonventilatory strategies. Chest 2010;137(6):1437–48.
9. Vender JS, Szokol JW, Murphy GS, et al. Sedation, analgesia, and neuromuscular blockade in sepsis: an evidence-based review. Crit Care Med 2004; 32(11 Suppl):S554–61.
10. Needham CJ, Brindley PG. Best evidence in critical care medicine: the role of neuromuscular blocking drugs in early severe acute respiratory distress syndrome. Can J Anaesth 2012;59(1): 105–8.
11. Brower RG, Lanken PN, MacIntyre N, et al. Higher versus lower positive end-expiratory pressures in patients with the acute respiratory distress syndrome. N Engl J Med 2004;351(4):327–36.
12. Mercat A, Richard JC, Vielle B, et al. Positive end-expiratory pressure setting in adults with acute lung injury and acute respiratory distress syndrome: a randomized controlled trial. JAMA 2008; 299(6):646–55.
13. Mehta S, Granton J, MacDonald RJ, et al. High-frequency oscillatory ventilation in adults: the Toronto experience. Chest 2004;126(2):518–27.
14. Murray MJ, Cowen J, DeBlock H, et al. Clinical practice guidelines for sustained neuromuscular blockade in the adult critically ill patient. Crit Care Med 2002;30(1):142–56.
15. Stark AR, Bascom R, Frantz ID III. Muscle relaxation in mechanically ventilated infants. J Pediatr 1979;94(3):439–43.
16. Bishop MJ. Hemodynamic and gas exchange effects of pancuronium bromide in sedated patients with respiratory failure. Anesthesiology 1984; 60(4):369–71.
17. Coggeshall JW, Marini JJ, Newman JH. Improved oxygenation after muscle relaxation in adult respiratory distress syndrome. Arch Intern Med 1985; 145(9):1718–20.
18. Conti G, Vilardi V, Rocco M, et al. Paralysis has no effect on chest wall and respiratory system mechanics of mechanically ventilated, sedated patients. Intensive Care Med 1995;21(10):808–12.
19. Westbrook PR, Stubbs SE, Sessler AD, et al. Effects of anesthesia and muscle paralysis on respiratory mechanics in normal man. J Appl Physiol 1973;34(1):81–6.
20. Hunter JM. New neuromuscular blocking drugs. N Engl J Med 1995;332(25):1691–9.
21. De JB, Lacherade JC, Sharshar T, et al. Intensive care unit-acquired weakness: risk factors and prevention. Crit Care Med 2009;37(10 Suppl):S309–15.
22. Lagneau F, D'honneur G, Plaud B, et al. A comparison of two depths of prolonged neuromuscular blockade induced by cisatracurium in mechanically ventilated critically ill patients. Intensive Care Med 2002;28(12):1735–41.
23. Gainnier M, Roch A, Forel JM, et al. Effect of neuromuscular blocking agents on gas exchange in patients presenting with acute respiratory distress syndrome. Crit Care Med 2004;32(1):113–9.
24. Forel JM, Roch A, Marin V, et al. Neuromuscular blocking agents decrease inflammatory response in patients presenting with acute respiratory distress syndrome. Crit Care Med 2006;34(11): 2749–57.
25. Alhazzani W, Alshahrani M, Jaeschke R, et al. Neuromuscular blocking agents in acute respiratory distress syndrome: a systematic review and meta-analysis of randomized controlled trials. Crit Care 2013;17(2):R43.
26. Neto AS, Pereira VG, Esposito DC, et al. Neuromuscular blocking agents in patients with acute respiratory distress syndrome: a summary of the current evidence from three randomized controlled trials. Ann Intensive Care 2012;2(1):33.
27. Steingrub JS, Lagu T, Rothberg MB, et al. Treatment with neuromuscular blocking agents and the

risk of in-hospital mortality among mechanically ventilated patients with severe sepsis. Crit Care Med 2014;42(1):90–6.

28. Tokics L, Hedenstierna G, Svensson L, et al. V/Q distribution and correlation to atelectasis in anesthetized paralyzed humans. J Appl Physiol (1985) 1996;81(4):1822–33.

29. Slutsky AS. Neuromuscular blocking agents in ARDS. N Engl J Med 2010;363(12):1176–80.

30. Yoshida T, Uchiyama A, Matsuura N, et al. Spontaneous breathing during lung-protective ventilation in an experimental acute lung injury model: high transpulmonary pressure associated with strong spontaneous breathing effort may worsen lung injury. Crit Care Med 2012;40(5):1578–85.

31. Latronico N, Bolton CF. Critical illness polyneuropathy and myopathy: a major cause of muscle weakness and paralysis. Lancet Neurol 2011;10(10):931–41.

32. Bolton CF. The discovery of critical illness polyneuropathy: a memoir. Can J Neurol Sci 2010;37(4):431–8.

33. De JB, Sharshar T, Lefaucheur JP, et al. Paresis acquired in the intensive care unit: a prospective multicenter study. JAMA 2002;288(22):2859–67.

34. Witt NJ, Zochodne DW, Bolton CF, et al. Peripheral nerve function in sepsis and multiple organ failure. Chest 1991;99(1):176–84.

35. Latronico N, Peli E, Botteri M. Critical illness myopathy and neuropathy. Curr Opin Crit Care 2005;11(2):126–32.

36. Van den Berghe G, Schoonheydt K, Becx P, et al. Insulin therapy protects the central and peripheral nervous system of intensive care patients. Neurology 2005;64(8):1348–53.

37. Sharshar T, Bastuji-Garin S, Stevens RD, et al. Presence and severity of intensive care unit-acquired paresis at time of awakening are associated with increased intensive care unit and hospital mortality. Crit Care Med 2009;37(12):3047–53.

38. Weber-Carstens S, Deja M, Koch S, et al. Risk factors in critical illness myopathy during the early course of critical illness: a prospective observational study. Crit Care Med 2010;14(3):R119.

39. Griffiths RD, Hall JB. Intensive care unit-acquired weakness. Crit Care Med 2010;38(3):779–87.

40. Hansen-Flaschen J, Cowen J, Raps EC. Neuromuscular blockade in the intensive care unit. More than we bargained for. Am Rev Respir Dis 1993;147(1):234–6.

41. Testelmans D, Maes K, Wouters P, et al. Infusions of rocuronium and cisatracurium exert different effects on rat diaphragm function. Intensive Care Med 2007;33(5):872–9.

42. Kress JP, Pohlman AS, O'Connor MF, et al. Daily interruption of sedative infusions in critically ill patients undergoing mechanical ventilation. N Engl J Med 2000;342(20):1471–7.

43. Girard TD, Kress JP, Fuchs BD, et al. Efficacy and safety of a paired sedation and ventilator weaning protocol for mechanically ventilated patients in intensive care (awakening and breathing controlled trial): a randomised controlled trial. Lancet 2008;371(9607):126–34.

44. Kaplan LJ, Bailey H, Formosa V. Airway pressure release ventilation increases cardiac performance in patients with acute lung injury/adult respiratory distress syndrome. Crit Care 2001;5(4):221–6.

45. Levine S, Nguyen T, Taylor N, et al. Rapid disuse atrophy of diaphragm fibers in mechanically ventilated humans. N Engl J Med 2008;358(13):1327–35.

46. Jaber S, Petrof BJ, Jung B, et al. Rapidly progressive diaphragmatic weakness and injury during mechanical ventilation in humans. Am J Respir Crit Care Med 2011;183(3):364–71.

47. Putensen C, Mutz NJ, Putensen-Himmer G, et al. Spontaneous breathing during ventilatory support improves ventilation-perfusion distributions in patients with acute respiratory distress syndrome. Am J Respir Crit Care Med 1999;159(4 Pt 1):1241–8.

48. Putensen C, Zech S, Wrigge H, et al. Long-term effects of spontaneous breathing during ventilatory support in patients with acute lung injury. Am J Respir Crit Care Med 2001;164(1):43–9.

49. Varpula T, Valta P, Niemi R, et al. Airway pressure release ventilation as a primary ventilatory mode in acute respiratory distress syndrome. Acta Anaesthesiol Scand 2004;48(6):722–31.

50. Varpula T, Jousela I, Niemi R, et al. Combined effects of prone positioning and airway pressure release ventilation on gas exchange in patients with acute lung injury. Acta Anaesthesiol Scand 2003;47(5):516–24.

51. Daoud EG, Farag HL, Chatburn RL. Airway pressure release ventilation: what do we know? Respir Care 2012;57(2):282–92.

52. Yoshida T, Uchiyama A, Matsuura N, et al. The comparison of spontaneous breathing and muscle paralysis in two different severities of experimental lung injury. Crit Care Med 2013;41(2):536–45.

53. Artigas A, Bernard GR, Carlet J, et al. The American-European Consensus Conference on ARDS, part 2: Ventilatory, pharmacologic, supportive therapy, study design strategies, and issues related to recovery and remodeling. Acute respiratory distress syndrome. Am J Respir Crit Care Med 1998;157(4 Pt 1):1332–47.

Extracorporeal Circulatory Approaches to Treat Acute Respiratory Distress Syndrome

Darryl Abrams, MD, Daniel Brodie, MD*

KEYWORDS

- Acute respiratory distress syndrome • Extracorporeal membrane oxygenation
- Extracorporeal carbon dioxide removal • Respiratory failure • Lung-protective ventilation

KEY POINTS

- In patients with severe acute respiratory distress syndrome (ARDS), extracorporeal membrane oxygenation (ECMO) is most commonly used as rescue therapy, providing adequate oxygenation for profound hypoxemia.
- Extracorporeal carbon dioxide removal ($ECCO_2R$) is a version of ECMO that provides minimal oxygenation support yet efficiently removes carbon dioxide from the blood via smaller, safer cannulae.
- $ECCO_2R$ may facilitate the use of standard-of-care lung-protective ventilation when respiratory system compliance is low.
- Evidence suggests that a very low-volume, low-pressure ventilation strategy (ultra–lung-protective ventilation) may offer additional benefit in ARDS of varying severity; however, this has yet to be proved.
- Rigorously designed studies, including cost-benefit analyses, should be undertaken before the broader application of ECMO for ARDS, particularly for less severe forms of the syndrome.

INTRODUCTION

Extracorporeal membrane oxygenation (ECMO) has a long history in the management of acute respiratory distress syndrome (ARDS), although early versions of the technology had high complication rates resulting in poor outcomes. More recent advances in technology, along with improved management strategies, have led to a more favorable risk-benefit profile and improved rates of survival in observational studies, when ECMO is used as salvage therapy for patients traditionally expected to have a high mortality. However, the benefit of ECMO over conventional standard-of-care ventilation has yet to be demonstrated in rigorously designed randomized controlled trials.

Funding Sources: None.
Conflicts of Interest: Research support from Maquet Cardiovascular including travel expenses for research meetings and compensation paid to Columbia University for research consulting (Dr D. Brodie). He receives no direct compensation from Maquet. Dr D. Brodie is a member of the Medical Advisory Board for ALung Technologies. Compensation is paid to Columbia University. Dr D. Brodie receives no direct compensation from ALung Technologies; None (Dr D. Abrams).
Division of Pulmonary, Allergy and Critical Care, Columbia University College of Physicians and Surgeons, PH 8E 101, New York, NY 10032, USA
* Corresponding author.
E-mail address: hdb5@cumc.columbia.edu

Clin Chest Med 35 (2014) 765–779
http://dx.doi.org/10.1016/j.ccm.2014.08.013
0272-5231/14/$ – see front matter © 2014 Elsevier Inc. All rights reserved.

As extracorporeal technology continues to evolve, there is potential to have a greater impact on the management of ARDS by both facilitating and enhancing lung-protective ventilatory strategies. This article reviews the implementation of, evidence behind and the rationale for ECMO in ARDS, along with potential future directions awaiting further clinical investigation.

EXTRACORPOREAL MEMBRANE OXYGENATION CANNULATION AND CONFIGURATIONS

ECMO consists of an extracorporeal circuit with a gas exchange device, referred to as an oxygenator, which directly oxygenates and removes carbon dioxide from the blood across a semipermeable membrane (**Fig. 1**).[1] Because it is more than simply oxygenation, a more precise term is extracorporeal gas exchange, although the acronym ECMO remains far more commonly used. Deoxygenated blood is withdrawn through a drainage cannula via an external pump, passes through the oxygenator, and is returned to the patient through a reinfusion cannula. When blood is both withdrawn from and returned to a central vein, it is referred to as venovenous ECMO (**Fig. 2**). Venovenous ECMO provides gas exchange only. By contrast, when blood is drained from a central vein and returned to an artery, it is referred to as venoarterial ECMO (**Fig. 3**). Venoarterial ECMO provides both respiratory and circulatory support. Because most cases of ARDS

involve respiratory failure alone, this article focuses primarily on the application of venovenous ECMO. However, it is important to consider the need for venoarterial ECMO if ARDS is accompanied by cardiogenic shock, as has been reported, for instance, in cases of ARDS complicating septic shock with an associated sepsis-induced cardiomyopathy.[2] In situations where severe hypoxemia results in isolated, severe right ventricular dysfunction, venovenous ECMO is typically adequate to support the patient without a need for venoarterial ECMO, with increases in oxygenation improving pulmonary vascular resistance, coronary perfusion, and right ventricular function. However, patients who have concomitant pulmonary hypertension that is unrelated to hypoxemic vasoconstriction may require a venoarterial configuration.[3]

- Venovenous ECMO provides only respiratory support
- Venoarterial ECMO provides both respiratory and circulatory support
- Isolated right heart dysfunction from hypoxemic respiratory failure is typically supported with venovenous ECMO alone

The amount of extracorporeal blood flow relative to total cardiac output, the fraction of oxygen delivered through the circuit, and the contribution of native lung function are the main determinants of blood oxygenation.[1] Of importance is that changes in the patient's cardiac output, at a given

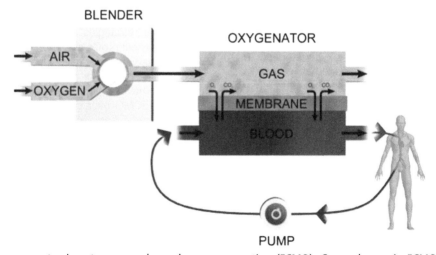

Fig. 1. The oxygenator in extracorporeal membrane oxygenation (ECMO). Gas exchange in ECMO is accomplished by pumping blood through an oxygenator, consisting of 2 chambers divided by a semipermeable membrane. Venous blood passes along one side of the membrane and fresh gas, referred to as sweep gas, passes along the other side. Oxygen uptake and carbon dioxide elimination occur across the membrane. The fraction of oxygen delivered through the gas chamber is determined by a blender, which typically mixes oxygen with room air. (*Courtesy of* www.collectedmed.com; with permission.)

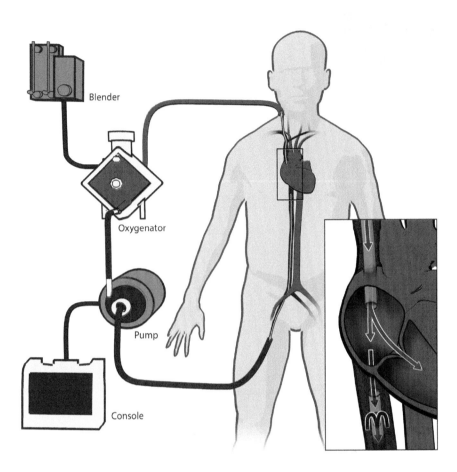

Fig. 2. Two-site venovenous ECMO. In venovenous ECMO, venous blood is withdrawn from a central vein, pumped through an oxygenator, and reinfused into a central vein. Venovenous ECMO only supports gas exchange, without providing any hemodynamic support. (*Inset*) When drainage and reinfusion ports are in close approximation, some reinfused, oxygenated blood may be drawn back into the circuit without having entered the systemic circulation, referred to as recirculation (*purple arrow*). Recirculation does not contribute to systemic oxygenation. (*Courtesy of* www.collectedmed.com; with permission.)

extracorporeal blood flow rate, will alter the proportion of the patient's blood volume passing through the oxygenator. If a greater proportion of blood is oxygenated by the circuit before mixing with blood that returns to the heart without passing through the circuit, systemic oxygenation will improve, and vice versa. This scenario should be considered when choosing the size of the cannulae that are inserted in the patient for ECMO. The choice of cannula size is based, in part, on the physiologic needs of the patient, with particular consideration given to the patient's estimated cardiac output.

The primary determinant of carbon dioxide removal is the rate of gas flow through the oxygenator, referred to as the sweep gas flow rate. Modern extracorporeal circuits are very efficient at carbon dioxide removal, doing so at blood flow rates in the range of 200 to 1500 mL/min, which is much lower than is typically needed to support oxygenation.[4] Therefore, when the focus is extracorporeal carbon dioxide removal (ECCO$_2$R), smaller cannulae can be used, which may minimize the risk and complexity of insertion and maintenance of the circuit.[5,6] ECCO$_2$R may be used to eliminate carbon dioxide in ARDS to permit lung-protective ventilation strategies. An alternative configuration used primarily for carbon dioxide removal is arteriovenous ECCO$_2$R, which utilizes the patient's native cardiac output to generate extracorporeal blood flow, negating the need for an external pump.[7,8] This configuration is associated with additional complications related to the arterial cannulation, including limb ischemia and

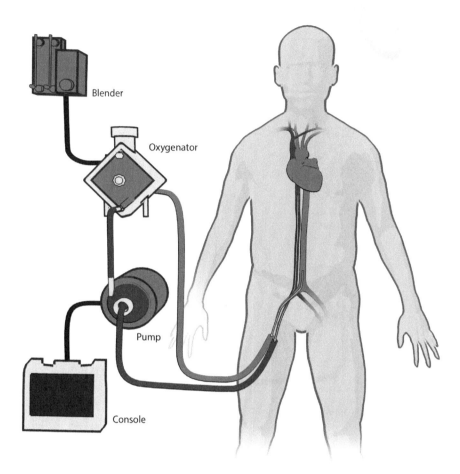

Fig. 3. Venoarterial ECMO. In venoarterial ECMO, venous blood is withdrawn from a central vein, pumped through an oxygenator, and reinfused into an artery. Venoarterial ECMO provides both respiratory and circulatory support. (*Courtesy of* www.collectedmed.com; with permission.)

compartment syndrome, making it less advantageous than venovenous $ECCO_2R$ in many clinical scenarios.[7,9]

- Extracorporeal oxygenation correlates with the amount of blood flow through the ECMO circuit, usually requiring large cannulae to achieve oxygenation goals
- Carbon dioxide removal can be achieved at very low blood flow rates, allowing for the use of smaller cannulae

Traditional venovenous ECMO configurations involve cannulation at 2 distinct venous access points for drainage and reinfusion of blood.[1] Such a 2-site configuration, whereby the ports of the drainage and reinfusion cannulae can be in close proximity, may lend itself to recirculation, whereby oxygenated blood is withdrawn back into the circuit without passing through the patient

or contributing to systemic oxygenation (see **Fig. 2**). In addition, a 2-site configuration requires femoral venous access. With the advent of a bicaval dual-lumen cannula, the internal jugular vein can be used as the sole venous access site to provide venovenous extracorporeal support, avoiding femoral cannulation and minimizing recirculation (**Fig. 4**).[10,11] This approach requires the proper positioning of the dual-lumen cannula with the reinfusion jet directed toward the tricuspid valve.[11]

- A 2-site venovenous configuration requires femoral cannulation and may increase the likelihood of recirculation
- Bicaval, dual-lumen cannulae, when properly positioned, minimize the amount of recirculation

Placement of bicaval dual-lumen cannulae typically requires fluoroscopic or transesophageal

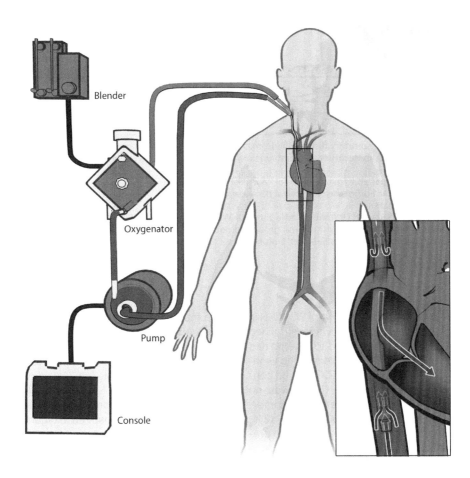

Fig. 4. Single-site venovenous ECMO. Bicaval, dual-lumen cannulae permit the use of venovenous ECMO via a single venous access point. (*Inset*) When the cannula is properly positioned, reinfused, oxygenated blood is directed toward the tricuspid valve, minimizing recirculation. (*Courtesy of* www.collectedmed.com; with permission.)

echocardiographic guidance.[12] For those patients in whom some form of mobilization is anticipated, a configuration that avoids femoral cannulation is preferred.

THE HISTORY OF EXTRACORPOREAL SUPPORT FOR ACUTE RESPIRATORY DISTRESS SYNDROME

The first use of ECMO as salvage therapy for severe hypoxemic respiratory failure was described in a case report by Hill and colleagues[13] in 1972. A subsequent randomized trial (published in 1979) attempted to define which patients with respiratory failure might benefit from ECMO, but the results failed to show a survival benefit from the addition of ECMO to conventional mechanical ventilation.[14] Survival was very poor in both groups (9.5% and 8.3%, respectively) (**Table 1**).

ECCO$_2$R, by contrast, was first observed as an unanticipated consequence of early hemodialysis membranes.[15] Gattinoni and colleagues[5,16–19] investigated its potential as a means of providing nearly all of the ventilation in cases of severe hypoxemic respiratory failure, minimizing the need for and complications from continuous positive-pressure ventilation, a strategy referred to as lung rest, while oxygenation was achieved passively (apneic oxygenation). This strategy of low-frequency positive-pressure ventilation and ECCO$_2$R resulted in 48.8% survival in an uncontrolled study of subjects whose gas-exchange abnormalities were similar to those of the participants in the 1979 trial. This significantly higher rate of

Table 1
Prospective randomized trials of ECLS for ARDS

Authors,[Ref.] Year	No. of Patients	Pao$_2$/Fio$_2$[a]	Modality	ECLS Survival (%)	Non-ECLS Survival (%)	Duration of ECLS Support (d)
Zapol et al,[14] 1979	90	<83	ECMO	9.5[b]	8.3	6.5[c,d]
Morris et al,[20] 1994	40	63	ECCO$_2$R	33[b]	42	8.7 ± 1.7[c]
Peek et al,[50] 2009	180	75	ECMO	63[e,f]	47	9.0 (6.0–16.0)[g]

Abbreviations: ARDS, acute respiratory distress syndrome; ECCO$_2$R, extracorporeal carbon dioxide removal; ECLS, extracorporeal life support; ECMO, extracorporeal membrane oxygenation; Fio$_2$, fraction of inspired oxygen; Pao$_2$, partial pressure of arterial oxygen.
   [a] Threshold value for Zapol et al; mean value for Morris et al and Peek et al.
   [b] No statistically significant difference in survival between groups.
   [c] Mean ± standard deviation.
   [d] Personal communication with Dr Robert Bartlett and Dr Warren Zapol, April 15, 2014.
   [e] 22 of 90 patients (24%) within ECMO referral group did not receive ECMO.
   [f] Relative risk of death or severe disability at 6 months 0.69 (95% CI 0.05–0.97; $P = .03$) compared with non-ECMO group.
   [g] Median (interquartile range).

survival prompted a randomized trial of ECCO$_2$R in ARDS.[20] Subjects with what is nowadays defined as severe ARDS were randomized to a combined strategy of pressure-controlled inverse-ratio ventilation followed by venovenous ECCO$_2$R or conventional mechanical ventilation. There was no significant difference in survival between the intervention and control groups (33% and 42%, respectively); combined with the results of the previous randomized trial, these findings led to a waning interest in either ECMO or ECCO$_2$R as a supportive therapy for severe hypoxemic respiratory failure. However, these trials were conducted with outdated extracorporeal technology and mechanical ventilation techniques, among other issues.

- Early randomized trials of ECMO for acute hypoxemic respiratory failure were negative, with high mortality rates in both intervention and control arms

MODERN-DAY EXTRACORPOREAL MEMBRANE OXYGENATION FOR SEVERE ACUTE RESPIRATORY DISTRESS SYNDROME

In the interval since those early trials, nonrandomized observational studies have suggested a survival rate of 49% to 81% for selected patients with severe ARDS.[21–29] More recently, there have been significant advances in extracorporeal technology, including the use of centrifugal pumps, polymethylpentene oxygenators, biocompatible circuit components, and single-site dual-lumen cannulae.[10,30]

In the era of modern extracorporeal circuitry, a resurgence of interest accompanied reports of success using ECMO for patients with severe ARDS during the 2009 influenza A (H1N1) pandemic, most notably the 75% survival among a subset of patients in Australia and New Zealand with a median partial pressure of arterial oxygen (Pao$_2$) to fraction of inspired oxygen (Fio$_2$) ratio of 56.[31–35] However, comparable rates of survival among patients with H1N1-related ARDS and similar degrees of hypoxemia (median Pao$_2$/Fio$_2$ ratio of 61) were observed at a center whose management strategy did not include ECMO.[36] There were no randomized trials of ECMO during the H1N1 pandemic. However, one study examined the effect of ECMO referral on survival by matching patients from the United Kingdom with H1N1-related ARDS who were referred to a center capable of providing ECMO, with a separate cohort of patients with H1N1-associated ARDS who were not referred for ECMO.[37] Analysis of matched pairs from each cohort demonstrated significantly improved survival in favor of referral for ECMO (relative risk 0.45–0.51), although the effect of unmeasured confounders may have contributed to these findings. By contrast, a matched propensity analysis by the French Réseau Européen de Recherche en Ventilation Artificielle (REVA) research network demonstrated no difference in intensive care unit mortality between patients who received ECMO for H1N1-associated ARDS and non-ECMO control subjects (odds ratio 1.48, 95% confidence interval 0.68–3.23; $P = .32$), with a matching strategy that avoided duplication of control subjects in the analysis.[38] An important limitation of this study was the inability to match 51 ECMO patients who were younger and more hypoxemic, had higher end-inspiratory plateau pressures, and had a lower mortality (22% vs 50%, $P<.01$) than the 52 ECMO patients who were able to be matched.

- Nonrandomized observational studies show conflicting results about the survival benefit of ECMO in severe ARDS

The trend of improved survival as reported in observational studies of ECMO in severe ARDS may also have been influenced by improvements in general critical care and mechanical ventilation management over the same interval.[39–46] Mortality among patients with acute lung injury and ARDS has declined from the ARDS Network's ARMA trial (ventilation with lower tidal volumes in comparison with traditional tidal volumes for acute lung injury and ARDS) (39.8% in the 12 mL/kg arm, 31% in 6 mL/kg arm) to the more recent FACTT, ALTA, and OMEGA trials (25.5%, 20.5%, and 21.7%, respectively), which may, in part, be reflective of these changes.[40,42,47–49]

The only controlled clinical trial of ECMO for ARDS using modern technology is the Conventional Ventilation or ECMO for Severe Adult Respiratory Failure (CESAR) trial, in which 180 subjects with severe but potentially reversible respiratory failure were randomized to receive conventional management at designated treatment centers or referral to a specialized center with a standardized treatment protocol, which included a strategy of lung-protective ventilation and consideration of ECMO.[50] The primary outcome of death or severe disability at 6 months occurred in 37% of the subjects referred for consideration for ECMO, compared with 53% in the conventional management group (relative risk 0.69, 95% confidence interval 0.05–0.97; $P - .03$). However, because the conventional management arm did not mandate a protocol for the delivery of mechanical ventilation and only recommended a low-volume, low-pressure ventilation strategy, only 70% of the conventional management subjects received lung-protective ventilation at any time in the study. With the conventional arm not guaranteed standard-of-care management, the results may have been biased in favor of the intervention arm. Conclusions that may be drawn about the survival benefit of the use of ECMO for patients with severe cases of ARDS, based on this trial, are limited. However, referral of patients with severe forms of ARDS to a center capable of performing ECMO as part of a standardized management protocol seems to be beneficial.[37,50]

- Because of limitations in the study design, the CESAR trial is insufficient for defining the clinical role of ECMO in patients with severe ARDS
- Referral of patients with severe ARDS to an ECMO-capable center may be beneficial

LONG-TERM IMPACT OF EXTRACORPOREAL MEMBRANE OXYGENATION ON SURVIVORS OF SEVERE ACUTE RESPIRATORY DISTRESS SYNDROME

The potential benefit of ECMO in severe ARDS, if any, may extend beyond survival. In a 12-month follow-up study of a subset of survivors from the Fluid and Catheter Treatment Trial (FACTT), cognitive impairment and psychiatric morbidity correlated with lower Pao_2 during the initial trial, arguing in favor of interventions that minimize hypoxemia, although this can only be considered a hypothesis at this time.[51]

There are few reports on the long-term physical, psychiatric, and neurocognitive outcomes in survivors of severe ARDS who received ECMO.[52] In one assessment of long-term outcomes among survivors of H1N1-associated severe ARDS in the REVA registry, those who received extracorporeal support (n = 12), compared with traditionally managed ARDS patients (n = 25), had similar rates of anxiety (50% vs 56%), depression (28% in each group), and posttraumatic stress disorder (41% vs 44%), with lower health-related quality of life (HRQoL) scores in both groups compared with age-matched and sex-matched healthy controls, although the ECMO-supported patients had a higher rate of returning to work at 1 year.[38] Analysis of long-term outcomes of an Australian cohort of 18 patients with severe ARDS who received ECMO revealed high rates of survival to discharge (86%), but low HRQoL scores across all domains compared with healthy controls, and lower scores in the domains of mental health, general health, vitality, and social function compared with separate cohorts of ARDS survivors who did not receive ECMO support.[53] However, the patients in the ECMO cohort had a higher average severity of illness than those in the non-ECMO cohorts.

- Randomized trials are necessary to define the impact of ECMO on long-term physical, neurocognitive, and psychiatric outcomes in survivors of ARDS

Despite the rapid growth of ECMO and its potential to improve outcomes in patients with severe ARDS, there is currently a lack of high-level evidence supporting its use. A randomized trial of ECMO versus standard-of-care ventilator management in severe ARDS is currently being undertaken (ECMO to Rescue Lung Injury in Severe ARDS [EOLIA], ClinicalTrials.gov Identifier: NCT01470703). Additional longitudinal physical, psychological, and neurocognitive assessments of survivors from this trial would provide valuable insight into the effect of ECMO on these important clinical outcomes.

FUTURE DIRECTIONS OF EXTRACORPOREAL MEMBRANE OXYGENATION AND EXTRACORPOREAL CARBON DIOXIDE REMOVAL FOR ACUTE RESPIRATORY DISTRESS SYNDROME

Extracorporeal Carbon Dioxide Removal for Less Severe Forms of Acute Respiratory Distress Syndrome

Although severe ARDS is the most commonly reported indication for ECMO in acute respiratory failure (**Boxes 1** and **2**),[1,54] its incidence occurs infrequently.[55] The more widespread application of ECMO or $ECCO_2R$ may likely be related to their use in moderate forms of ARDS, particularly with regard to the management of severe hypercapnia and acidemia in the context of instituting lung-protective ventilatory strategies.

- Although it is the most common indication for ECMO for respiratory failure, severe ARDS occurs infrequently
- Extracorporeal support may have its greatest impact in ARDS by facilitating lung-protective ventilation

In the setting of ARDS, the ability to use low-volume, low-pressure ventilation may be limited by reductions in lung compliance, resulting in intolerable levels of hypercapnia and acidemia. Although the precise threshold for an acceptable pH is undefined, low-volume ventilation must ultimately be limited, at some point, by respiratory acidosis. In such cases, lung-protective ventilation must be sacrificed to maintain adequate pH. The removal of carbon dioxide directly from the blood with an extracorporeal circuit, by contrast, could permit the use of lung-protective ventilation in these patients by maintaining pH even at low tidal volumes. Beyond this, further removal of carbon dioxide could permit the use of tidal volumes and end-inspiratory plateau pressures below the current standard of care. If low tidal volume ventilation improves mortality, then perhaps very low tidal volume ventilation may provide additional benefit.

- $ECCO_2R$ can mitigate disturbances in pH and carbon dioxide when applying lung-protective ventilation in the setting of reduced respiratory system compliance

---

Box 1
Suggested indications and contraindications for ECMO in ARDS

Indications

Severe hypoxemia (eg, ratio of Pao_2 to Fio_2 <80) despite the application of high levels of PEEP, typically 15 to 20 cm H_2O, in patients with potentially reversible respiratory failure

Uncompensated hypercapnia with acidemia (pH <7.15) despite optimal ventilator management

Excessively high plateau airway pressures (>35–45 cm H_2O, depending on the patient's body size) despite optimal ventilator management

Relative contraindications

Prolonged use (>7 days) of high-pressure ventilation (plateau pressure >30 cm H_2O)

Prolonged use (>7 days) of high amounts of Fio_2 (>0.8)

Limited vascular access

Any condition or organ dysfunction that would limit the likelihood of overall benefit from ECMO, such as severe, irreversible brain injury or untreatable metastatic cancer

Contraindication to anticoagulation

Absolute contraindications

ECMO for irreversible, end-stage respiratory failure if transplantation will not be considered

Abbreviations: ARDS, acute respiratory distress syndrome; ECMO, extracorporeal membrane oxygenation; Fio_2, fraction of inspired oxygen; Pao_2, partial pressure of arterial oxygen; PEEP, positive end-expiratory pressure.

- The same approach can facilitate reductions in lung volumes and pressures beyond the current standard of care, which may have additional clinical benefits

Importance of Lung-Protective Ventilation

A volume-limited and pressure-limited ventilatory strategy has been shown to improve survival in the ARMA trial,[40] and additional studies have confirmed that ventilator-associated lung injury can be minimized by implementing lung-protective ventilation.[56–58] Of importance is that lung-protective ventilation may have a survival benefit that endures well beyond the initial event.[59] A prospective cohort study by Needham and colleagues[59] assessing the impact of lung-protective ventilation on acute lung injury showed

overestimating tidal volume, which, in turn, may worsen ventilator-associated lung injury and negatively affect survival.

Physicians generally have a misperception of their adherence to low tidal volume ventilation, as evidenced by a survey of critical care physicians across 214 intensive care units in Germany. Perceived adherence to low tidal volume ventilation was 79.9% in sepsis-induced ARDS, but the actual use of a tidal volume of 6 mL/kg or less of predicted body weight was only 2.6%, between 6 and 8 mL/kg 17.1%, and greater than 8 mL/kg 80.3%. Mean tidal volume was 10 mL/kg.[61] Reasons cited for nonadherence to a low tidal volume ventilatory strategy have included the presence of uncompensated hypercapnia and acidemia.[62,63] The addition of $ECCO_2R$, in the general ARDS population, could facilitate the application of lung-protective ventilation, not to mention serving as a reminder to clinicians of the importance of lowering tidal volumes and end-inspiratory plateau pressures.

that for every additional ventilator setting adherent to a volume-limited and pressure-limited strategy, there was a 3% reduction in mortality at the end of 2 years of follow-up, and for every additional milliliter per kilogram of tidal volume delivered, there was a direct correlation with increasing mortality. However, only 41% of the eligible ventilator settings in 485 consecutive patients over a 4-year period were adherent to lung-protective ventilation. Thirty-seven percent of patients never received lung-protective ventilation at any time.

- Despite definitive evidence of the survival benefit of lung-protective ventilation in ARDS, actual adherence rates remain relatively low

Because lung-protective ventilation is predicated on the use of predicted body weight, tidal volume may be overestimated in women and those with short stature, when actual body weight is used. In 421 patients with sepsis-related acute lung injury across 7 teaching hospitals, low tidal volume ventilation was correctly applied in only 53% of patients within the first 48 hours after diagnosis (women 46%, men 59%).[60] In multivariate analysis, the factors that were significantly associated with receiving low tidal volume ventilation were severity of illness and height. Adherence to low tidal volume ventilation was higher when patients' actual body weights were used (73%), but actual body weight exceeded predicted body weight by an average of 18 kg (84 vs 66 kg). Such discrepancies highlight the importance of using predicted body weight to avoid

Role of Very Low Tidal Volume Ventilation

Results from some, but not all, animal models of acute lung injury suggest an incremental reduction in ventilator-associated lung injury by achieving lower tidal volumes and end-inspiratory plateau pressures than were targeted in the ARMA trial.[64–69] In rats with hydrochloric acid–induced acute lung injury, a tidal volume of 3 mL/kg, with a corresponding end-inspiratory plateau pressure of 16 cm H_2O, resulted in significantly less extravascular lung water than tidal volumes of 6 mL/kg (end-inspiratory plateau pressure of 21 cm H_2O) and 12 mL/kg (end-inspiratory plateau pressure of 30 cm H_2O).

Secondary analysis of the ARDSnet database from the ARMA trial demonstrates a linear relationship between lower end-inspiratory plateau pressure on day 1 of enrollment and decreased mortality that holds true at end-inspiratory plateau pressures well below 30 cm H_2O, suggesting that there may not be a safe end-inspiratory plateau pressure.[70] When subjects were stratified by quartile of day-1 end-inspiratory plateau pressure, the lower plateau pressure quartiles had a lower mortality than the higher plateau pressure quartiles. Likewise, the lower tidal volume strategy was associated with decreased mortality within each quartile, consistent with the conclusion drawn from the original analysis of the ARMA trial. Multivariable logistic regression analysis showed that lower tidal volume, lower plateau pressure quartile, and lower severity of illness all predicted decreased mortality. The lack of significant interaction between tidal volume assignment and plateau pressure quartile suggests that subjects in the higher tidal volume group would have benefited from reduction in tidal volume, regardless of plateau pressure quartile. However, lower end-inspiratory plateau pressures in the study were achieved with a tidal volume of 6 mL/kg when respiratory system compliance was relatively high. The effect of reducing tidal volumes to lower than 6 mL/kg could not be evaluated.

- Lower tidal volumes and plateau pressures beyond those investigated in the ARMA trial may have an incremental survival benefit

Extracorporeal Carbon Dioxide Removal–Assisted Very Low Tidal Volume Ventilation

Terragni and colleagues[71] attempted to address this very issue by reducing tidal volumes to lower than 6 mL/kg of predicted body weight (to an average of around 4 mL/kg) in patients with ARDS to reduce end-inspiratory plateau pressures from a range of 28 to 30 cm H_2O to 25 to 27 cm H_2O. At very low tidal volume ventilation with the lower range of end-inspiratory plateau pressures, inflammatory markers indicating lung injury (interleukin-6, interleukin-8, interleukin-1β, and interleukin-1 receptor antagonist) were significantly reduced in comparison with baseline levels measured at end-inspiratory plateau pressures of 28 to 30 cm H_2O. Tidal volumes of around 4 mL/kg could only be achieved with the use of $ECCO_2R$ to maintain what they defined as adequate pH (>7.25), requiring blood flows of only 5% to 10% of cardiac output via a 14F dual-lumen cannula in the femoral vein. Without $ECCO_2R$, hypercapnia and acidemia were considered unacceptably severe. There were no significant adverse events related to the use of $ECCO_2R$. The lack of a conventionally managed control group with end-inspiratory plateau pressures of 28 to 30 cm H_2O limits the interpretation of this study. However, the decrease in inflammatory markers in the intervention group to levels comparable with those of subjects with baseline end-inspiratory plateau pressures of 25 to 27 cm H_2O suggests that lower volumes and pressures than the ARDSnet ARMA protocol would further minimize ventilator-associated lung injury. A subsequent randomized trial compared $ECCO_2R$-assisted very low tidal volume ventilation (approximately 3 mL/kg predicted body weight) with standard-of-care lung-protective ventilation in patients with moderate to severe ARDS.[72] Although there was no statistically significant difference in the number of ventilator-free days within 60 days between the 2 groups (33 vs 29, $P = .469$), post

hoc analysis demonstrated more ventilator-free days at 60 days in subjects with more severe hypoxemia (40.9 vs 28.2, $P = .033$).

- $ECCO_2R$ is necessary to consistently achieve very low tidal volume ventilation
- Additional data are necessary to determine the risks and benefits of very low tidal volume ventilation in managing ARDS

Based on the existing literature, a reduction in tidal volume to significantly less than 6 mL/kg seems to be technically feasible when an extracorporeal circuit is implemented. Randomized controlled trials are still needed to clarify the role of $ECCO_2R$ in facilitating the current standard-of-care volume-limited and pressure-limited ventilation strategy when intolerable acidemia and hypercapnia are present. Additional studies will be necessary to evaluate the efficacy of $ECCO_2R$-assisted very low tidal volume ventilation in enhancing lung-protective ventilation beyond current practice.

EXTUBATION DURING EXTRACORPOREAL SUPPORT

If minimization of ventilator-associated lung injury is believed to be fundamental to the management of patients with ARDS, then, theoretically, removal of invasive mechanical ventilation from a patient receiving ECMO would eliminate that mechanism of injury entirely. In addition, extubation may allow for the reduction in or avoidance of sedatives that might otherwise be necessary for patient-ventilator synchrony and elimination of ventilator-associated pneumonia. However, spontaneous breathing may exacerbate lung injury by increasing mechanical stress.[73,74] There is limited experience with spontaneous breathing, with or without invasive mechanical ventilation, during extracorporeal support for severe ARDS,[74–76] and further study is needed before any recommendations can be made.

- Elimination of invasive mechanical ventilation may be possible in ARDS with the assistance of ECMO, although there are insufficient data to recommend this practice

ACTIVE PHYSICAL THERAPY DURING EXTRACORPOREAL SUPPORT

Physical therapy, including ambulation, is increasingly being recognized as an important component of critical care management,[46,77,78] and such activity is being reported with increased frequency among patients receiving ECMO for respiratory failure.[79] However, these data are mostly limited to the population receiving extracorporeal support as a bridge to lung transplantation.[80–83] Although most patients with severe ARDS requiring ECMO are currently believed to be too critically ill to participate in active rehabilitation, a subset of patients may be appropriate for such interventions.[79] Any program focusing on active physical therapy in this complex patient population should involve a carefully designed, multidisciplinary approach to ensure both safety and efficacy.[79]

- Physical therapy is an important intervention in optimizing outcomes in critically ill patients
- A multidisciplinary team approach may allow for the safe implementation of active rehabilitation in selected ARDS patients receiving ECMO

COMPLICATIONS OF EXTRACORPOREAL SUPPORT

Any potential benefit from ECMO must be balanced against its risks. Hemorrhage, thrombosis, hemolysis, and infection are among the more commonly reported complications from extracorporeal support (**Table 2**).[84–88] With advances in extracorporeal technology, the rates of many of these complications have been decreasing over time.[89]

ECONOMIC CONSIDERATIONS

There are few cost-benefit analyses of ECMO use in ARDS. The CESAR trial included an economic assessment of extracorporeal support in ARDS,[50,90] but this was limited to a particular

health care system within the confines of a randomized trial. Careful economic evaluations will be necessary to determine whether the potential benefit of a resource-intensive intervention such as ECMO is worth the health care costs, particularly before more widespread application of the technology.

ETHICAL CONSIDERATIONS

The ability of ECMO to support patients with respiratory failure creates the potential for unique ethical dilemmas.[91] Patients dependent on ECMO are necessarily confined to an intensive care unit. There is no destination device therapy for ECMO for respiratory failure. If there is no expectation of recovery after an appropriate course of medical therapy, the patient may effectively have no end point, often referred to as a "bridge to nowhere." Careful selection of patients who are most likely to have favorable outcomes from ECMO-supported ARDS may help avoid such scenarios.[92,93]

SUMMARY

In the absence of high-quality data from rigorously designed trials, ECMO is viewed by many clinicians exclusively as salvage therapy for severe, refractory hypoxemia, and even that use remains controversial.[94] The impact of ECMO on the management of severe ARDS may be clarified with a modern-day randomized controlled trial. The ability of ECCO$_2$R to facilitate lung-protective ventilation, or ultra–lung-protective ventilation beyond the currently accepted standard of care, if shown to improve clinically meaningful outcomes, may further broaden the role of ECMO in ARDS.

Table 2 Complications associated with ECMO	
Complication	**Rate (%)[a]**
Hemorrhage	
Cannula site	13.5
Surgical site	10.6
Gastrointestinal	7.2
CNS	2.5
Circuit thrombosis	25.2
Infection	10.4
Hemolysis	6.8
Disseminated intravascular coagulopathy	2.0

Abbreviations: CNS, central nervous system; ECMO, extracorporeal membrane oxygenation.
[a] Percentages of complications of ECMO for respiratory failure in 2013 in the United States as reported by the Extracorporeal Life Support Organization.[89]

REFERENCES

1. Brodie D, Bacchetta M. Extracorporeal membrane oxygenation for ARDS in adults. N Engl J Med 2011;365(20):1905–14.
2. Brechot N, Luyt CE, Schmidt M, et al. Venoarterial extracorporeal membrane oxygenation support for refractory cardiovascular dysfunction during severe bacterial septic shock. Crit Care Med 2013; 41(7):1616–26.
3. Abrams D, Brodie D, Bacchetta M, et al. Upper-body extracorporeal membrane oxygenation as a strategy in decompensated pulmonary arterial hypertension. Pulm Circ 2013;3(2):432–5.
4. Schmidt M, Tachon G, Devilliers C, et al. Blood oxygenation and decarboxylation determinants during venovenous ECMO for respiratory failure in adults. Intensive Care Med 2013;39(5):838–46.

5. Gattinoni L, Kolobow T, Damia G, et al. Extracorporeal carbon dioxide removal ($ECCO_2R$): a new form of respiratory assistance. Int J Artif Organs 1979; 2(4):183–5.

6. Abrams D, Brodie D. Emerging indications for extracorporeal membrane oxygenation in adults with respiratory failure. Ann Am Thorac Soc 2013; 10(4):371–7.

7. Bein T, Weber F, Philipp A, et al. A new pumpless extracorporeal interventional lung assist in critical hypoxemia/hypercapnia. Crit Care Med 2006; 34(5):1372–7.

8. Fischer S, Simon AR, Welte T, et al. Bridge to lung transplantation with the novel pumpless interventional lung assist device NovaLung. J Thorac Cardiovasc Surg 2006;131(3):719–23.

9. Aziz F, Brehm CE, El-Banyosy A, et al. Arterial complications in patients undergoing extracorporeal membrane oxygenation via femoral cannulation. Ann Vasc Surg 2014;28:178–83.

10. Wang D, Zhou X, Liu X, et al. Wang-Zwische double lumen cannula-toward a percutaneous and ambulatory paracorporeal artificial lung. ASAIO J 2008;54(6):606–11.

11. Javidfar J, Brodie D, Wang D, et al. Use of bicaval dual-lumen catheter for adult venovenous extracorporeal membrane oxygenation. Ann Thorac Surg 2011;91(6):1763–8 [discussion: 1769].

12. Javidfar J, Wang D, Zwischenberger JB, et al. Insertion of bicaval dual lumen extracorporeal membrane oxygenation catheter with image guidance. ASAIO J 2011;57(3):203–5.

13. Hill JD, O'Brien TG, Murray JJ, et al. Prolonged extracorporeal oxygenation for acute post-traumatic respiratory failure (shock-lung syndrome). Use of the Bramson membrane lung. N Engl J Med 1972;286(12):629–34.

14. Zapol WM, Snider MT, Hill JD, et al. Extracorporeal membrane oxygenation in severe acute respiratory failure. A randomized prospective study. JAMA 1979;242(20):2193–6.

15. Sherlock JE, Yoon Y, Ledwith JW, et al. Respiratory gas exchange during hemodialysis. Proc Clin Dial Transplant Forum 1972;2:171–4.

16. Gattinoni L, Kolobow T, Agostoni A, et al. Clinical application of low frequency positive pressure ventilation with extracorporeal CO_2 removal (LFPPV-$ECCO_2R$) in treatment of adult respiratory distress syndrome (ARDS). Int J Artif Organs 1979;2(6):282–3.

17. Gattinoni L, Agostoni A, Pesenti A, et al. Treatment of acute respiratory failure with low-frequency positive-pressure ventilation and extracorporeal removal of CO_2. Lancet 1980;2(8189):292–4.

18. Gattinoni L, Pesenti A, Caspani ML, et al. The role of total static lung compliance in the management of severe ARDS unresponsive to conventional treatment. Intensive Care Med 1984;10(3):121–6.

19. Gattinoni L, Pesenti A, Mascheroni D, et al. Low-frequency positive-pressure ventilation with extracorporeal CO_2 removal in severe acute respiratory failure. JAMA 1986;256(7):881–6.

20. Morris AH, Wallace CJ, Menlove RL, et al. Randomized clinical trial of pressure-controlled inverse ratio ventilation and extracorporeal CO_2 removal for adult respiratory distress syndrome. Am J Respir Crit Care Med 1994;149(2 Pt 1):295–305.

21. Wagner PK, Knoch M, Sangmeister C, et al. Extracorporeal gas exchange in adult respiratory distress syndrome: associated morbidity and its surgical treatment. Br J Surg 1990;77(12):1395–8.

22. Brunet F, Belghith M, Mira JP, et al. Extracorporeal carbon dioxide removal and low-frequency positive-pressure ventilation. Improvement in arterial oxygenation with reduction of risk of pulmonary barotrauma in patients with adult respiratory distress syndrome. Chest 1993;104(3):889–98.

23. Kolla S, Awad SS, Rich PB, et al. Extracorporeal life support for 100 adult patients with severe respiratory failure. Ann Surg 1997;226(4):544–64 [discussion: 565–6].

24. Lewandowski K, Rossaint R, Pappert D, et al. High survival rate in 122 ARDS patients managed according to a clinical algorithm including extracorporeal membrane oxygenation. Intensive Care Med 1997;23(8):819–35.

25. Manert W, Haller M, Briegel J, et al. Venovenous extracorporeal membrane oxygenation (ECMO) with a heparin-lock bypass system. An effective addition in the treatment of acute respiratory failure (ARDS). Anaesthesist 1996;45(5):437–48 [in German].

26. Linden V, Palmer K, Reinhard J, et al. High survival in adult patients with acute respiratory distress syndrome treated by extracorporeal membrane oxygenation, minimal sedation, and pressure supported ventilation. Intensive Care Med 2000; 26(11):1630–7.

27. Peek GJ, Moore HM, Moore N, et al. Extracorporeal membrane oxygenation for adult respiratory failure. Chest 1997;112(3):759–64.

28. Schmid C, Philipp A, Hilker M, et al. Venovenous extracorporeal membrane oxygenation for acute lung failure in adults. J Heart Lung Transplant 2012;31(1):9–15.

29. Bartlett RH, Roloff DW, Custer JR, et al. Extracorporeal life support: the University of Michigan experience. JAMA 2000;283(7):904–8.

30. Bottrell S, Bennett M, Augustin S, et al. A comparison study of haemolysis production in three contemporary centrifugal pumps. Perfusion 2014; 29(5):411–6.

31. Davies A, Jones D, Bailey M, et al. Extracorporeal membrane oxygenation for 2009 influenza A(H1N1) acute respiratory distress syndrome. JAMA 2009;302(17):1888–95.

32. Patroniti N, Zangrillo A, Pappalardo F, et al. The Italian ECMO network experience during the 2009 influenza A(H1N1) pandemic: preparation for severe respiratory emergency outbreaks. Intensive Care Med 2011;37(9):1447–57.

33. Roch A, Lepaul-Ercole R, Grisoli D, et al. Extracorporeal membrane oxygenation for severe influenza A (H1N1) acute respiratory distress syndrome: a prospective observational comparative study. Intensive Care Med 2010;36(11):1899–905.

34. Holzgraefe B, Broome M, Kalzen H, et al. Extracorporeal membrane oxygenation for pandemic H1N1 2009 respiratory failure. Minerva Anestesiol 2010; 76(12):1043–51.

35. Davies A, Jones D, Gattas D. Extracorporeal membrane oxygenation for ARDS due to 2009 influenza A(H1N1) [reply]. JAMA 2010;303(10):941–2.

36. Miller RR 3rd, Markewitz BA, Rolfs RT, et al. Clinical findings and demographic factors associated with ICU admission in Utah due to novel 2009 influenza A(H1N1) infection. Chest 2010;137(4): 752–8.

37. Noah MA, Peek GJ, Finney SJ, et al. Referral to an extracorporeal membrane oxygenation center and mortality among patients with severe 2009 influenza A(H1N1). JAMA 2011;306(15): 1659–68.

38. Pham T, Combes A, Rozo H, et al. Extracorporeal membrane oxygenation for pandemic influenza A(H1N1)-induced acute respiratory distress syndrome: a cohort study and propensity-matched analysis. Am J Respir Crit Care Med 2013;187(3): 276–85.

39. Amato MB, Barbas CS, Medeiros DM, et al. Effect of a protective-ventilation strategy on mortality in the acute respiratory distress syndrome. N Engl J Med 1998;338(6):347–54.

40. Ventilation with lower tidal volumes as compared with traditional tidal volumes for acute lung injury and the acute respiratory distress syndrome. The Acute Respiratory Distress Syndrome Network. N Engl J Med 2000;342(18):1301–8.

41. Villar J, Kacmarek RM, Perez-Mendez L, et al. A high positive end expiratory pressure, low tidal volume ventilatory strategy improves outcome in persistent acute respiratory distress syndrome: a randomized, controlled trial. Crit Care Med 2006; 34(5):1311–8.

42. Wiedemann HP, Wheeler AP, Bernard GR, et al. Comparison of two fluid-management strategies in acute lung injury. N Engl J Med 2006;354(24): 2564–75.

43. Girou E, Brun-Buisson C, Taille S, et al. Secular trends in nosocomial infections and mortality associated with noninvasive ventilation in patients with exacerbation of COPD and pulmonary edema. JAMA 2003;290(22):2985–91.

44. Srinivasan A, Wise M, Bell M, et al, Centers for Disease Control and Prevention (CDC). Vital signs: central line-associated blood stream infections–United States, 2001, 2008, and 2009. MMWR Morb Mortal Wkly Rep 2011;60(8):243–8.

45. Girard TD, Kress JP, Fuchs BD, et al. Efficacy and safety of a paired sedation and ventilator weaning protocol for mechanically ventilated patients in intensive care (awakening and breathing controlled trial): a randomised controlled trial. Lancet 2008; 371(9607):126–34.

46. Schweickert WD, Pohlman MC, Pohlman AS, et al. Early physical and occupational therapy in mechanically ventilated, critically ill patients: a randomised controlled trial. Lancet 2009;373(9678):1874–82.

47. Matthay MA, Brower RG, Carson S, et al. Randomized, placebo-controlled clinical trial of an aerosolized beta(2)-agonist for treatment of acute lung injury. Am J Respir Crit Care Med 2011;184(5):561–8.

48. Rice TW, Wheeler AP, Thompson BT, et al. Enteral omega-3 fatty acid, gamma-linolenic acid, and antioxidant supplementation in acute lung injury. JAMA 2011;306(14):1574–81.

49. Matthay MA, Ware LB, Zimmerman GA. The acute respiratory distress syndrome. J Clin Invest 2012; 122(8):2731–40.

50. Peek GJ, Mugford M, Tiruvoipati R, et al. Efficacy and economic assessment of conventional ventilatory support versus extracorporeal membrane oxygenation for severe adult respiratory failure (CESAR): a multicentre randomised controlled trial. Lancet 2009;374(9698):1351–63.

51. Mikkelsen ME, Christie JD, Lanken PN, et al. The adult respiratory distress syndrome cognitive outcomes study: long-term neuropsychological function in survivors of acute lung injury. Am J Respir Crit Care Med 2012;185(12):1307–15.

52. Abrams D, Brodie D, Combes A. What is new in extracorporeal membrane oxygenation for ARDS in adults? Intensive Care Med 2013;39:2028–30.

53. Hodgson CL, Hayes K, Everard T, et al. Long-term quality of life in patients with acute respiratory distress syndrome requiring extracorporeal membrane oxygenation for refractory hypoxaemia. Crit Care 2012;16(5):R202.

54. Extracorporeal Life Support Organization. ECLS registry report, international summary, 2013. Accessed April 14, 2014.

55. Rubenfeld GD, Caldwell E, Peabody E, et al. Incidence and outcomes of acute lung injury. N Engl J Med 2005;353(16):1685–93.

56. Parsons PE, Eisner MD, Thompson BT, et al. Lower tidal volume ventilation and plasma cytokine markers of inflammation in patients with acute lung injury. Crit Care Med 2005;33(1):1–6 [discussion: 230–2].

57. Ranieri VM, Suter PM, Tortorella C, et al. Effect of mechanical ventilation on inflammatory mediators in patients with acute respiratory distress syndrome: a randomized controlled trial. JAMA 1999; 282(1):54–61.

58. Putensen C, Theuerkauf N, Zinserling J, et al. Meta-analysis: ventilation strategies and outcomes of the acute respiratory distress syndrome and acute lung injury. Ann Intern Med 2009;151(8):566–76.

59. Needham DM, Colantuoni E, Mendez-Tellez PA, et al. Lung protective mechanical ventilation and two year survival in patients with acute lung injury: prospective cohort study. BMJ 2012;344:e2124.

60. Han S, Martin GS, Maloney JP, et al. Short women with severe sepsis-related acute lung injury receive lung protective ventilation less frequently: an observational cohort study. Crit Care 2011;15(6): R262.

61. Brunkhorst FM, Engel C, Ragaller M, et al. Practice and perception–a nationwide survey of therapy habits in sepsis. Crit Care Med 2008;36(10): 2719–25.

62. Rubenfeld GD, Cooper C, Carter G, et al. Barriers to providing lung-protective ventilation to patients with acute lung injury. Crit Care Med 2004;32(6): 1289–93.

63. Mikkelsen ME, Dedhiya PM, Kalhan R, et al. Potential reasons why physicians underuse lung-protective ventilation: a retrospective cohort study using physician documentation. Respir Care 2008; 53(4):455–61.

64. Frank JA, Gutierrez JA, Jones KD, et al. Low tidal volume reduces epithelial and endothelial injury in acid-injured rat lungs. Am J Respir Crit Care Med 2002;165(2):242–9.

65. Savel RH, Yao EC, Gropper MA. Protective effects of low tidal volume ventilation in a rabbit model of *Pseudomonas aeruginosa*-induced acute lung injury. Crit Care Med 2001;29(2):392–8.

66. Tsuno K, Prato P, Kolobow T. Acute lung injury from mechanical ventilation at moderately high airway pressures. J Appl Physiol (1985) 1990;69(3):956–61.

67. Parker JC, Townsley MI, Rippe B, et al. Increased microvascular permeability in dog lungs due to high peak airway pressures. J Appl Physiol Respir Environ Exerc Physiol 1984;57(6):1809–16.

68. Parker JC, Hernandez LA, Longenecker GL, et al. Lung edema caused by high peak inspiratory pressures in dogs. Role of increased microvascular filtration pressure and permeability. Am Rev Respir Dis 1990;142(2):321–8.

69. Carlton DP, Cummings JJ, Scheerer RG, et al. Lung overexpansion increases pulmonary microvascular protein permeability in young lambs. J Appl Physiol (1985) 1990;69(2):577–83.

70. Hager DN, Krishnan JA, Hayden DL, et al. Tidal volume reduction in patients with acute lung injury when plateau pressures are not high. Am J Respir Crit Care Med 2005;172(10):1241–5.

71. Terragni PP, Del Sorbo L, Mascia L, et al. Tidal volume lower than 6 ml/kg enhances lung protection: role of extracorporeal carbon dioxide removal. Anesthesiology 2009;111(4):826–35.

72. Bein T, Weber-Carstens S, Goldmann A, et al. Lower tidal volume strategy (approximately 3 ml/kg) combined with extracorporeal CO(2) removal versus 'conventional' protective ventilation (6 ml/kg) in severe ARDS: the prospective randomized Xtravent-study. Intensive Care Med 2013;39:847–56.

73. Yoshida T, Torsani V, Gomes S, et al. Spontaneous effort causes occult pendelluft during mechanical ventilation. Am J Respir Crit Care Med 2013; 188(12):1420–7.

74. Guldner A, Pelosi P, Gama de Abreu M. Spontaneous breathing in mild and moderate versus severe acute respiratory distress syndrome. Curr Opin Crit Care 2014;20(1):69–76.

75. Nosotti M, Rosso L, Tosi D, et al. Extracorporeal membrane oxygenation with spontaneous breathing as a bridge to lung transplantation. Interact Cardiovasc Thorac Surg 2013;16(1):55–9.

76. Mauri T, Bellani G, Grasselli G, et al. Patient-ventilator interaction in ARDS patients with extremely low compliance undergoing ECMO: a novel approach based on diaphragm electrical activity. Intensive Care Med 2013;39(2):282–91.

77. Bailey P, Thomsen GE, Spuhler VJ, et al. Early activity is feasible and safe in respiratory failure patients. Crit Care Med 2007;35(1):139–45.

78. Needham DM, Korupolu R. Rehabilitation quality improvement in an intensive care unit setting: implementation of a quality improvement model. Top Stroke Rehabil 2010;17(4):271–81.

79. Abrams D, Javidfar J, Farrand E, et al. Early mobilization of patients receiving extracorporeal membrane oxygenation: a retrospective cohort study. Critical Care 2014;18:R38.

80. Turner DA, Cheifetz IM, Rehder KJ, et al. Active rehabilitation and physical therapy during extracorporeal membrane oxygenation while awaiting lung transplantation: a practical approach. Crit Care Med 2011;39(12):2593–8.

81. Rehder KJ, Turner DA, Hartwig MG, et al. Active rehabilitation during extracorporeal membrane oxygenation as a bridge to lung transplantation. Respir Care 2013;58(8):1291–8.

82. Javidfar J, Brodie D, Iribarne A, et al. Extracorporeal membrane oxygenation as a bridge to lung transplantation and recovery. J Thorac Cardiovasc Surg 2012;144(3):716–21.

83. Abrams DC, Brenner K, Burkart KM, et al. Pilot study of extracorporeal carbon dioxide removal to facilitate extubation and ambulation in exacerbations of chronic obstructive pulmonary disease. Ann Am Thorac Soc 2013;10(4):307–14.

84. Paden ML, Conrad SA, Rycus PT, et al. Extracorporeal life support organization registry report 2012. ASAIO J 2013;59(3):202–10.

85. Schmidt M, Brechot N, Hariri S, et al. Nosocomial infections in adult cardiogenic shock patients supported by venoarterial extracorporeal membrane oxygenation. Clin Infect Dis 2012;55(12): 1633–41.

86. Heilmann C, Geisen U, Beyersdorf F, et al. Acquired von Willebrand syndrome in patients with extracorporeal life support (ECLS). Intensive Care Med 2012;38(1):62–8.

87. Cheng R, Hachamovitch R, Kittleson M, et al. Complications of extracorporeal membrane oxygenation for treatment of cardiogenic shock and cardiac arrest: a meta-analysis of 1,866 adult patients. Ann Thorac Surg 2014;97(2):610–6.

88. Johnson SM, Itoga N, Garnett GM, et al. Increased risk of cardiovascular perforation during ECMO with a bicaval, wire-reinforced cannula. J Pediatr Surg 2014;49(1):46–50.

89. Extracorporeal Life Support Organization Registry Report. US complications January 2014. Accessed April 14, 2014.

90. Peek GJ, Elbourne D, Mugford M, et al. Randomised controlled trial and parallel economic evaluation of conventional ventilatory support versus extracorporeal membrane oxygenation for severe adult respiratory failure (CESAR). Health Technol Assess 2010;14(35):1–46.

91. Abrams D, Prager K, Blinderman C, et al. Ethical dilemmas encountered with the use of ECMO in adults. Chest 2014;145:876–82.

92. Schmidt M, Zogheib E, Roze H, et al. The PRESERVE mortality risk score and analysis of long-term outcomes after extracorporeal membrane oxygenation for severe acute respiratory distress syndrome. Intensive Care Med 2013;39(10):1704–13.

93. Pappalardo F, Pieri M, Greco T, et al. Predicting mortality risk in patients undergoing venovenous ECMO for ARDS due to influenza A (H1N1) pneumonia: the ECMOnet score. Intensive Care Med 2013;39(2):275–81.

94. Morris AH. Exciting new ECMO technology awaits compelling scientific evidence for widespread use in adults with respiratory failure. Intensive Care Med 2012;38(2):186–8.

Steroids for Acute Respiratory Distress Syndrome?

Catherine L. Hough, MD, MSc

KEYWORDS

• ARDS • Corticosteroids • Prevention • Treatment • Outcomes

KEY POINTS

- No studies support the use of corticosteroids for the prevention of acute respiratory distress syndrome (ARDS).
- High-dose and short-course treatment with steroids does not improve the outcomes of patients with ARDS.
- There are compelling data that low-dose and prolonged treatment with steroids improves pulmonary physiology in patients with ARDS, but additional studies are needed to recommend treatment with steroids for ARDS.

INTRODUCTION: WHY TALK ABOUT STEROIDS AND ACUTE RESPIRATORY DISTRESS SYNDROME?

The first report in the literature of the acute respiratory distress syndrome (ARDS) presents 12 patients who developed acute hypoxemic respiratory failure in response to overwhelming illness or injury, and concludes with the statement that, "Corticosteroids appeared to have value in the treatment of fat emboli and possibly viral pneumonia."[1]

It has been nearly 50 years since this initial description of ARDS, during which time much has been learned about pathogenesis, epidemiology, supportive care, and long-term outcomes.[2] However, the search for pharmacologic therapy has been disappointing, without convincing proof of a single agent to decrease the mortality of patients with ARDS. However, it seems so compelling that this syndrome, which is defined by overexuberant inflammation, should be treated with corticosteroids (powerful antiinflammatory agents that are part of the body's endogenous response to stress) that clinicians continue to maintain hope. Do corticosteroids have value in the treatment of ARDS, or possibly in specific settings?

This article discusses the pathogenesis of ARDS and reviews the mechanism of action of corticosteroids. It then reviews clinical data from studies of corticosteroids across the spectrum of ARDS (prevention, early, and late), focusing on the results of randomized trials. Studies of corticosteroids in specific settings associated with ARDS, such as septic shock and pneumonia, are also discussed. In addition, the article concludes by making some recommendations for clinical practice and by identifying gaps that require future research.

Financial Disclosure: My work in this area has been funded by the NHLBI grants (T32 HL 007287, K23 HL074294 HHSN268200536173C) and the Francis Family Foundation.
Division of Pulmonary and Critical Care Medicine, Harborview Medical Center, University of Washington, 325 Ninth Avenue, Mailstop 359762, Seattle, WA 98104, USA
E-mail address: cterrlee@uw.edu

chestmed.theclinics.com

INFLAMMATION, FIBROSIS, AND THE PATHOPHYSIOLOGY OF ACUTE RESPIRATORY DISTRESS SYNDROME

Histology early in the course of ARDS reveals interstitial and alveolar edema, infiltration of cells into the alveolar spaces (neutrophils, macrophages, and red blood cells), and alveolar epithelial and endothelial injury. The alveolar basement membranes often become denuded; hyaline membranes form.[3] Dysregulated inflammation, both in the endothelial and epithelial spaces, is a key driver of the pathogenesis of ARDS. Ventilator-induced lung injury may further perpetuate both pulmonary and systemic inflammation.[4] Alveolar macrophages release proinflammatory cytokines, including neutrophil chemoattractants that promote neutrophilic activation and migration into the interstitial and alveolar spaces. These activated neutrophils release proinflammatory molecules, which contribute to and perpetuate the inflammatory environment.[5] Vascular permeability increases as these products released by neutrophils interrupt tight junctions and promote alveolar cell death, with loss of the normal function of the endothelial barrier.[6] There is also activation of local fibroblasts. Key homeostatic mechanisms to prevent injury caused by uncontrolled inflammation, such as endogenous glucocorticoid secretion and the release of antiinflammatory cytokines, are overwhelmed.[7] Degree of pulmonary and systemic inflammation, as measured by cytokine concentrations in the alveolar compartment and in serum, has been shown to be associated with severity and outcome in ARDS.[8,9]

After the initial phase of ARDS, recovery may occur quickly, with reabsorption of the edema fluid, removal of the cellular infiltrates, and reparative epithelial proliferation with restoration of the alveolar barrier.[2] However, for some patients with ARDS, recovery is complicated by persistent inflammation and fibroproliferation. Along with capillaries, fibroblasts proliferate in the alveolar and interstitial spaces, leading to collagen deposition and fibrosis.[10] The presence and magnitude of fibrosis in ARDS have been shown to be associated with outcome, using measurement of procollagen peptide III in bronchoalveolar lavage fluid as a marker of collagen deposition in the alveolar space.[11]

PHARMACOLOGIC EFFECTS OF CORTICOSTEROIDS

Synthetic corticosteroids, such as methylprednisolone and hydrocortisone, exert their clinical effects by mimicking natural glucocorticoids.[12]

Glucocorticoids are potent antiinflammatories that act primarily by binding to cytoplasmic glucocorticoid receptors. Once bound, the glucocorticoid-receptor complexes regulate the transcription of glucocorticoid-response elements such as nuclear factor receptor-κβ (NF-κβ). The transcription of many proinflammatory cytokines (including interleukins 1α, 1β, 2, 3, 5, 6, 8, and 12; tumor necrosis factor alpha; and interferon gamma) is modulated by NF-κβ.[13] In addition, glucocorticoids act synergistically with natural antiinflammatory cytokines, such as interleukins 4, 10, 13, and interleukin-1 receptor antagonist.[14] Glucocorticoids also have actions on fibrotic pathways, inhibiting fibroblast proliferation and decreasing collagen deposition.[15]

Regulated by the hypothalamic-pituitary-adrenal axis, endogenous glucocorticoids are key effectors in the natural response to stress. Stressful stimuli, such as infection or injury, lead to hypothalamic release of corticotropin-releasing hormone, which then acts on the anterior pituitary to produce adrenocorticotropic hormone (ACTH). The adrenal cortex is stimulated by ACTH to release glucocorticoids into the blood. Glucocorticoids, such as cortisol, have myriad cardiovascular effects, including increasing vascular adrenergic receptor function, decreasing cytokine-induced nitric oxide synthetase, increasing endothelial integrity, decreasing vascular permeability, and increasing myocardial contractility, all of which help maintain blood pressure and cardiac output under stress.[13] In addition to antiinflammatory and cardiovascular effects, glucocorticoids have profound metabolic effects, including inducing gluconeogenesis; increasing serum glucose levels; and altering protein, fat, and bone metabolism.[12]

CLINICAL TRIALS OF STEROIDS IN PREVENTION AND TREATMENT OF ACUTE RESPIRATORY DISTRESS SYNDROME

In the 1970s, many clinical and animal studies showed beneficial effects of corticosteroids on intermediate physiologic outcomes in the setting of sepsis and ARDS. Steroids were shown to reduce inflammation by decreasing complement activation[16] and neutrophil aggregation,[17] and were found to have potentially advantageous effects on oxyhemoglobin dissociation,[18] cardiac output,[19] pulmonary vascular pressure,[20] and alveolocapillary permeability.[21] In combination with case reports describing improved outcomes of patients with sepsis and ARDS after receipt of steroids, there was enough evidence to spur randomized clinical trials.

Note that all randomized trials discussed here were conducted in the 1980s and 1990s, before low-tidal-volume ventilation,[4] which was an era with much higher ARDS-associated mortality.[2] While considering each of these studies, it is also relevant to question whether findings can be generalized to the current treatment of ARDS.

Clinical Trials for Acute Respiratory Distress Syndrome Prevention

There have been 4 randomized trials of corticosteroids that assessed the outcome of prevention of ARDS,[22–25] as shown in **Table 1**. High-dose methylprednisolone (30 mg/kg) was used in all trials, with number of doses ranging from 1 to 8 over a period of up to 48 hours. Three studies enrolled only patients with septic shock with similar but not identical definitions; 1 study enrolled patients with respiratory failure at high risk for ARDS. ARDS was the primary outcome measure for all studies, although definitions for ARDS were highly variable between the 4 studies.

The first study by Schein and colleagues[24] began enrollment in 1979, and included patients with septic shock, both with and without ARDS at the time of enrollment. Patients were randomized into 3 arms: methylprednisolone (30 mg/kg), dexamethasone (6 mg/kg), or no therapy (no placebo described). If shock persisted after 4 hours, a second dose of study drug was administered. This study found similar rates of ARDS across all 3 arms, and no difference in the intermediate outcome measure of plasma complement levels.

Around the same time, Weigelt and colleagues[23] enrolled 81 patients with hypoxemic respiratory failure (PaO$_2$/fractional inspired oxygen [FiO$_2$] <350) into a single-centered randomized controlled trial of methylprednisolone for the prevention of ARDS. The primary cause of respiratory failure was sepsis and shock for three-quarters of all patients enrolled. Patients received 30 mg/kg of intravenous methylprednisolone every 6 hours for a total of 8 doses in the intervention group; control subjects received mannitol. There was no evidence for benefit of steroids; ARDS, infectious complications, and death were all significantly more common among patients randomized to methylprednisolone.

Between 1982 and 1985, Luce and colleagues[25] randomized patients with septic shock to high-dose methylprednisolone or placebo within 2 hours of meeting criteria. This study was stopped early for safety.[26] Eight-seven patients were enrolled and treated, but only the 75 patients with positive culture results were included in the analysis. There was no difference in proportion of patients

meeting ARDS criteria between randomization groups, nor was there a difference in hospital mortality, which was more than 50% for both groups. There was no significant association between development of ARDS and hospital mortality; there also was no association between randomization to corticosteroids and plasma complement levels.

A large multicenter study was conducted simultaneously by Bone and colleagues[26] testing the efficacy of methylprednisolone on reducing mortality in patients with septic shock. This study found no benefit of high-dose steroids on mortality, and a subgroup analysis found an association between randomization to steroids and increased mortality if serum creatinine was greater than 2 mg/dL (which led to the decision for early stopping in the Luce and colleagues[25] study). A secondary analysis was performed including patients who did not meet ARDS criteria before study enrollment; this analysis did not find that methylprednisolone either prevented ARDS or decreased its associated mortality.[22]

Several methodological issues complicate interpretation of these studies, both alone and in combination. Because these studies used different durations of therapy and varying definitions of ARDS, there is significant heterogeneity between trials. None of the 3 studies that prospectively sought to determine the effect of methylprednisolone on ARDS were adequately powered; to show a reduction in ARDS incidence from 40% to 20% in a 2-arm study with 80% power would require a sample size of more than 180 patients. When combined, these studies and the secondary analysis of the Bone and colleagues[26] trial suggest that there is no role for high-dose methylprednisolone early in septic shock for the prevention of ARDS.[27] Recent meta-analysis by Peter and colleagues[27] showed that there is an 86.6% probability that high-dose steroid therapy will instead increase the incidence of ARDS.

There have been no recent randomized trials to inform the utility of corticosteroids for ARDS prevention. However, 2 recent cohort studies investigated the role of prehospital inhaled or systemic corticosteroid use on the subsequent development of ARDS in patients at risk.[28,29] Investigators found no significant independent association between either inhaled or systemic corticosteroids on ARDS development.

Clinical Trials for Treatment of Early Acute Respiratory Distress Syndrome

The first randomized controlled trial of corticosteroids for decreasing mortality in patients with established ARDS was conducted in the early

Table 1
Randomized trials of methylprednisolone for ARDS prevention

Author (Dates)	Patients	Intervention (Drug, Dose, Duration)	ARDS Definition	Number Enrolled	Outcome: Steroids	Outcome: Control	Notes
Schein et al,[24] (1979–1982)	Septic shock	MP 30 mg/kg; DX 6 m/kg, redosed after 4 h if shock persisted	CXR: diffuse bilateral infiltrates; Hypoxemia: PaO_2/FiO_2 ratio <160; PAOP <15 mm Hg	59 enrolled, 42 without ARDS at time of first study drug	ARDS: 4 of 16 (MP), 3 of 13 (DX)	ARDS: 2 of 13	Steroid treatment did not affect complement levels
Weigelt et al,[23] (1980–1983)	Hypoxemic respiratory failure	MP 30 mg/kg q6 h for 48 h	Pulmonary failure and ARDS, including hypoxemia, shunt, and CXR infiltrates	81 enrolled	ARDS: 25 of 39; Died: 18 of 39	ARDS: 14 of 42; Died: 13 of 42	Increased infectious complication in MP group
Bone et al,[22] (1982–1985)	Septic shock	MP 30 mg/kg q6 h for 24 h	CXR: bilateral infiltrates; Hypoxemia: PaO_2 <70 mm Hg on FiO_2 ≥40%; PAOP <18 mm Hg	304 enrolled	ARDS 50 of 152; Died by day 14, 26 of 50 (ARDS only)	ARDS 38 of 152; Died by day 14, 23 of 38 (ARDS only)	Secondary analysis of study with primary end point of mortality
Luce et al,[25] (1983–1986)	Septic shock	MP 30 mg/kg q6 h for 24 h	CXR: 4 quadrant infiltrates; Hypoxemia: arterial to alveolar oxygen tension <0.3; PAOP ≤18 mm Hg	87 enrolled, 75 confirmed with sepsis and analyzed	ARDS: 13 of 38; Died: 22 of 38	ARDS: 14 of 37; Died: 20 of 37	Stopped early (safety)

Abbreviations: CXR, chest radiograph; DX, dexamethasone; FiO_2, fractional inspired oxygen; MP, methylprednisolone; PAOP, pulmonary artery occlusion pressure; q, every.

1980s. Bernard and colleagues[30] used a similar protocol as the prevention trials: 30 mg/kg of intravenous methylprednisolone every 6 hours for a total of 4 doses, with the hypothesis that this treatment would reduce 45-day mortality. This study was stopped early for futility, with 60% mortality in the methylprednisolone group and 63% in the control group, after enrolling 99 patients. There was no increase in infectious complications noted in the steroid group, and no significant benefits in reduction of infiltrates on chest radiograph, lung compliance, or oxygenation.

The end of the 1980s brought a close to the era of studies of high-dose methylprednisolone both for ARDS prevention and early treatment. However, interest was renewed after the publication of Annane and colleagues'[31] randomized controlled trial of treatment of refractory septic shock with low-dose hydrocortisone and fludrocortisone. This study investigated the effect of 50 mg of intravenous hydrocortisone given every 6 hours for 1 week, in combination with 50 μg of enteral fludrocortisone once daily, on 28-day mortality. The investigators hypothesized that there would be significant benefit in patients with critical illness-related adrenal insufficiency,[32] diagnosed by nonresponse to a short corticotropin test (nonresponders). Although overall there was no significant effect on 28-day mortality, treatment with steroids was associated with decreased mortality among nonresponders (53% vs 63%; P = .04). Of the 300 patients in the study, 177 met criteria for ARDS[33] at study entry (59%), 129 of whom were nonresponders.

A post-hoc analysis of this study tested the hypothesis that randomization to steroids was associated with decreased mortality among nonresponders with ARDS; nonresponders with ARDS had lower mortality if randomized to steroids (53% vs 75%; P = .021).[34] However, there was no mortality reduction associated with randomization to steroids among all ARDS patients. A large subsequent study of hydrocortisone for septic shock found no mortality benefit, either among nonresponders or in the group as a whole. There has been no post-hoc analysis published to date of the ARDS subgroup in this study (Table 2).[35]

In the late 1990s, Meduri and colleagues[36] conducted a pilot randomized controlled trial to investigate the effect of a longer course of low-dose methylprednisolone on pulmonary outcomes, including lung injury score[37] and ventilator-free days.[38] This study enrolled 91 patients within the first 72 hours of onset of ARDS and randomized in a 2:1 ratio to 1 mg/kg of methylprednisolone followed by a prolonged infusion at 1 mg/kg/d or placebo. Most patients had pneumonia, aspiration, or nonpulmonary sepsis. Randomization to steroids improved pulmonary outcomes, with a dramatic increase in ventilator-free days and improvement in lung injury score. Twelve of 28 patients in the placebo group died before hospital discharge (43%), compared with 15 of 63 in the steroid group (24%; P = .07).

There have been no other randomized studies published to date that investigate the efficacy of low-dose steroids in decreasing hospital mortality for patients with early ARDS, although pilot studies in closely related groups, such as patients with severe community-acquired pneumonia, may show promise.[39] Despite the lack of clear evidence, the American College of Critical Care Medicine issued a recommendation in 2008 that moderate-dose glucocorticoids should be considered in the management strategy of patients with early severe ARDS ($PaO_2/FiO_2 < 200$), with a grade 2B.[32] In the recent Surviving Sepsis Campaign guidelines, no recommendations were made regarding the use of steroids in ARDS, despite 12 other recommendations specific to clinical management of ARDS in sepsis.[40]

Clinical Trials for Treatment of Late Acute Respiratory Distress Syndrome

While evidence was mounting against high-dose, short-term treatment with corticosteroids for prevention and early treatment of ARDS, there were several case reports and small series describing treatment of established ARDS with longer courses and lower doses.[41–45] These studies showed remarkable improvements in lung function and patient outcome after treatment with steroids. Meduri and colleagues[46] were early champions of this work and they conducted a small randomized controlled trial of patients who had unresolving ARDS, defined as meeting ARDS criteria, requiring greater than 7 days of mechanical ventilation, and without significant improvement of lung injury since onset. Patients were excluded if they met ARDS criteria for more than 3 weeks, or if they had untreated infection. Patients were randomized in a 2:1 ratio to methylprednisolone or placebo. Methylprednisolone was given with an initial loading dose of 2 mg/kg, which was followed by 14 days of 2 mg/kg/d at 6-hour intervals, which was then tapered over an additional 18 days. The protocol included a crossover, wherein patients without improvement in lung injury score by at least 1 point by the 10th day of treatment were blindly switched to the alternate treatment group. Primary outcomes were intensive care unit (ICU) survival and improvement in lung injury score.

Table 2
Randomized trials of corticosteroids for treatment of early ARDS

Author (Dates)	Patients	Intervention (Drug, Dose, Duration)	ARDS Definition	Number Enrolled	Outcome: Steroids	Outcome: Control	Notes
Bernard et al,[30] (1982–1985)	ARDS, risk factor, no shock	MP 30 mg/kg every 6 h for 24 h	CXR: bilateral infiltrates Hypoxemia: PaO_2 <70 mm Hg on FiO_2 ≥40%, or arterial to alveolar oxygen tension <0.3 PAOP <18 mm Hg	99	45-d mortality: 30 of 50	45-d mortality: 31 of 49	Stopped early for futility No difference in infectious complications; MP associated with hyperglycemia
Annane et al,[34] (1995–1999)	Septic shock, ARDS	HC 50 mg q6 h for 7 d, plus FC 50 μg qd	AECC criteria with PaO_2/FiO_2 ratio <200	300 with sepsis, 177 with ARDS, 129 nonresponders	28-d mortality: 49 of 85, 33 of 62 (nonresponders)	28-d mortality: 62 of 92, 50 of 75 (nonresponders)	Post-hoc secondary analysis of RCT
Meduri et al,[36] (1997–2002)	ARDS, first 72 h	MP 1 mg/kg load then 1 mg/kg/d infusion for 14 d or until extubation, then tapered over 14 d	AECC definition	91	Hospital mortality: 15 of 63 VFDs at 28 days: 16.5 (10.1)	Hospital mortality: 12 of 28 VFDs at 28 days: 8.7 (10.2)	Primary end point: reduction in lung injury score 2:1 randomization protocol

Abbreviations: AECC, American European Consensus Conference; FC, fludrocortisone; HC, hydrocortisone; qd, every day; RCT, randomized controlled trial; VFD, ventilator-free day.

This study was stopped after enrollment of 24 patients when ICU mortality was significantly different between the groups: none of the 16 patients in the initial steroid group died before ICU discharge compared with 5 of 8 in the placebo group (0% vs 63%; *P* = .002) (**Table 3**).

Despite a marked difference in ICU mortality between groups, several aspects of trial design give pause to clinical application of their results. First, the sample size is small, with only 8 patients in the placebo group, which brings into question the statistical stability of the results, raising the likelihood of false-positives. Second, half of the placebo group were crossed over and began receiving methylprednisolone on study day 10, late in the course of ARDS. All deaths in the placebo group occurred after crossover; it is unclear what role very late treatment with methylprednisolone might have played in patient outcome. Third, an ICU mortality of more than 60% is considerably higher than expected from a late-ARDS population.

In follow-up, the National Institutes of Health National Heart Lung and Blood Institute (NHLBI) ARDS Network conducted a multicenter randomized controlled trial of patients meeting ARDS criteria for at least 7 days, with continuous mechanical ventilation and persistent infiltrates on chest radiograph at study entry.[47] Patients meeting ARDS criteria for longer than 28 days were excluded. The intervention was intravenous methylprednisolone, given as a 2-mg/kg loading dose, then 2 mg/kg/d in 4 divided doses for 14 days, then tapered over 11 days. If a patient achieved 48 hours of unassisted breathing, study drug was tapered early, over 4 days. The primary outcome was 60-day mortality. It was estimated that the intervention would decrease mortality from 40% to 20%, with a sample size of 180% and 85% power. Sixty-day mortality was lower than anticipated (29%) and was equal in both study groups.

There were interesting differences between the treatment groups. Patients randomized to steroids liberated from mechanical ventilation sooner than those on placebo (14 days vs 23 days; *P* = .006) and had significantly more ventilator-free days at both 28 and 180 days. However, there was no difference in ICU length of stay between the groups, and return to mechanical ventilation was significantly more likely among patients randomized to steroids (20 vs 6; *P* = .008). All 9 serious adverse events of neuromyopathy were in the steroid group, but there was no significant difference between clinician recognition of neuromyopathy during the hospitalization between the two groups. There was no difference in infectious complications. However, hyperglycemia was more common in the steroid group.

Two planned subgroup analyses were hypothesis generating. First, there was a significant interaction between duration of ARDS and randomization group. Among patients enrolled after day 13 of ARDS, mortality was 12% in the placebo group compared with 44% in steroid group, suggesting that steroids may be harmful if begun too late in the course of ARDS. In contrast, benefit of steroids may be greatest while inflammation and fibroproliferation are still active. Supporting this theory, a second subgroup analysis identified significant effect modification between treatment group and level of procollagen peptide III (PIIIP) in bronchoalveolar lavage fluid at study baseline. Patients with high levels of PIIIP who were randomized to steroids were less likely to die (4% vs 24% in placebo).

These findings raise at least 3 important questions. First, is there an identifiable subgroup of patients with late ARDS who may benefit from treatment with corticosteroids? Both studies suggest that treatment may be beneficial earlier and harmful later, inferring from the higher mortality in the ARDS Network treatment group enrolled after day 14,[47] as well as in the placebo group of Meduri and colleagues'[46] study after late crossover to steroids. However, the evidence is sparse enough that a new randomized controlled trial targeting persistent ARDS between days 7 and 13 is required before recommending this treatment clinically. It is possible that biomarkers, such as PIIIP, could help identify the subgroup, but ideally such a biomarker would be available clinically with rapid turnaround. Also, measurement of the biomarker in the alveolar compartment significantly limits its clinical utility, because resource limitation and patient stability prevent widespread use. Even in the trial setting, only half of the patients in the ARDS Network study had bronchoalveolar lavages performed at study entry.

Second, why did so many patients in the steroid group develop recurrent respiratory failure requiring return to mechanical ventilation? It has been suggested that tapering methylprednisolone early after liberation from the ventilator led to recrudescence of lung inflammation and fibroproliferation, deteriorating compliance and oxygenation, increased work of breathing, and subsequent need for mechanical ventilation.[47,48] Perhaps a protocol that continued treatment with steroids well beyond liberation from mechanical ventilation would prevent this mechanism of recurrent respiratory failure. However, a competing hypothesis is that complications from steroid therapy were responsible for return to mechanical ventilation, such as infection or neuromuscular weakness. Although there is no compelling evidence

Table 3
Randomized trials of corticosteroids for treatment of late ARDS

Author (Dates)	Patients	Intervention (Drug, Dose, Duration)	ARDS Definition	Number Enrolled	Outcome: Steroids	Outcome: Control	Notes
Meduri et al,[46] (1994–1996)	ARDS on ventilator for ≥7 d, no improvement in lung injury score	MP: 2 mg/kg/d × 14 d, then tapered over 18 d	AECC	24	Died in ICU: 0 of 16	Died in ICU: 5 of 8	Met early stopping rules on second look. 4 of 8 placebo patients crossed to MP treatment on day 10
Steinberg et al,[47] (1997–2003)	ARDS criteria, on ventilator 7–28 d	MP: 2 mg/kg/d × 14 d, then tapered over 11 d (or over 4 d after 2 d off ventilator)	AECC	180	60-d mortality: 26 of 91 VFDs at day 28: 11.2 (9.4)	60-d mortality: 26 of 89 VFDs at day 28: 6.8 (8.5)	—

to suggest higher infection rates, recognition of neuromyopathy was higher in the steroid group, particularly within the first 28 days of the study.[49] If weakness was a direct contributor to recurrent respiratory failure, then extending the course of steroids seems an unlikely solution.

The relationship between steroids and ICU-acquired neuromyopathy remains uncertain. Clinical evidence of neuromyopathy (weakness, deconditioning, myopathy, and neuropathy) was common in both arms of the ARDS Network trial (43 of 128 hospital survivors; 34%), with no significant increase in patients randomized to steroids (odds ratio, 1.5; 95% confidence interval, 0.7–3.2).[49] Cohort studies have yielded conflicting results with regard to the association between steroids and ICU-acquired neuromyopathy.[50] In the setting of intensive insulin therapy, which controls hyperglycemia and promotes muscle anabolism,[51] steroids may reduce the risk of ICU-acquired neuromyopathy.[52] Conflicting findings may reflect the complicated roles that steroids may play in muscle and nerve disorder and recovery.[53]

Third, given the consistent increase in ventilator-free days across both the Meduri and colleagues and ARDS Network studies, is there enough evidence to recommend widespread clinical use of corticosteroids for late ARDS? The problem is that ventilator-free days may not represent a truly patient-centered outcome; despite a nearly 5-day difference in ventilator-free days between the groups, there was no significant difference in mortality or even ICU length of stay. Although decreasing duration of mechanical ventilation among survivors is a positive outcome, the associated long-term risks are not known. There are concerns that long-term physical function may be worse among patients treated with steroids in the ICU.[54,55] The relationship between steroids and long-term mental health is also unclear, with studies suggesting beneficial actions of steroids on depression[56] and posttraumatic stress.[57]

Although the American College of Critical Care Medicine recommends consideration of steroid treatment of unresolving ARDS before day 14,[32] new randomized controlled trials are needed to increase certainty of efficacy, and to inform patient choice and timing of treatment, duration of therapy, and approach to taper, and to provide evidence of the effect of treatment on long-term patient outcomes.[13,58] In addition, information is needed regarding the clinical utility of steroids in the era of low-tidal-volume ventilation.[4] Ventilator-induced lung injury is an important contributor to both inflammation and fibrosis,[59–62] which are mitigated by treatment with steroids.[63–65] It may be that the beneficial effects of steroids are diminished in patients managed with low-tidal-volume ventilation. The effects of low-tidal-volume ventilation on the natural history are still largely undescribed, but it may be that preventing ventilator-induced lung injury decreases fibroproliferation. If so, the incidence of unresolving ARDS may be declining, benefiting patients but complicating future attempts to study the effect of steroids (or anything else) in this population.

META-ANALYSES OF STEROIDS FOR ACUTE RESPIRATORY DISTRESS SYNDROME

Meta-analytical techniques are often useful for integrating information across small or conflicting studies. However, the approach to meta-analysis may introduce additional heterogeneity, because each author may incorporate different definitions, different studies, and different subgroups; this is the case for the 5 meta-analyses of steroids for ARDS published in the last decade.[27,48,66–68] **Table 4** presents the inclusion criteria, eligible studies, primary findings, and conclusions from each of these recent meta-analyses; conclusion differ markedly based on studies and subgroups included in each report. These meta-analyses found high degrees of heterogeneity among studies, and significant quality issues, such as inclusion of studies with frequent and early stopping. It is notable that several of these conclusions include estimates that rely on post-hoc subgroup analyses, because they may be inconsistent and imprecise.[67] However, a recent survey suggests that clinicians may recognize the limitations of current evidence, with only 12% endorsing that they sometimes use systemic corticosteroids for treatment of ARDS.[67]

SPECIFIC ACUTE RESPIRATORY DISTRESS SYNDROME CAUSES AND STEROIDS

In general, clinical trials provide little evidence supporting the use of steroids for the prevention of ARDS and for early treatment. However, ARDS is heterogeneous; steroids may be beneficial for some causes of ARDS, and not for others. For example, ARDS associated with *Pneumocystis carinii* (*jirovecii*) pneumonia should be treated with steroids, because high-quality randomized controlled trials have shown that steroid treatment decreases both the risk of respiratory failure and death.[73–75] However, this level of evidence is lacking for most other causes of ARDS. It has been suggested that steroids improve outcomes from ARDS associated with acute monocytic leukemia,[76] but no randomized trials have been

Table 4
Overview of meta-analyses of steroids and ARDS

Author	Inclusion Criteria	Strata	Studies Included	Effects of Steroids on Outcome	Conclusion
Agarwal et al,[66] 2007	RCT or observational cohorts of patients with ARDS treated with steroids	Early and late ARDS	Early: Bernard et al[30], Annane et al[34]; Lee et al[69] Late: Meduri et al[46], Steinberg et al[47], Keel et al[70]	Early: OR 0.57 (0.25–1.32) Late: OR 0.58 (0.22–1.53)	Current evidence does not support a role for corticosteroids in the early or late stages of the disease
Meduri et al,[48] 2008	RCT of ≥7 d of treatment with steroids for ARDS	Study size, duration of ARDS <14 d and duration of therapy >7 d (including subgroups)	Meduri et al[46], Confalonieri et al[39], Annane et al[34], Steinberg et al[47], Meduri et al[36]	Larger: OR 0.84 (0.68–1.04) ARDS <14 d: OR 0.78 (0.64–0.96) ARDS <14 d and Rx >7 d: OR 0.62 (0.43–0.90)	Prolonged glucocorticoid treatment substantially and significantly improves meaningful patient-centered outcome variable, and has a distinct survival benefit when initiated before day 14 of ARDS
Peter et al,[27] 2008	RCT of steroid for ARDS prevention or treatment between 1966 and 2007	Prevention and treatment	Weigelt et al[23], Bone et al[22], Schein et al[24], Luce et al[25], Bernard et al[30], Meduri et al[46], Steinberg et al[47], Annane et al[34], Meduri et al[36]	Prevention: OR 1.55 (0.58–4.05) Treatment: 0.62 (0.23–1.26)	A definitive role of corticosteroids in the treatment of ARDS is not established. A possibility of reduced mortality and increased VFDs with steroids started after the onset of ARDS was suggested

| Tang et al,[68] 2009 | RCTs and cohort studies that used low-dose steroids to treat ARDS | Cohort and RCT | Keel et al[70], Varpula et al[71], Huh et al[72], Lee et al[69], Annane et al[34], Meduri et al[46], Confalonieri et al[39], Steinberg et al[47], Meduri et al[36] | Overall: OR 0.62 (0.43–0.91) Cohort: OR 0.66 (0.43–1.02) RCT: 0.51 (0.24–1.09) | The use of low-dose corticosteroids was associated with improved mortality and morbidity outcomes without increased adverse reactions. The consistency of results in both study designs and all outcomes suggests they are effective treatments of ARDS |
| Lamontagne et al,[57] 2010 | RCTs of steroids for ARDS, limited to ARDS <14 d at enrollment | Definition of ARDS | Annane et al[34], Bernard et al[30], Meduri et al[46], Meduri et al[36], Steinberg et al[47] | OR 0.79 (0.61–1.01) | Analysis suggests that low-dose corticosteroid therapy administered within 14 d of disease onset may reduce all-cause mortality in patients with ARDS, but the mortality benefits rely on analyses of subgroups, which are both inconsistent and imprecise |

Abbreviation: OR, odds ratio.

published to support this observation. Clinical trials of steroids for treatment of sepsis[77] and pneumonia,[78] which are among the most common ARDS risk factors, are inconclusive to date. In addition, despite significant interest in the use of steroids in treatment of pandemic H1N1 influenza–associated ARDS, most reports from careful observation in cohort studies suggest that such treatment was associated with harm.[79–81]

SUMMARY

Should steroids ever be given for treatment of ARDS? In a word: maybe… but not yet. There is no evidence to suggest that a short course of high-dose steroids is helpful for either prevention or treatment of ARDS. Work still needs to be done to determine whether there are benefits to prolonged treatment with low-dose corticosteroids for unresolving ARDS in the current era, with well-designed randomized controlled trials. These trials must determine whether potential benefits outweigh short-term and long-term risks, including delayed recovery and impairments in physical function and health-related quality of life.

REFERENCES

1. Ashbaugh DG, Bigelow DB, Petty TL, et al. Acute respiratory distress in adults. Lancet 1967; 2(7511):319–23.
2. Matthay MA, Ware LB, Zimmerman GA. The acute respiratory distress syndrome. J Clin Invest 2012; 122(8):2731–40.
3. Katzenstein AL, Bloor CM, Liebow AA. Diffuse alveolar damage: the role of oxygen, shock, and related factors. Am J Pathol 1976;85:209–28.
4. Ventilation with lower tidal volumes as compared with traditional tidal volumes for acute lung injury and the acute respiratory distress syndrome. The Acute Respiratory Distress Syndrome Network. N Engl J Med 2000;342(18):1301–8.
5. Ware LB, Matthay MA. The acute respiratory distress syndrome. N Engl J Med 2000;342(18): 1334–49.
6. Matthay MA, Zemans RL. The acute respiratory distress syndrome: pathogenesis and treatment. Annu Rev Pathol 2011;6:147–63.
7. Pittet JF, Mackersie RC, Martin TR, et al. Biological markers of acute lung injury: prognostic and pathogenetic significance. Am J Respir Crit Care Med 1997;155(4):1187–205.
8. Barnett N, Ware LB. Biomarkers in acute lung injury–marking forward progress. Crit Care Clin 2011;27(3):661–83.
9. Ware LB, Koyama T, Billheimer DD, et al. Prognostic and pathogenetic value of combining clinical and biochemical indices in patients with acute lung injury. Chest 2010;137(2):288–96.
10. Martin C, Papazian L, Payan MJ, et al. Pulmonary fibrosis correlates with outcome in adult respiratory distress syndrome. A study in mechanically ventilated patients. Chest 1995;107(1):196–200.
11. Clark JG, Milberg JA, Steinberg KP, et al. Type III procollagen peptide in the adult respiratory distress syndrome. Association of increased peptide levels in bronchoalveolar lavage fluid with increased risk for death. Ann Intern Med 1995; 122(1):17–23.
12. Newton R. Molecular mechanisms of glucocorticoid action: what is important? Thorax 2000;55(7):603–13.
13. Thompson BT. Corticosteroids for ARDS. Minerva Anestesiol 2010;76(6):441–7.
14. Wiegers GJ, Reul JM. Induction of cytokine receptors by glucocorticoids: functional and pathological significance. Trends Pharmacol Sci 1998;19(8): 317–21.
15. Thompson BT. Glucocorticoids and acute lung injury. Crit Care Med 2003;31(Suppl 4):S253–7.
16. Wollersheim T, Woehlecke J, Krebs M, et al. Dynamics of myosin degradation in intensive care unit-acquired weakness during severe critical illness. Intensive Care Med 2014;40:528–38.
17. Wieske L, Witteveen E, Petzold A, et al. Neurofilaments as a plasma biomarker for ICU-acquired weakness: an observational pilot study. Crit Care 2014;18(1):R18.
18. Sharshar T, Citerio G, Andrews PJ, et al. Neurological examination of critically ill patients: a pragmatic approach. Report of an ESICM expert panel. Intensive Care Med 2014;40:484–95.
19. Balas MC, Vasilevskis EE, Olsen KM, et al. Effectiveness and safety of the awakening and breathing coordination, delirium monitoring/management, and early exercise/mobility bundle. Crit Care Med 2014;42(5):1024–36.
20. Argov Z, Latronico N. Neuromuscular complications in intensive care patients. Handb Clin Neurol 2014;121:1673–85.
21. Sibbald WJ, Anderson RR, Reid B, et al. Alveolocapillary permeability in human septic ARDS. Effect of high-dose corticosteroid therapy. Chest 1981;79(2):133–42.
22. Bone RC, Fisher CJ Jr, Clemmer TP, et al. Early methylprednisolone treatment for septic syndrome and the adult respiratory distress syndrome. Chest 1987;92(6):1032–6.
23. Weigelt JA, Norcross JF, Borman KR, et al. Early steroid therapy for respiratory failure. Arch Surg 1985;120(5):536–40.
24. Schein RM, Bergman R, Marcial EH, et al. Complement activation and corticosteroid therapy in the development of the adult respiratory distress syndrome. Chest 1987;91(6):850–4.

25. Luce JM, Montgomery AB, Marks JD, et al. Ineffec-tiveness of high-dose methylprednisolone in pre-venting parenchymal lung injury and improving mortality in patients with septic shock. Am Rev Re-spir Dis 1988;138(1):62–8.

26. Bone RC, Fisher CJ Jr, Clemmer TP, et al. A controlled clinical trial of high-dose methylpred-nisolone in the treatment of severe sepsis and sep-tic shock. N Engl J Med 1987;317(11):653–8.

27. Peter JV, John P, Graham PL, et al. Corticosteroids in the prevention and treatment of acute respiratory distress syndrome (ARDS) in adults: meta-analysis. BMJ 2008;336(7651):1006–9.

28. Wieske L, Chan Pin Yin DR, Verhamme C, et al. Autonomic dysfunction in ICU-acquired weakness: a prospective observational pilot study. Intensive Care Med 2013;39(9):1610–7.

29. Winkelman C. Mechanisms for muscle health in the critically ill patient. Crit Care Nurs Q 2013;36(1):5–16.

30. Bernard GR, Luce JM, Sprung CL, et al. High-dose corticosteroids in patients with the adult respiratory distress syndrome. N Engl J Med 1987;317(25): 1565–70.

31. Annane D, Sebille V, Charpentier C, et al. Effect of treatment with low doses of hydrocortisone and flu-drocortisone on mortality in patients with septic shock. JAMA 2002;288(7):862–71.

32. Marik PE, Pastores SM, Annane D, et al. Recom-mendations for the diagnosis and management of corticosteroid insufficiency in critically ill adult pa-tients: consensus statements from an international task force by the American College of Critical Care Medicine. Crit Care Med 2008;36(6):1937–49.

33. Bernard GR, Artigas A, Brigham KL, et al. The American-European Consensus Conference on ARDS. Definitions, mechanisms, relevant out-comes, and clinical trial coordination. Am J Respir Crit Care Med 1994;149(3 Pt 1):818–24.

34. Annane D, Sebille V, Bellissant E, Ger-Inf-05 Study Group. Effect of low doses of corticosteroids in septic shock patients with or without early acute respiratory distress syndrome. Crit Care Med 2006;34(1):22–30.

35. Sprung CL, Annane D, Keh D, et al. Hydrocortisone therapy for patients with septic shock. N Engl J Med 2008;358(2):111–24.

36. Meduri GU, Golden E, Freire AX, et al. Methylpred-nisolone infusion in early severe ARDS: results of a randomized controlled trial. Chest 2007;131(4): 954–63.

37. Murray JF, Matthay MA, Luce JM, et al. An expanded definition of the adult respiratory distress syndrome. Am Rev Respir Dis 1988; 138(3):720–3.

38. Schoenfeld DA, Bernard GR. Statistical evaluation of ventilator-free days as an efficacy measure in clinical trials of treatments for acute respiratory distress syndrome. Crit Care Med 2002;30(8): 1772–7.

39. Confalonieri M, Urbino R, Potena A, et al. Hydrocor-tisone infusion for severe community-acquired pneumonia: a preliminary randomized study. Am J Respir Crit Care Med 2005;171(3):242–8.

40. Trees DW, Smith JM, Hockert S. Innovative mobility strategies for the patient with intensive care unit-acquired weakness: a case report. Phys Ther 2013;93(2):237–47.

41. Meduri GU, Belenchia JM, Estes RJ, et al. Fibropro-liferative phase of ARDS. Clinical findings and ef-fects of corticosteroids. Chest 1991;100(4):943–52.

42. Meduri GU, Chinn AJ, Leeper KV, et al. Corticoste-roid rescue treatment of progressive fibroprolifera-tion in late ARDS. Patterns of response and predictors of outcome. Chest 1994;105(5):1516–27.

43. Meduri GU. Pulmonary fibroproliferation and death in patients with late ARDS. Chest 1995;107(1):5–6.

44. Hooper RG, Kearl RA. Established adult respiratory distress syndrome successfully treated with corti-costeroids. South Med J 1996;89(4):359–64.

45. Ashbaugh DG, Maier RV. Idiopathic pulmonary fibrosis in adult respiratory distress syndrome. Diagnosis and treatment. Arch Surg 1985;120(5): 530–5.

46. Meduri GU, Headley AS, Golden E, et al. Effect of prolonged methylprednisolone therapy in unresolv-ing acute respiratory distress syndrome: a random-ized controlled trial. JAMA 1998;280(2):159–65.

47. Steinberg KP, Hudson LD, Goodman RB, et al. Ef-ficacy and safety of corticosteroids for persistent acute respiratory distress syndrome. N Engl J Med 2006;354(16):1671–84.

48. Meduri GU, Marik PE, Chrousos GP, et al. Steroid treatment in ARDS: a critical appraisal of the ARDS network trial and the recent literature. Inten-sive Care Med 2008;34(1):61–9.

49. Hough CL, Steinberg KP, Taylor Thompson B, et al. Intensive care unit-acquired neuromyopathy and corticosteroids in survivors of persistent ARDS. Intensive Care Med 2009;35(1):63–8.

50. Stevens RD, Dowdy DW, Michaels RK, et al. Neuro-muscular dysfunction acquired in critical illness: a systematic review. Intensive Care Med 2007; 33(11):1876–91.

51. Semmler A, Okulla T, Kaiser M, et al. Long-term neuromuscular sequelae of critical illness. J Neurol 2013;260(1):151–7.

52. Hermans G, Wilmer A, Meersseman W, et al. Impact of intensive insulin therapy on neuromus-cular complications and ventilator dependency in the medical intensive care unit. Am J Respir Crit Care Med 2007;175(5):480–9.

53. Hudson LD, Hough CL. Therapy for late-phase acute respiratory distress syndrome. Clin Chest Med 2006;27(4):671–7 [abstract: ix–x].

54. De Jonghe B, Sharshar T, Lefaucheur JP, et al. Paresis acquired in the intensive care unit: a prospective multicenter study. JAMA 2002;288(22): 2859–67.

55. Herridge MS, Cheung AM, Tansey CM, et al. One-year outcomes in survivors of the acute respiratory distress syndrome. N Engl J Med 2003;348(8):683–93.

56. Davydow DS, Kohen R, Hough CL, et al. A pilot investigation of the association of genetic polymorphisms regulating corticotrophin-releasing hormone with posttraumatic stress and depressive symptoms in medical-surgical intensive care unit survivors. J Crit Care 2014;29(1):101–6.

57. Schelling G, Stoll C, Kapfhammer HP, et al. The effect of stress doses of hydrocortisone during septic shock on posttraumatic stress disorder and health-related quality of life in survivors. Crit Care Med 1999;27(12):2678–83.

58. Iwashyna TJ, Angus DC. Declining case fatality rates for severe sepsis: good data bring good news with ambiguous implications. JAMA 2014; 311:1295–7.

59. Ranieri VM, Suter PM, Tortorella C, et al. Effect of mechanical ventilation on inflammatory mediators in patients with acute respiratory distress syndrome: a randomized controlled trial. JAMA 1999; 282(1):54–61.

60. Cabrera-Benitez NE, Parotto M, Post M, et al. Mechanical stress induces lung fibrosis by epithelial-mesenchymal transition. Crit Care Med 2012; 40(2):510–7.

61. Tremblay L, Valenza F, Ribeiro SP, et al. Injurious ventilatory strategies increase cytokines and c-fos m-RNA expression in an isolated rat lung model. J Clin Invest 1997;99(5):944–52.

62. Ricard JD, Dreyfuss D, Saumon G. Production of inflammatory cytokines in ventilator-induced lung injury: a reappraisal. Am J Respir Crit Care Med 2001;163(5):1176–80.

63. Nalayanda DD, Fulton WB, Colombani PM, et al. Pressure induced lung injury in a novel in vitro model of the alveolar interface: protective effect of dexamethasone. J Pediatr Surg 2014;49(1):61–5 [discussion: 65].

64. Hegeman MA, Hennus MP, Cobelens PM, et al. Dexamethasone attenuates VEGF expression and inflammation but not barrier dysfunction in a murine model of ventilator-induced lung injury. PLoS One 2013;8(2):e57374.

65. Hegeman MA, Cobelens PM, Kamps J, et al. Liposome-encapsulated dexamethasone attenuates ventilator-induced lung inflammation. Br J Pharmacol 2011;163(5):1048–58.

66. Agarwal R, Nath A, Aggarwal AN, et al. Do glucocorticoids decrease mortality in acute respiratory distress syndrome? A meta-analysis. Respirology 2007;12(4):585–90.

67. Lamontagne F, Briel M, Guyatt GH, et al. Corticosteroid therapy for acute lung injury, acute respiratory distress syndrome, and severe pneumonia: a meta-analysis of randomized controlled trials. J Crit Care 2010;25(3):420–35.

68. Tang BM, Craig JC, Eslick GD, et al. Use of corticosteroids in acute lung injury and acute respiratory distress syndrome: a systematic review and meta-analysis. Crit Care Med 2009;37(5): 1594–603.

69. Lee HS, Lee JM, Kim MS, et al. Low-dose steroid therapy at an early phase of postoperative acute respiratory distress syndrome. Ann Thorac Surg 2005;79(2):405–10.

70. Keel JB, Hauser M, Stocker R, et al. Established acute respiratory distress syndrome: benefit of corticosteroid rescue therapy. Respiration 1998; 65(4):258–64.

71. Varpula T, Pettila V, Rintala E, et al. Late steroid therapy in primary acute lung injury. Intensive Care Med 2000;26:526–31.

72. Huh J, Lim CM, Jegal Y. The effect of steroid therapy in patients with late ARDS. Tuberc Respir Dis (Seoul) 2002;52:376–84.

73. Gagnon S, Boota AM, Fischl MA, et al. Corticosteroids as adjunctive therapy for severe *Pneumocystis carinii* pneumonia in the acquired immunodeficiency syndrome: a double-blind, placebo-controlled trial. N Engl J Med 1990;323(21): 1444–50.

74. Kovacs JA, Masur H. Are corticosteroids beneficial as adjunctive therapy for *Pneumocystis* pneumonia in AIDS? Ann Intern Med 1990;113(1):1–3.

75. Montaner JS, Lawson LM, Levitt N, et al. Corticosteroids prevent early deterioration in patients with moderately severe *Pneumocystis carinii* pneumonia and the acquired immunodeficiency syndrome (AIDS). Ann Intern Med 1990;113(1): 14–20.

76. Azoulay E, Canet E, Raffoux E, et al. Dexamethasone in patients with acute lung injury from acute monocytic leukaemia. Eur Respir J 2012;39(3): 648–53.

77. Cronin L, Cook DJ, Carlet J, et al. Corticosteroid treatment for sepsis: a critical appraisal and meta-analysis of the literature. Crit Care Med 1995;23(8):1430–9.

78. Nie W, Zhang Y, Cheng J, et al. Corticosteroids in the treatment of community-acquired pneumonia in adults: a meta-analysis. PLoS One 2012;7(10): e47926.

79. Brun-Buisson C, Richard JC, Mercat A, et al, REVA-SRLF A/H1N1v 2009 Registry Group. Early corticosteroids in severe influenza A/H1N1 pneumonia and acute respiratory distress syndrome. Am J Respir Crit Care Med 2011; 183(9):1200–6.

80. Kim SH, Hong SB, Yun SC, et al. Corticosteroid treatment in critically ill patients with pandemic influenza A/H1N1 2009 infection: analytic strategy using propensity scores. Am J Respir Crit Care Med 2011;183(9):1207–14.

81. Martin-Loeches I, Lisboa T, Rhodes A, et al. Use of early corticosteroid therapy on ICU admission in patients affected by severe pandemic (H1N1)v influenza A infection. Intensive Care Med 2011; 37(2):272–83.

Endogenous and Exogenous Cell-Based Pathways for Recovery from Acute Respiratory Distress Syndrome

Jeffrey E. Gotts, MD, PhD, Michael A. Matthay, MD*

KEYWORDS

- Acute respiratory distress syndrome • Lung progenitor cells • Mesenchymal stem/stromal cells

KEY POINTS

- Acute respiratory distress syndrome (ARDS) occurs when protein-rich fluid accumulates in the air spaces because of a breakdown of the alveolar-capillary barrier following endothelial and epithelial damage and dysfunction.
- Endogenous lung progenitor populations are mobilized differentially in various animal models of lung injury.
- Exogenous cell therapies for ARDS hold substantial promise for improving the endogenous response, and clinical trials are ongoing.

ACUTE RESPIRATORY DISTRESS SYNDROME. DISRUPTION OF THE ALVEOLAR-CAPILLARY BARRIER

Acute respiratory distress syndrome (ARDS) develops when the normal capacity of the alveoli to remain dry and participate in gas exchange is overwhelmed by a cascade of insults to the delicate alveolar-capillary barrier, resulting in airspace fluid accumulation. In health, pulmonary capillary endothelial cells form a relatively tight membrane resistant to the paracellular movement of proteinaceous fluid and inflammatory cells. This barrier depends on adherens junctions held together by VE-cadherin, as shown by studies specifically targeting this molecule with a metalloproteinase.[1] Endothelial adherens junctions can be disrupted by tumor necrosis factor α, vascular endothelial growth factor (VEGF), and other cytokines from activated leukocytes,[2] in addition to thrombin, complement activation, and toll-like receptor 4 signaling.[3] Furthermore, lung endothelial cells can be damaged or killed by bacterial products,[4] activated platelets,[5,6] and neutrophils.[7]

Increased permeability of lung endothelium is necessary but not sufficient for the development of pulmonary edema. Clearance of extravasated fluid from the interstitial space by lymphatics is normally rapid.[8] Similarly to the lung endothelium, alveolar epithelial cells are joined together by tight junctions, but this barrier can be disrupted by toxic mediators from activated neutrophils[9] or macrophages,[10] pathogens including influenza,[11] and

The authors have no relevant financial disclosures.
This work was supported by NHLBI grants R37HL51856, R01HL51854, and F32HL117549.
Departments of Medicine and Anesthesia, Cardiovascular Research Institute, University of California, San Francisco, 505 Parnassus Avenue, San Francisco, CA 94143-0624, USA
* Corresponding author. 505 Parnassus Avenue, Moffitt, Room M-917, San Francisco, CA 94143-0624.
E-mail address: Michael.matthay@ucsf.edu

Clin Chest Med 35 (2014) 797–809
http://dx.doi.org/10.1016/j.ccm.2014.08.015

excessive mechanical stretch.[12] In addition, the alveolar epithelium is normally capable of actively transporting fluid from the alveolar lumen to the interstitial space as a final defense against alveolar flooding. The rate of alveolar fluid clearance can be increased by mild insults[13] but has been shown to be reduced by high tidal volume mechanical ventilation, inflammatory cytokines, and infection.[14] Not surprisingly, pathologic[15] and clinical studies[16] of patients with ARDS have revealed evidence of combined endothelial and epithelial dysfunction, including impaired alveolar fluid clearance. Furthermore, damage to alveolar type II cells along with extravasated plasma proteins and cellular debris disrupts the normal secretion and function of pulmonary surfactant.[17]

ENDOGENOUS CELL-BASED PATHWAYS FOR RECOVERY
General Mechanisms of Recovery

Returning the alveolus to a functional state is the obvious imperative for survival and recovery from ARDS (**Fig. 1**). Repair and/or replacement of most damaged alveoli must occur in patients, given the relatively mild pulmonary physiologic abnormalities measured in long-term survivors.[18] The processes whereby this occurs remain largely unknown, but some key insights have been generated over the last several decades. Broadly speaking, there must be resolution of edema fluid, removal of inflammatory cells and debris, and repair of the structural integrity and function of the alveolar epithelium and lung endothelium.

As recovery begins, aided by the resolution of the triggering event and prevention of further mechanical injury with lung-protective ventilation, there is a shift away from proinflammatory signaling.

Interleukin (IL)-10, secreted by CD4 T cells, macrophages, and dendritic cells, is present even early during acute inflammation and acts primarily on macrophages to reduce proinflammatory mediator secretion and antigen presentation while enhancing scavenger function and production of other anti-inflammatory molecules, such as IL-1 receptor antagonist (IL-1ra).[19] Thus, IL-10 is thought to be crucial in balancing pathogen clearance and tissue homeostasis. Its importance in this regard is highlighted by the existence of pathogen mimics such as Epstein-Barr virus encoded BCRF1.[19] A subset of CD4 T cells termed regulatory T cells (Tregs), major secretors of IL-10 in a variety of disease states,[20] are present in the air spaces of patients with ARDS, and are critical in the resolution of endotoxin-induced acute lung injury in mice, in part through increasing the anti-inflammatory molecule transforming growth factor (TGF)-β.[21]

IL-10, IL-1ra, and TGF-β notwithstanding, it had generally been thought that resolution of inflammatory injury occurs primarily because of the passive decline of dozens of proinflammatory mediators. More recently, however, several investigators have defined a new paradigm of active resolution of inflammation. A complex class of highly potent fatty-acid derivatives including lipoxins, resolvins, protectins, and maresins are now known to be generated during resolution. These lipid mediators bind to specific immune and resident cell receptors with high affinity, and inhibit granulocyte recruitment and tissue activation, induce phagocytosis of apoptotic cells and bacteria, and aid in clearance of mucosal leukocytes.[22] Apoptotic neutrophils and other cells are removed mostly by macrophages in a phagocytic process termed efferocytosis.[23] The act of ingesting apoptotic cells is itself a stimulus to further

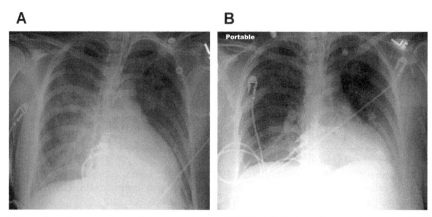

Fig. 1. Resolution of acute respiratory distress syndrome (ARDS). (*A*) Typical chest radiography findings in a patient with ARDS include patchy bilateral air-space opacities. (*B*) During resolution, these changes improve significantly.

anti-inflammatory signaling, helping to propel a feed-forward process of resolution.[24]

Endogenous Lung Progenitors

As the air spaces begin to clear, the damaged alveolar epithelium must replace lost cells and re-form tight junctions. How this occurs is an active and controversial area of investigation, but has particular relevance to understanding the potential for stem and progenitor cell therapies in ARDS. As one moves in the lung from proximal to distal, settled fact yields progressively to confusion and uncertainty, and so what follows is merely the current state of the evidence (**Table 1**).

Based primarily on studies in mice there is now general agreement that, in the large airways, basal cells self-renew and produce both ciliated and secretory cell types following epithelial damage incurred by various insults, including acid and naphthalene.[25,26] In the smaller intralobar airways, Clara cells, secretory cells that express secretoglobin 1a1 (Scgb1a1 or CCSP) can self-renew and also produce ciliated cells.[27] The subset of Scgb1a1+ cells at the bronchioloalveolar duct junction (BADJ) that also express surfactant protein C (SPC) has been termed bronchioalveolar stem cells (BASCs). In 2005, Kim and colleagues[28] reported that BASCs proliferated in situ following injury with naphthalene (kills Clara cells) or bleomycin (kills alveolar epithelial cells [AECs]) and showed multipotency in clonal assays in vitro. Subsequently, Rawlins and colleagues[29] performed lineage tracing of cells expressing Scgb1a1 and reported no contribution to the alveolar epithelium following hyperoxia (which damages terminal bronchioles and alveoli). Following bleomycin injury, cells expressing Scgb1a1 do indeed produce AECs, as reported by multiple investigators.[30,31] This finding demonstrates, perhaps not surprisingly, that the injury model itself is crucial in identifying which progenitor populations become active and how repair occurs.

To add to the complexity, there are at least 2 other cell types that can reportedly produce AECs:

- Integrin α6β4-expressing alveolar cells (not expressing other known epithelial markers) generate airway and alveolar epithelia in vitro[32] and impressively produce alveolar-like structures abutting vascular elements in lung "organoids" when implanted into the kidney capsule of adult mice.[33]
- Kajstura and colleagues[34] reported that c-kit–expressing cells derived from adult human lungs and injected into a 2-mm^2 region of mouse lung destroyed by cryoinjury produced airways, alveoli, and blood vessels bearing

human lineage tracer; these results await confirmation.

Several other reports add to the theme of progenitor response being dependent on injury type. Barkauskas and colleagues[35] found with lineage tracing that SPC-expressing type II AECs self-renew and produce types I and II AECs slowly during adult life, but rapidly following specific ablation of type II AECs with diphtheria toxin. That type II AECs could repopulate alveoli had been suspected since the 1970s,[36] but these results provided the best evidence to date. Similarly, Desai and colleagues[37] recently reported that type II AECs repopulate alveoli slowly during healthy adulthood, but rapidly after hyperoxia-mediated alveolar injury.

In contrast to these relatively mild, mostly alveolar-specific injuries, Kumar and colleagues[38] reported that H1N1 influenza in mice induced massive areas of lung destruction followed by the appearance of p63+, keratin-5+ (Krt5) pods of cells that appeared to migrate from airways into injured lung parenchyma and potentially give rise to new alveoli, although the ultimate fate of these cells has not yet been determined convincingly by lineage tracing. This phenomenon had not been reported following the comparatively milder injury models in common use, and demonstrates that lung progenitor populations may respond to injury in a graded fashion.

Coordination of Endogenous Progenitor Responses

With such flexibility in the response of lung epithelial progenitors, 2 recent reports deserve special attention because they illustrate potentially important regulatory mechanisms. In 2011, Ding and colleagues[39] performed pneumonectomies (PTX) on adult mice, and reproduced the finding that the intact lobes of the lung undergo rapid expansion with apparent formation of new alveoli.[40] By flow analysis, proliferating epithelial cells 3 days after PTX were similar phenotypically to BASCs. Of note, disrupting VEGF signaling only within pulmonary endothelium blocked the epithelial progenitor response. In a series of elegant experiments, the investigators showed that VEGF signaling in lung endothelium triggers the production of matrix metalloproteinase 14, which in turn releases EGF-receptor ligands that drive epithelial progenitor proliferation and alveologenesis.

Lee and colleagues[41] cocultured single BASCs with primary lung or liver endothelial cells, and found that only lung endothelia supported BASC multilineage differentiation into airway and AECs. Thrombospondin 1 (Tsp1), an inhibitor of angiogenesis expressed developmentally during

Table 1
Summary of lung progenitor studies

Reported Stem/Progenitor[a]	Injury Model	Injured Cells	Finding	Authors,[Ref.] Year
Type II AECs in rats	Nitrogen dioxide	AECs	Electron microscopy and autoradiography suggested that type II AECs self-renew and produce type I AECs	Evans et al,[36] 1973
Type II AECs	Bleomycin; targeted diphtheria toxin	Type I and II AECs; type II AECs	SPC lineage tracing showed replacement of both types I and II AECs	Barkauskas et al,[35] 2013
Fraction of type II AECs	Hyperoxia	Type I AECs	Replacement of both types I and II AECs via EGFR/KRAS signaling	Desai et al,[37] 2014
BASC expressing Scgb1a1 and SPC	Naphthalene; bleomycin	Clara cells; AECs	These cells at the junction of bronchioles and alveoli self-renewed and had multipotent differentiation in culture	Kim et al,[28] 2005
BASC	Naphthalene; hyperoxia	Clara cells; terminal bronchioles and type I AECs	Scgb1a1 lineage tracing showed that BASCs replace airway but not alveolar epithelium	Rawlins et al,[29] 2009
BASC	Bleomycin	AECs	Scgb1a1 lineage tracing showed that BASCs produce types I and II AECs	Tropea et al,[30] 2012; Rock et al,[31] 2011
Basal cells	Naphthalene	Clara cells	KRT5 lineage tracing showed basal cells self-renew and make new Clara and ciliated cells in the airways	Rock et al,[26] 2009
Human c-kit–expressing cells	Cryoinjury	All epithelial cell types	C-kit+ cells engraft into mouse lung and produce airways, alveoli, and blood vessels	Kajstura et al,[34] 2011
P63-expressing bronchiolar cells	Influenza	All epithelial cell types	Massive wave of Krt-5 expressing cells appeared to migrate from airways and form new alveoli	Kumar et al,[38] 2011

Abbreviations: AECs, alveolar epithelial cells; BASC, bronchioalveolar stem cell; EGFR, epidermal growth factor receptor; KRT5, keratin 5; Scgb1a1, secretoglobin 1a1; SPC, surfactant protein C.

[a] All murine unless otherwise specified.

alveolization,[42] was found to be central to this supportive role, as mice deficient in this molecule had impaired epithelialization of airways (following naphthalene) and alveoli (following bleomycin). Remarkably, alveolar repair in Tsp1 knockout mice could be rescued by the conditioned media of primary lung endothelial cells. Taken together, these results suggest an important role of the lung vasculature in guiding the expansion and differentiation of epithelial progenitors, similar to what is thought to occur in lung development[43] and in other adult tissues harboring multipotent progenitors, including the brain[44] and bone marrow.[45] Given the intricate structural and functional relationships between alveoli and lung capillaries required for effective gas exchange, this interaction during repair is not surprising. Further insights into how these vascular and epithelial processes are coordinated will clearly be important in optimizing endogenous lung repair and in developing exogenous repair strategies.

Enhancement of Epithelial and Endothelial Barrier Function

Once reconstituted as a tight membrane, the alveolar epithelial barrier can resume effective active edema fluid transport and clearance in addition to surfactant secretion. Although little is known about endogenous mechanisms controlling epithelial barrier tightening, several key signaling pathways are now known to regulate endothelial barrier function. Abbasi and Garcia[46] have discovered an important role for the sphingolipid sphingosine-1-phosphate (S1P) in rapidly enhancing lung endothelial barrier function by altering the cytoskeleton to increase cell overlap, and inducing adherens and tight junction assembly. S1P or its synthetic analogues have shown therapeutic efficacy in murine[47] and canine[48] models of endotoxin-induced acute lung injury, ischemia/reperfusion,[49] radiation-induced lung injury,[50] and influenza.[51] Angiopoietin-1 is produced by a variety of cells and acts on endothelial Tie2 receptors to promote barrier integrity.[52] Adrenomedullin binds calcitonin receptor-like receptor on lung endothelial cells and promotes intercellular adherence.[53] Administration of adrenomedullin improves endothelial barrier function in rodent models of ventilator-induced[54] and endotoxin-mediated lung injury.[55] Finally, London and colleagues[56] reported that Slit acts on lung endothelial Robo4 receptors to reduce vascular leakage in response to intratracheal endotoxin and H5N1 influenza, likely by promoting VE-cadherin expression.

EXOGENOUS CELL–BASED PATHWAYS FOR RECOVERY

As many of the mechanisms of lung injury have been worked out over the last several decades, researchers have tested a variety of targeted pharmacologic interventions in patients with ARDS, including antioxidants, β-agonists, surfactant, and IL-10.[57] However, the results have been uniformly disappointing, probably in part because ARDS is heterogeneous and is characterized by multiple injurious cascades operating simultaneously. Mortality has declined as lung-protective ventilation and fluid management strategies have been implemented,[58] and additional clinical benefits from paralysis[59] and prone positioning[60] may improve outcomes further. Nevertheless, there remains a compelling need to develop therapies that directly target the complex pathophysiology of ARDS. Exogenous cell–based therapies may hold special promise in this regard, as recent research has shown that these cells are capable of affecting multiple pathways of lung injury and repair.

Endothelial Progenitor Cells

Given the derangement of endothelial barrier function known to characterize ARDS, endothelial progenitor cells (EPCs) have intuitive appeal as a potential therapy. EPCs were originally described in the late 1990s as circulating CD34$^+$ cells that differentiated into endothelial cells in vitro and localized to sites of angiogenesis in adult animals.[61] In 2005, Yamada and colleagues[62] found that circulating EPCs were increased in patients with bacterial pneumonia, and that lower EPC counts were associated with persistent lung fibrosis following pneumonia resolution. Burnham and colleagues[63] then isolated EPCs in patients with ARDS, finding that the number of EPC colonies predicted improved survival. In 2008, Lam and colleagues[64] reported that administering autologous EPCs to rabbits 30 minutes following oleic acid injury improved endothelial barrier function and reduced lung edema, hemorrhage, and inflammation. Mao and colleagues[65] treated rats with autologous EPCs or saline 30 minutes after intravenous endotoxin, finding that EPC-treated rats had improved survival, reduced lung edema, and increased IL-10. Interestingly there was evidence of modest engraftment into the injured lung endothelium up to 14 days later. Such engraftment may be model-specific, however, as these cells do not seem to contribute to lung endothelial expansion after pneumonectomy.[66] Autologous EPCs are now the subject of clinical trials in cirrhosis (NCT01333228), ischemic stroke

(NCT01468064), and critical limb ischemia (NCT01595776). However, given that EPCs circulate at low levels, autologous transplantation is unlikely to be an option in the acute phase of ARDS, and the safety of allogeneic EPC transplantation remains unknown.

Mesenchymal Stem/Stromal Cells

In contrast to EPCs, mesenchymal stem/stromal cells (MSCs) are relatively immunoprivileged and known to be well tolerated after allogeneic transplantation.[67] These cells were first described in the 1960s as plastic-adherent, spindle-like cells that can be isolated from bone marrow, fat, umbilical cord blood, placenta, and connective tissues.[68] Although defined in part by the capacity to differentiate into osteoblasts, chondroblasts, and adipocytes, the overwhelming balance of evidence is that they rarely integrate and survive long term in adult tissues after allogeneic transplantation.[69] These cells have been studied extensively in models of acute inflammation in many different organ systems, and have been found to have remarkable therapeutic effects across a range of murine models of acute lung injury, including

bleomycin,[70] intratracheal[71-73] or intraperitoneal[74] endotoxin, cecal ligation and puncture,[75,76] pseudomonal abdominal sepsis,[77] and *Escherichia coli* pneumonia.[78] Recently, human bone marrow–derived MSCs were shown to reduce inflammation and improve alveolar fluid clearance in ex vivo human lungs injured with live *E coli*.[79] At least some of their therapeutic properties can be recapitulated by the microvesicles they actively secrete in culture.[80-82]

MSCs are thought to work by multiple mechanisms in these models (**Fig. 2**), including: (1) reducing alveolar-capillary barrier permeability,[72,75,76,83] in part by secretion of angiopoietin-1[84]; (2) increasing alveolar fluid clearance, at least in part by secretion of keratinocyte growth factor[79,85]; (3) shifting cytokines and resident macrophages from proinflammatory to anti-inflammatory[86]; (4) improving bacterial clearance by enhancing phagocytosis and secreting antibacterial peptides[77,78,83]; and, remarkably, (5) transferring mitochondria to AECs, rescuing adenosine triphosphate generation.[73]

Another intriguing possible mechanism has come to light recently. When postnatal rodents are exposed to high oxygen concentrations, they

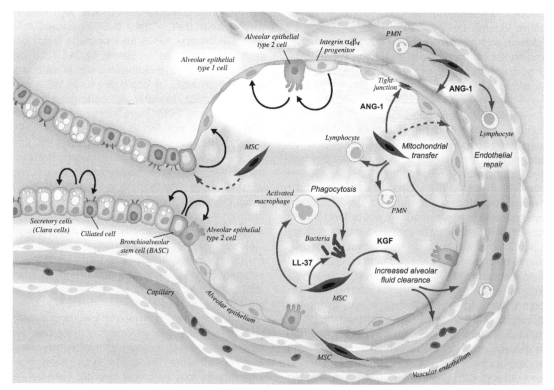

Fig. 2. An injured alveolus and adjacent alveolar duct. Potential mechanisms of MSC therapeutic effects in ARDS are shown with brown arrows. Black arrows depict lineage relationships during cell turnover. ANG-1, angiopoietin-1; KGF, keratinocyte growth factor; LL-37, cathelicidin; MSC, mesenchymal stem cell; PMN, polymorphonuclear leukocyte.

develop pulmonary hypertension from a dramatic simplification of lung architecture, modeling human bronchopulmonary dysplasia (BPD). In 2009, MSCs were shown to largely normalize lung capillary and alveolar growth when given by airway or blood in mouse and rat BPD models, but without any evidence of significant engraftment.[87,88] In 2012, Tropea and colleagues[30] reported that MSCs increased BASCs in the BPD model by a paracrine mechanism. This work suggests that MSCs, like lung endothelium, may help orchestrate epithelial progenitor responses to injury. Indeed, in other experimental systems, MSCs have been shown to interact with endothelial cells to establish a hematopoietic microenvironment after heterotopic transplantation,[89] to increase the proliferation and survival of hippocampal neural progenitors,[90] and to increase c-kit[+] cardiac stem cells in a porcine model of myocardial infarction.[91]

With this in mind, there is considerable optimism following the recently completed Korean phase 1 clinical trial of MSCs in neonates at high risk for BPD.[92] In this dose-escalation study, 9 patients with a mean gestational age of 25 weeks (mean birth weight 790 g) received either 1×10^7 or 2×10^7 allogeneic umbilical cord blood–derived MSCs/kg by airway at an average of 10 days after birth. There were no adverse events, and although the study was not designed to test efficacy, BPD severity appeared lower in treated patients than in a matched comparison group. A 2-year follow-up study of these patients is planned (NCT01632475).

Given the encouraging preclinical results from MSCs in rodent, sheep (Asmussen and colleagues, unpublished data 2014, under revision at *Thorax*), and ex vivo perfused human lung models of acute lung injury, an NHLBI-supported phase 1/2 (NCT01775774/NCT02097641) clinical trial of bone marrow–derived allogeneic MSCs in patients with moderate to severe ARDS is now under way. START (*ST*em cells for *A*RDS *T*reatment) targets a total enrollment of 69 patients, 9 in phase 1 and 60 in phase 2. In phase 1, 3 cohorts of patients received 1×10^6, 5×10^6, or 10×10^6 cells/kg intravenously, and there were no significant adverse events at the highest dose. In phase 2, patients will be randomized 2:1 to receive 10×10^6 MSCs/kg or plasmalyte control. The primary end point of phase 2 will be safety, but secondary end points will include the lung injury score, ratio of partial pressure of arterial oxygen/fraction of inspired oxygen, oxygenation index, Sequential Organ Failure Assessment score at day 3, ventilator-free days, 60-day mortality, plasma biomarkers of lung epithelial injury, endothelial injury and inflammation, and protein in a mini-bronchoalveolar lavage at 48 hours.

BARRIERS TO DEVELOPING CELL-BASED THERAPIES IN PATIENTS WITH ACUTE RESPIRATORY DISTRESS SYNDROME

As with all trials in critical care, the complex nature of the patients and the importance of logistical speed pose formidable hurdles in the design and implementation of exogenous cell–based therapies for ARDS. Beyond these difficulties, additional challenges, many summarized in a recent report from an National Institutes of Health/National Heart, Lung, and Blood Institute workshop,[93] include (**Table 2**):

- Ensuring consistent cell therapy product. This activity involves strict screening of donors and Good Manufacturing Practice for sterility, use of animal-derived products, and passage number.
- Quality control. Standard testing for cultured cell products includes screening for blood-borne pathogens, post-thaw cell viability, bacterial endotoxin, and cytogenetics.

Table 2
Challenges to the implementation of exogenous cell-based therapies for ARDS

Potential Barrier	Details
Consistency of the cell product	Cell handling, passage number, reagents (especially animal-derived)
Quality control	Screening for blood-borne pathogens, endotoxin limits, viability after thaw, cytogenetics
Potency	Assay should be simple, fast, reliable, and predictive of therapeutic effects in patients
IND-enabling animal data	GMP and GLP practices, standardized procedures for shipping, storing, freezing, thawing, diluting, washing, and administering; use of large animal models
Best delivery route	Airway or intravenous
IND submission	Highly technical and labor intensive

Abbreviations: GLP, good laboratory practice; GMP, good manufacturing practice; IND, investigational new drug.

- Assessing potency, ideally with a rapid, simple, reliable assay that can be run at multiple sites and correlates well with observed therapeutic effects. Potency assessment is a challenging but critical barrier to upscaling any new promising cell-based therapy for widespread use (as for phase 3 trials and beyond); an effective potency assay is essential in fine-tuning donor selection, manufacturing processes, and final preparation of the product.
- Developing preclinical (animal) data that adequately mirror the phase 1 safety studies required by the Food and Drug Administration (FDA). This development might require a shift in mindset for basic science investigators, as it requires careful attention to logistics including cell storage, shipment, packaging, freezing and thawing procedures (including method of cryoprotection), dilution, washing, and method and speed of administration. In addition, supportive animal studies must follow Good Laboratory Practice guidelines.
- Determining the optimal dosage, route, and timing of cell delivery. Intratracheal administration bypasses the vasculature and theoretically offers more direct access to injured lung tissue,[92] although it may pose additional hazards to gas exchange in the acute and often dynamic respiratory failure that characterizes ARDS.
- Careful consideration should be given to using large animal models, given that such studies may (1) provide important additional information on efficacy, and (2) permit monitoring of salient physiologic safety end points, especially during and immediately after cell administration.
- Filing an Investigational New Drug application. For this challenging process, it is helpful to elicit initial feedback from the FDA[94] during the planning stages of the animal experiments, and to obtain institutional support for the writing and submission of this highly technical document.

REMAINING QUESTIONS AND RESEARCH PRIORITIES

Regenerative medicine has entered an era of intense discovery, as evidenced by exponential growth in clinical trials targeting a wide range of human diseases with cellular therapies; this promise holds true for those of us engaged in developing better therapies for ARDS. However, key questions remain, and many obstacles may yet prevent effective cell-based therapies from becoming a reality.

Understanding the Endogenous Response

The importance of the type of injury in determining the endogenous progenitor cell response (highlighted in detail earlier) cannot be overstated. Going forward, it will be increasingly important to use clinically relevant models of lung injury, including bacterial and viral pneumonia, which together account for most cases of ARDS.[95] These models are challenged by a tendency to be variable in the severity of lung injury, to cause severe systemic illness, and to produce a robust immune response with a complex cellular infiltrate, all of which complicate the kinds of lineage-tracing studies that are now the accepted scientific standard.

Looking forward, researchers must advance the level of evidence of endogenous repair from a simple qualitative demonstration of expression of mature epithelial markers to a richer anatomic and temporal understanding of how newly formed epithelial-lined structures interface with lung capillaries and become (or fail to become) functional alveolar units. It may well be that simultaneous mechanisms are at work, including the diffuse growth of uninjured lung (as occurs following pneumonectomy[39]) and the more dramatic progenitor migratory events reported after influenza.[38] Insights generated from this research have obvious relevance for ARDS, but also hold promise for improving our understanding of endogenous repair processes in diseases as diverse as chronic obstructive pulmonary disease (COPD) and interstitial lung disease.

Safety of Exogenous Cell-Based Therapies

The perils of developing new classes of therapies for patients are well known from gene-therapy trials in the 1990s.[96] Potential complications of allogeneic cell therapy include infections (caused by contaminated product, immunomodulation, or even zoonoses, as prions can theoretically be carried by cell-culture reagents), worsened inflammation from immune rejection of transplanted cells, and, for intravenous administration, embolic load on the right ventricle (because most cells deposit at least temporarily in the lung[97]). A recent review[98] reported that MSC therapy in children and adults with left heart failure, myocardial infarction, spinal cord injury, stroke, hematologic malignancies, and Crohn disease seems to be safe, with only transient fever being occasionally noted. Given the concern for possible embolic insult to a pulmonary vasculature and right heart already stressed from the acute hypoxemia of ARDS, it is reassuring that a recent placebo-controlled randomized clinical trial of MSCs in moderate to severe COPD[99] showed no acute changes in hemodynamics or oxygenation, and no measurable difference in diffusing capacity, ambulatory oxygenation saturation, or echocardiographic estimate of right-sided pressures through 2 years of follow-up. The recent phase 1 data from MSC administration by airway to neonates at risk for BPD[92] and intravenously to patients with moderate to severe ARDS (NCT01775774) are similarly reassuring.

Neoplasia is another significant safety concern. In the MSC literature, there is some evidence that murine bone marrow–derived MSCs have genetic instability even at low passage number, with reports of tumor formation following intravenous administration in models of myocardial infarction and diabetic neuropathy.[100] Fortunately, this seems to be unique to murine MSCs, as human MSCs cultured for prolonged periods do not appear to transform.[101] A review of more than 500 large animals treated with MSCs for the treatment of myocardial infarction failed to reveal any evidence of malignancy for up to 3 months.[102] Finally, autopsy material from heavily immunosuppressed patients who had previously received allogeneic MSCs revealed minimal long-term engraftment and no evidence of ectopic tissue formation.[103]

Off-Target Effects

Given that ARDS is frequently associated with multiorgan failure, might exogenous cell therapies prove to have favorable effects outside the lung, for example in acute kidney injury[104] or sepsis?[105] Ideally, trial design for cell therapy in critical illness will incorporate clinical and biological end points that can help inform both efficacy and mechanism of action across related organ systems and scientific disciplines. Could cell therapies that effectively dampen the acute inflammatory response in ARDS unexpectedly impair the endogenous lung repair processes highlighted herein? Or might they accelerate them? These and other questions should become more tractable in the coming years as more data from clinical trials become available, and as the basic science research toolkit continues to expand.

ACKNOWLEDGMENTS

The authors thank Diana Lim for her excellent assistance in preparing **Fig. 2**.

REFERENCES

1. Schulz B, Pruessmeyer J, Maretzky T, et al. ADAM10 regulates endothelial permeability and T-cell transmigration by proteolysis of vascular endothelial cadherin. Circ Res 2008;102(10): 1192–201.

2. Vestweber D, Winderlich M, Cagna G, et al. Cell adhesion dynamics at endothelial junctions: VE-cadherin as a major player. Trends Cell Biol 2009;19(1):8–15.

3. Müller-Redetzky HC, Suttorp N, Witzenrath M. Dynamics of pulmonary endothelial barrier function in acute inflammation: mechanisms and therapeutic perspectives. Cell Tissue Res 2014;355:657–73.

4. Wiener-Kronish JP, Pittet JF. Therapies against virulence products of Staphylococcus aureus and Pseudomonas aeruginosa. Semin Respir Crit Care Med 2011;32(2):228–35.

5. Dixon JT, Gozal E, Roberts AM. Platelet-mediated vascular dysfunction during acute lung injury. Arch Physiol Biochem 2012;118(2):72–82.

6. Caudrillier A, Kessenbrock K, Gilliss BM, et al. Platelets induce neutrophil extracellular traps in transfusion-related acute lung injury. J Clin Invest 2012;122(7):2661–71.

7. Scheiermann C, Kunisaki Y, Jang JE, et al. Neutrophil microdomains: linking heterocellular interactions with vascular injury. Curr Opin Hematol 2010;17(1):25–30.

8. Wiener-Kronish JP, Broaddus VC, Albertine KH, et al. Relationship of pleural effusions to increased permeability pulmonary edema in anesthetized sheep. J Clin Invest 1988;82(4):1422–9.

9. Zemans RL, Colgan SP, Downey GP. Transepithelial migration of neutrophils: mechanisms and implications for acute lung injury. Am J Respir Cell Mol Biol 2009;40(5):519–35.

10. Frank JA, Wray CM, McAuley DF, et al. Alveolar macrophages contribute to alveolar barrier dysfunction in ventilator-induced lung injury. Am J Physiol Lung Cell Mol Physiol 2006;291(6):L1191–8.

11. Short KR, Kroeze EJ, Fouchier RA, et al. Pathogenesis of influenza-induced acute respiratory distress syndrome. Lancet Infect Dis 2014;14(1):57–69.

12. Davidovich N, DiPaolo BC, Lawrence GG, et al. Cyclic stretch-induced oxidative stress increases pulmonary alveolar epithelial permeability. Am J Respir Cell Mol Biol 2013;49(1):156–64.

13. Garat C, Rezaiguia S, Meignan M, et al. Alveolar endotoxin increases alveolar liquid clearance in rats. J Appl Physiol (1985) 1995;79(6):2021–8.

14. Folkesson HG, Matthay MA. Alveolar epithelial ion and fluid transport: recent progress. Am J Respir Cell Mol Biol 2006;35(1):10–9.

15. Bachofen M, Weibel ER. Alterations of the gas exchange apparatus in adult respiratory insufficiency associated with septicemia. Am Rev Respir Dis 1977;116(4):589–615.

16. Ware LB, Matthay MA. Alveolar fluid clearance is impaired in the majority of patients with acute lung injury and the acute respiratory distress

syndrome. Am J Respir Crit Care Med 2001;163(6): 1376–83.

17. Zasadzinski JA, Stenger PC, Shieh I, et al. Overcoming rapid inactivation of lung surfactant: analogies between competitive adsorption and colloid stability. Biochim Biophys Acta 2010;1798(4): 801–28.

18. Herridge MS, Tansey CM, Matté A, et al. Functional disability 5 years after acute respiratory distress syndrome. N Engl J Med 2011;364(14):1293–304.

19. Iyer SS, Cheng G. Role of interleukin 10 transcriptional regulation in inflammation and autoimmune disease. Crit Rev Immunol 2012;32(1):23–63.

20. Peterson RA. Regulatory T-cells: diverse phenotypes integral to immune homeostasis and suppression. Toxicol Pathol 2012;40(2):186–204.

21. D'Alessio FR, Tsushima K, Aggarwal NR, et al. CD4+CD25+Foxp3+ Tregs resolve experimental lung injury in mice and are present in humans with acute lung injury. J Clin Invest 2009;119(10): 2898–913.

22. Levy BD, Serhan CN. Resolution of acute inflammation in the lung. Annu Rev Physiol 2014;76:467–92.

23. Janssen WJ, Henson PM. Cellular regulation of the inflammatory response. Toxicol Pathol 2012;40(2): 166–73.

24. Fadok VA, Bratton DL, Konowal A, et al. Macrophages that have ingested apoptotic cells in vitro inhibit proinflammatory cytokine production through autocrine/paracrine mechanisms involving TGF-beta, PGE2, and PAF. J Clin Invest 1998; 101(4):890–8.

25. Wansleeben C, Barkauskas CE, Rock JR, et al. Stem cells of the adult lung: their development and role in homeostasis, regeneration, and disease. Wiley Interdiscip Rev Dev Biol 2013;2(1): 131–48.

26. Rock JR, Onaitis MW, Rawlins EL, et al. Basal cells as stem cells of the mouse trachea and human airway epithelium. Proc Natl Acad Sci U S A 2009;106(31):12771–5.

27. Giangreco A, Reynolds SD, Stripp BR. Terminal bronchioles harbor a unique airway stem cell population that localizes to the bronchoalveolar duct junction. Am J Pathol 2002;161(1):173–82.

28. Kim CF, Jackson EL, Woolfenden AE, et al. Identification of bronchioalveolar stem cells in normal lung and lung cancer. Cell 2005;121(6):823–35.

29. Rawlins EL, Okubo T, Xue Y, et al. The role of Scgb1a1+ Clara cells in the long-term maintenance and repair of lung airway, but not alveolar, epithelium. Cell Stem Cell 2009;4(6):525–34.

30. Tropea KA, Leder E, Aslam M, et al. Bronchioalveolar stem cells increase after mesenchymal stromal cell treatment in a mouse model of bronchopulmonary dysplasia. Am J Physiol Lung Cell Mol Physiol 2012;302(9):L829–37.

31. Rock JR, Barkauskas CE, Cronce MJ, et al. Multiple stromal populations contribute to pulmonary fibrosis without evidence for epithelial to mesenchymal transition. Proc Natl Acad Sci U S A 2011; 108(52):E1475–83.

32. McQualter JL, Yuen K, Williams B, et al. Evidence of an epithelial stem/progenitor cell hierarchy in the adult mouse lung. Proc Natl Acad Sci U S A 2010;107(4):1414–9.

33. Chapman HA, Li X, Alexander JP, et al. Integrin α6β4 identifies an adult distal lung epithelial population with regenerative potential in mice. J Clin Invest 2011;121(7):2855–62.

34. Kajstura J, Rota M, Hall SR, et al. Evidence for human lung stem cells. N Engl J Med 2011;364(19): 1795–806.

35. Barkauskas CE, Cronce MJ, Rackley CR, et al. Type 2 alveolar cells are stem cells in adult lung. J Clin Invest 2013;123(7):3025–36.

36. Evans MJ, Cabral LJ, Stephens RJ, et al. Renewal of alveolar epithelium in the rat following exposure to NO2. Am J Pathol 1973;70(2):175–98.

37. Desai TJ, Brownfield DG, Krasnow MA. Alveolar progenitor and stem cells in lung development, renewal and cancer. Nature 2014;507(7491):190–4.

38. Kumar PA, Hu Y, Yamamoto Y, et al. Distal airway stem cells yield alveoli in vitro and during lung regeneration following H1N1 influenza infection. Cell 2011;147(3):525–38.

39. Ding BS, Nolan DJ, Guo P, et al. Endothelial-derived angiocrine signals induce and sustain regenerative lung alveolarization. Cell 2011;147(3):539–53.

40. Cowan MJ, Crystal RG. Lung growth after unilateral pneumonectomy: quantitation of collagen synthesis and content. Am Rev Respir Dis 1975;111(3): 267–77.

41. Lee JH, Bhang DH, Beede A, et al. Lung stem cell differentiation in mice directed by endothelial cells via a BMP4-NFATc1-thrombospondin-1 axis. Cell 2014;156(3):440–55.

42. Sozo F, Hooper SB, Wallace MJ. Thrombospondin-1 expression and localization in the developing ovine lung. J Physiol 2007;584(Pt 2):625–35.

43. Thébaud B. Angiogenesis in lung development, injury and repair: implications for chronic lung disease of prematurity. Neonatology 2007;91(4):291–7.

44. Goldman SA, Chen Z. Perivascular instruction of cell genesis and fate in the adult brain. Nat Neurosci 2011;14(11):1382–9.

45. Colmone A, Sipkins DA. Beyond angiogenesis: the role of endothelium in the bone marrow vascular niche. Transl Res 2008;151(1):1–9.

46. Abbasi T, Garcia JG. Sphingolipids in lung endothelial biology and regulation of vascular integrity. Handb Exp Pharmacol 2013;(216):201–26.

47. Sammani S, Moreno-Vinasco L, Mirzapoiazova T, et al. Differential effects of sphingosine 1-phosphate

receptors on airway and vascular barrier function in the murine lung. Am J Respir Cell Mol Biol 2010; 43(4):394–402.

48. Szczepaniak WS, Zhang Y, Hagerty S, et al. Sphingosine 1-phosphate rescues canine LPS-induced acute lung injury and alters systemic inflammatory cytokine production in vivo. Transl Res 2008; 152(5):213–24.

49. Okazaki M, Kreisel F, Richardson SB, et al. Sphingosine 1-phosphate inhibits ischemia reperfusion injury following experimental lung transplantation. Am J Transplant 2007;7(4):751–8.

50. Mathew B, Jacobson JR, Berdyshev E, et al. Role of sphingolipids in murine radiation-induced lung injury: protection by sphingosine 1-phosphate analogs. FASEB J 2011;25(10):3388–400.

51. Teijaro JR, Walsh KB, Cahalan S, et al. Endothelial cells are central orchestrators of cytokine amplification during influenza virus infection. Cell 2011; 146(6):980–91.

52. Eklund L, Saharinen P. Angiopoietin signaling in the vasculature. Exp Cell Res 2013;319(9):1271–80.

53. Hocke AC, Temmesfeld-Wollbrueck B, Schmeck B, et al. Perturbation of endothelial junction proteins by Staphylococcus aureus alpha-toxin: inhibition of endothelial gap formation by adrenomedullin. Histochem Cell Biol 2006;126(3):305–16.

54. Müller HC, Witzenrath M, Tschernig T, et al. Adrenomedullin attenuates ventilator-induced lung injury in mice. Thorax 2010;65(12):1077–84.

55. Itoh T, Obata H, Murakami S, et al. Adrenomedullin ameliorates lipopolysaccharide-induced acute lung injury in rats. Am J Physiol Lung Cell Mol Physiol 2007;293(2):L446–52.

56. London NR, Zhu W, Bozza FA, et al. Targeting Robo4-dependent slit signaling to survive the cytokine storm in sepsis and influenza. Sci Transl Med 2010;2(23):23ra19.

57. Matthay MA, Ware LB, Zimmerman GA. The acute respiratory distress syndrome. J Clin Invest 2012; 122(8):2731–40.

58. Li G, Malinchoc M, Cartin-Ceba R, et al. Eight-year trend of acute respiratory distress syndrome: a population-based study in Olmsted County, Minnesota. Am J Respir Crit Care Med 2011;183(1):59–66.

59. Papazian L, Forel JM, Gacouin A, et al. Neuromuscular blockers in early acute respiratory distress syndrome. N Engl J Med 2010;363(12):1107–16.

60. Guérin C, Reignier J, Richard JC, et al. Prone positioning in severe acute respiratory distress syndrome. N Engl J Med 2013;368(23):2159–68.

61. Asahara T, Murohara T, Sullivan A, et al. Isolation of putative progenitor endothelial cells for angiogenesis. Science 1997;275(5302):964–7.

62. Yamada M, Kubo H, Ishizawa K, et al. Increased circulating endothelial progenitor cells in patients with bacterial pneumonia: evidence that bone marrow derived cells contribute to lung repair. Thorax 2005;60(5):410–3.

63. Burnham EL, Taylor WR, Quyyumi AA, et al. Increased circulating endothelial progenitor cells are associated with survival in acute lung injury. Am J Respir Crit Care Med 2005;172(7):854–60.

64. Lam CF, Liu YC, Hsu JK, et al. Autologous transplantation of endothelial progenitor cells attenuates acute lung injury in rabbits. Anesthesiology 2008; 108(3):392–401.

65. Mao M, Wang SN, Lv XJ, et al. Intravenous delivery of bone marrow-derived endothelial progenitor cells improves survival and attenuates lipopolysaccharide-induced lung injury in rats. Shock 2010;34(2):196–204.

66. Voswinckel R, Ziegelhoeffer T, Heil M, et al. Circulating vascular progenitor cells do not contribute to compensatory lung growth. Circ Res 2003; 93(4):372–9.

67. Le Blanc K, Rasmusson I, Sundberg B, et al. Treatment of severe acute graft-versus-host disease with third party haploidentical mesenchymal stem cells. Lancet 2004;363(9419):1439–41.

68. Friedenstein AJ, Petrakova KV, Kurolesova AI, et al. Heterotopic of bone marrow. Analysis of precursor cells for osteogenic and hematopoietic tissues. Transplantation 1968;6(2):230–47.

69. Prockop DJ, Kota DJ, Bazhanov N, et al. Evolving paradigms for repair of tissues by adult stem/progenitor cells (MSCs). J Cell Mol Med 2010;14(9): 2190–9.

70. Ortiz LA, Gambelli F, McBride C, et al. Mesenchymal stem cell engraftment in lung is enhanced in response to bleomycin exposure and ameliorates its fibrotic effects. Proc Natl Acad Sci U S A 2003;100(14):8407–11.

71. Gupta N, Su X, Popov B, et al. Intrapulmonary delivery of bone marrow-derived mesenchymal stem cells improves survival and attenuates endotoxin-induced acute lung injury in mice. J Immunol 2007;179(3):1855–63.

72. Mei SH, McCarter SD, Deng Y, et al. Prevention of LPS-induced acute lung injury in mice by mesenchymal stem cells overexpressing angiopoietin 1. PLoS Med 2007;4(9):e269.

73. Islam MN, Das SR, Emin MT, et al. Mitochondrial transfer from bone-marrow-derived stromal cells to pulmonary alveoli protects against acute lung injury. Nat Med 2012;18(5):759–65.

74. Xu J, Woods CR, Mora AL, et al. Prevention of endotoxin-induced systemic response by bone marrow-derived mesenchymal stem cells in mice. Am J Physiol Lung Cell Mol Physiol 2007;293(1): L131–41.

75. Mei SH, Haitsma JJ, Dos Santos CC, et al. Mesenchymal stem cells reduce inflammation while enhancing bacterial clearance and improving

survival in sepsis. Am J Respir Crit Care Med 2010;
182(8):1047–57.

76. Nemeth K, Mayer B, Mezey E. Modulation of bone marrow stromal cell functions in infectious diseases by toll-like receptor ligands. J Mol Med (Berl) 2010; 88(1):5–10.

77. Krasnodembskaya A, Samarani G, Song Y, et al. Human mesenchymal stem cells reduce mortality and bacteremia in gram negative sepsis in mice in part by enhancing the phagocytic activity of blood monocytes. Am J Physiol Lung Cell Mol Physiol 2012;302:L1003–13.

78. Gupta N, Krasnodembskaya A, Kapetanaki M, et al. Mesenchymal stem cells enhance survival and bacterial clearance in murine Escherichia coli pneumonia. Thorax 2012;67(6):533–9.

79. Lee JW, Krasnodembskaya A, McKenna DH, et al. Therapeutic effects of human mesenchymal stem cells in ex vivo human lungs injured with live bacteria. Am J Respir Crit Care Med 2013;187(7): 751–60.

80. Zhu YG, Feng XM, Abbott J, et al. Human mesenchymal stem cell microvesicles for treatment of Escherichia coli endotoxin-induced acute lung injury in mice. Stem Cells 2014;32(1):116–25.

81. Bruno S, Grange C, Deregibus MC, et al. Mesenchymal stem cell-derived microvesicles protect against acute tubular injury. J Am Soc Nephrol 2009;20(5):1053–67.

82. Sdrimas K, Kourembanas S. MSC microvesicles for the treatment of lung disease: a new paradigm for cell-free therapy. Antioxid Redox Signal 2014. [Epub ahead of print].

83. Krasnodembskaya A, Song Y, Fang X, et al. Antibacterial effect of human mesenchymal stem cells is mediated in part from secretion of the antimicrobial peptide LL-37. Stem Cells 2010; 28(12):2229–38.

84. Fang X, Neyrinck AP, Matthay MA, et al. Allogeneic human mesenchymal stem cells restore epithelial protein permeability in cultured human alveolar type II cells by secretion of angiopoietin-1. J Biol Chem 2010;285(34):26211–22.

85. Lee JW, Fang X, Gupta N, et al. Allogeneic human mesenchymal stem cells for treatment of E. coli endotoxin-induced acute lung injury in the ex vivo perfused human lung. Proc Natl Acad Sci U S A 2009;106(38):16357–62.

86. Prockop DJ, Youn Oh J. Mesenchymal stem/stromal cells (MSCs): role as guardians of inflammation. Mol Ther 2012;20(1):14–20.

87. Aslam M, Baveja R, Liang OD, et al. Bone marrow stromal cells attenuate lung injury in a murine model of neonatal chronic lung disease. Am J Respir Crit Care Med 2009;180(11):1122–30.

88. Van Haaften T, Byrne R, Bonnet S, et al. Airway delivery of mesenchymal stem cells prevents arrested alveolar growth in neonatal lung injury in rats. Am J Respir Crit Care Med 2009;180(11):1131–42.

89. Sacchetti B, Funari A, Michienzi S, et al. Self-renewing osteoprogenitors in bone marrow sinusoids can organize a hematopoietic microenvironment. Cell 2007;131(2):324–36.

90. Munoz JR, Stoutenger BR, Robinson AP, et al. Human stem/progenitor cells from bone marrow promote neurogenesis of endogenous neural stem cells in the hippocampus of mice. Proc Natl Acad Sci U S A 2005;102(50):18171–6.

91. Hatzistergos KE, Quevedo H, Oskouei BN, et al. Bone marrow mesenchymal stem cells stimulate cardiac stem cell proliferation and differentiation. Circ Res 2010;107(7):913–22.

92. Chang YS, Ahn SY, Yoo HS, et al. Mesenchymal stem cells for bronchopulmonary dysplasia: phase 1 dose-escalation clinical trial. J Pediatr 2014;164: 966–72.e6.

93. Matthay MA, Anversa P, Bhattacharya J, et al. Cell therapy for lung diseases. Report from an NIH-NHLBI workshop, November 13-14, 2012. Am J Respir Crit Care Med 2013;188(3):370–5.

94. Feigal EG, Tsokas K, Zhang J, et al. Perspective: communications with the Food and Drug Administration on the development pathway for a cell-based therapy: why, what, when, and how? Stem Cells Transl Med 2012;1(11):825–32.

95. Matthay MA, Zemans RL. The acute respiratory distress syndrome: pathogenesis and treatment. Annu Rev Pathol 2011;6:147–63.

96. Couzin J, Kaiser J. Gene therapy. As Gelsinger case ends, gene therapy suffers another blow. Science 2005;307(5712):1028.

97. Fischer UM, Harting MT, Jimenez F, et al. Pulmonary passage is a major obstacle for intravenous stem cell delivery: the pulmonary first-pass effect. Stem Cells Dev 2009;18(5):683–92.

98. Lalu MM, McIntyre L, Pugliese C, et al. Safety of cell therapy with mesenchymal stromal cells (safecell): a systematic review and meta-analysis of clinical trials. PLoS One 2012;7(10):e47559.

99. Weiss DJ, Casaburi R, Flannery R, et al. A placebo-controlled, randomized trial of mesenchymal stem cells in COPD. Chest 2013;143(6):1590–8.

100. Jeong JO, Han JW, Kim JM, et al. Malignant tumor formation after transplantation of short-term cultured bone marrow mesenchymal stem cells in experimental myocardial infarction and diabetic neuropathy. Circ Res 2011;108(11):1340–7.

101. Hatzistergos KE, Blum A, Ince T, et al. What is the oncologic risk of stem cell treatment for heart disease? Circ Res 2011;108(11):1300–3.

102. Van der Spoel TI, Jansen of Lorkeers SJ, Agostoni P, et al. Human relevance of pre-clinical studies in stem cell therapy: systematic review and meta-analysis of large animal models of

ischaemic heart disease. Cardiovasc Res 2011; 91(4):649–58.

103. Von Bahr L, Batsis I, Moll G, et al. Analysis of tissues following mesenchymal stromal cell therapy in humans indicates limited long-term engraftment and no ectopic tissue formation. Stem Cells 2012; 30(7):1575–8.

104. Erpicum P, Detry O, Weekers L, et al. Mesenchymal stromal cell therapy in conditions of renal ischaemia/reperfusion. Nephrol Dial Transplant 2014;29:1487–93.

105. Kusadasi N, Groeneveld AB. A perspective on mesenchymal stromal cell transplantation in the treatment of sepsis. Shock 2013;40(5):352–7.

Muscle Wasting and Early Mobilization in Acute Respiratory Distress Syndrome

CrossMark

Christopher J. Walsh, MD, FRCPC[a], Jane Batt, MD, FRCPC, PhD[a],
Margaret S. Herridge, MD, FRCPC, MPH[b],
Claudia C. Dos Santos, MD, FRCPC, MSc[a],*

KEYWORDS

- Muscle weakness • Neuromuscular disease • Critical illness • ARDS • Intensive care unit
- Early rehabilitation

KEY POINTS

- Patients with acute respiratory distress syndrome frequently develop persistent muscle weakness and poor functional outcome attributed to intensive care unit (ICU)–acquired weakness (ICUAW).
- Risk factors for ICUAW include sepsis, immobility, and hyperglycemia.
- Clinical diagnosis of ICUAW by physical examination has limitations, even in cooperative patients.
- Early rehabilitation programs in the ICU have been shown to be safe and feasible and have resulted in improved functional status after ICU discharge.
- Few interventions are available for prevention of ICUAW. Elucidating the molecular pathways that cause ICUAW is critical to develop novel targeted therapeutics.

INTRODUCTION

Survivors of acute respiratory distress syndrome (ARDS) frequently develop substantial and persistent muscle weakness associated with impairments in physical function and health-related quality of life.[1–4] Intensive care unit (ICU)–acquired weakness (ICUAW), well described in the acute phase of critical illness, is increasingly recognized to contribute to long-term disability in survivors of critical illness.[2,4–6] Skeletal muscle wasting and weakness acquired during critical illness may result from muscle dysfunction, loss of myosin and less commonly, frank myofiber necrosis (critical illness myopathy [CIM]), axonal sensory-motor axonopathy (critical illness polyneuropathy [CIP]), or a combination of both. Both processes manifest clinically as muscle weakness, induced by the resultant and variable combination of muscle wasting and impaired muscle contractility.[6]

In the acute phase, ICUAW is associated with failure of ventilator weaning, prolonged ICU stay, and increased mortality.[7–10] In patients who survive, ICUAW may resolve completely over several weeks.[11] However, a large proportion of patients

Funding Sources: This work was supported by the Canadian Institutes of Health Research (grant # MOP-106545), the Ontario Thoracic Society (grants OTS2010/2011/2012), the Physicians' Services Incorporated Foundation (grant # PSI 09–21), and the Early Research Award from the Ministry of Research and Innovation of Ontario (grant ERA/MRI 2011), Canada.
[a] Department of Medicine, Institute of Medical Sciences, Keenan Centre for Biomedical Science, Li Ka Shing Knowledge institute, St. Michael's Hospital, University of Toronto, 30 Bond Street, Toronto, Ontario M5B 1W8, Canada; [b] Interdepartmental Division of Critical Care, University of Toronto, Toronto General Hospital, NCSB 11C-1180, 585 University Avenue, Toronto, ON M5G 2N2, Canada
* Corresponding author.
E-mail address: dossantosc@smh.ca

Clin Chest Med 35 (2014) 811–826
http://dx.doi.org/10.1016/j.ccm.2014.08.016
0272-5231/14/$ – see front matter © 2014 Elsevier Inc. All rights reserved.

chestmed.theclinics.com

(40%–65%) have diminished functional capacity 5 years after ICU discharge (ie, reduced 6-minute walk [6MW]). The determinants of this persistent ICUAW remain inadequately defined.[2,9]

Inactivity has been shown to accelerate loss of muscle protein in severe illness and is a risk factor for ICUAW.[12,13] Early rehabilitation is hypothesized to prevent disuse atrophy and improve muscle strength in both short-term and long-term ICU survivors. An increasing number of interventional studies have emerged over the past decade examining muscle function and ICUAW as outcomes, notably trials implementing early rehabilitation in the ICU setting.

This article highlights the risk factors and molecular mechanisms associated with ICUAW and examines the current evidence for prevention and management of muscle weakness in critically ill patients, with a focus on early rehabilitation.

RISK FACTORS FOR INTENSIVE CARE UNIT–ACQUIRED WEAKNESS

Classification of ICU patients within clinical phenotypes has the potential to accurately stratify patients by likelihood of persistent weakness.[14] Several risks factors for ICUAW have been identified in multiple studies, including sepsis, immobility, and hyperglycemia. Age, burden of comorbid disease, and ICU length of stay have been recognized as major risk modifiers of

long-term recovery of function after critical illness (**Fig. 1**).

Patients with sepsis and multiorgan dysfunction syndrome (MODS) are at high risk for ICUAW; a recent systematic review found a nearly 50% incidence of ICUAW in this population.[12] The severity and duration of both systemic inflammatory response syndrome (SIRS) and MODS have been associated with ICUAW in several studies and several investigators have concluded that ICUAW is one manifestation of MODS.[11,15–19] ICUAW has been associated with immobilization in several studies using the duration of mechanical ventilation (MV) and ICU stay as indirect measures of immobility.[11,15,20]

Hyperglycemia, a frequent complication of critical illness and inactivity, has been linked to ICUAW in multiple observational studies[12] and in 2 large randomized controlled trials (RCTs) of insulin therapy that examined the effect of intensive insulin therapy (IIT) versus conventional insulin therapy (CIT) on ICUAW as a secondary outcome.[21,22] The first RCT screened for ICUAW by electromyography weekly in 363 surgical patients requiring ICU stay for 1 week or more. The trial found a reduced incidence of ICUAW (28.7% vs 51.9%; P<.001) and a faster resolution of ICUAW in the IIT group versus CIT.[22] The second RCT enrolled 420 medical ICU patients requiring more than 1 week in the ICU and found similar outcomes.[22] Both trials showed reduced

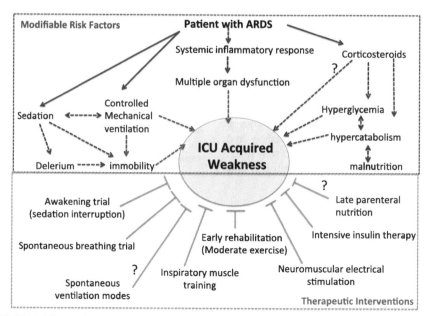

Fig. 1. Modifiable risk factors for muscle atrophy and ICUAW (*above*) and potential therapeutic interventions (*below*) in a mechanically ventilated patient with ARDS. Solid red arrows denote interventions for ARDS. Dashed arrows denote adverse effects of the intervention in addition to underlying critical illness/ARDS. Interventions with predominantly inconclusive or contradictory findings in the literature are denoted by a question mark (?).

180-day mortality, ICU stay, and duration of MV in the total population and the population screened for ICUAW.

It is unclear whether the shortened duration of MV and mortality benefit can be explained by fewer cases of ICUAW or reductions of other hyperglycemia-associated morbidities.[23] However, a large multicenter trial found increased mortality at 90 days (mostly from cardiovascular complications) in 6104 patients randomized to IIT versus CIT (number needed to harm of 38).[24] Although ICUAW was not formally evaluated in this study it did not find any difference in duration of MV or ICU stay. A significantly higher proportion of patients in the IIT arm received corticosteroids in this trial, which may have confounded the outcome measure. Nevertheless, the benefits of preventing ICUAW with an intensive insulin protocol must be weighed against the harms of potentially higher mortality.

There have been conflicting conclusions regarding the association of corticosteroids with ICUAW.[3,12,15,25] An ARDSnet RCT that compared methylprednisone versus placebo for severe persistent ARDS found that 9 patients in the intervention group developed serious adverse events associated with ICUAW versus none in the placebo group.[26] A secondary analysis of this trial found no difference in ICUAW among the 128 patients who survived 60 days after study enrollment by reviewing patient charts.[27] Another RCT found no difference in rate of ICUAW between prolonged administration of methylprednisolone (1 mg/kg/d) versus controls in early ARDS using a protocol that avoided neuromuscular blocking agents (NMBAs).[28] ICUAW was not a secondary outcome measure in these trials and patients were not systematically evaluated for ICUAW. It has been argued that although corticosteroids may increase the risk of myopathy, these agents may alternatively decrease the overall risk of ICUAW in the patients with ARDS by reducing the duration of shock and MV.[27]

NMBAs are commonly used in the management of ARDS to prevent patient-ventilator asynchrony and improve ventilation. These agents have been associated with ICUAW in a retrospective study of septic patients[25] and severe asthma[29]; however, these studies are confounded by the use of high-dose glucocorticoid therapy. A double-blind trial that randomized 340 patients with severe ARDS to 48-hour continuous infusion of cisatracurium or placebo resulted in decreased mortality at 28 days with no increased risk of ICUAW measured by physical examination (Medical Research Council [MRC] score) at day 28 and at time of ICU discharge.[30] Changes to the

administration of NMBA, including shorter duration and avoidance of agents associated with persistent drug effect, along with bedside monitoring to detect excessive blockage, may explain the lower risk of ICUAW in more recent trials.[15] Further studies are warranted assessing the incidence of ICUAW with NMBAs, as well as the interaction of NMBAs with corticosteroids using more sensitive methods to detect ICUAW.

Clinical Phenotyping to Assess Risk of Persistent Intensive Care Unit–acquired Weakness

Clinical data indicate that young, previously healthy patients with severe ARDS can have CIM that is rapidly reversible, whereas patients of advanced age or comorbidity are more likely to develop both acute and sustained CIM.[14] This finding has led to attempts to define phenotypes of ICUAW based on age, comorbid illness, ICU length of stay, and severity of critical illness. Each phenotype is likely to possess different degrees of muscle reserve and responses to injury, which predisposes to different functional outcomes. Older patients have less skeletal muscle reserve at baseline and lose a greater proportion of muscle with inactivity than younger patients.[31] Moreover, the resulting muscle atrophy may have more significant functional consequences in older patients.[14]

Studying patients classified by clinical phenotypes may be necessary to elucidate the specific molecular pathways that give rise to each phenotype and to direct future targeted therapies. Stratifying patients based on the extent of muscle atrophy (structural) and functional (contractile) impairment may also prove to be important to predict long-term outcomes and responsiveness to physical therapy.

EPIDEMIOLOGY OF INTENSIVE CARE UNIT–ACQUIRED WEAKNESS IN ACUTE RESPIRATORY DISTRESS SYNDROME

The rate of ICUAW in patients with severe ARDS was evaluated as a secondary prespecified outcome in a double-blind RCT comparing neuromuscular blockade with placebo using a validated measure (MRC score) to screen for ICUAW.[30] ICUAW occurred in 37.7% (61 of 162) of patients receiving placebo on day 28 or at time of hospital discharge. A secondary analysis of 128 patients with ARDS surviving more than 60 days after enrollment in a prospective trial found that 34% were diagnosed with ICUAW, although the investigators speculated that some cases likely went undetected.[27]

A retrospective study of 50 consecutive patients with ARDS screened for ICUAW using electrophysiologic studies and physical examination (MRC score) found that nearly two-thirds (27 of 50) of patients were diagnosed with ICUAW. At the time of admission, all patients with ARDS fulfilled sepsis/SIRS criteria and 38 of 50 patients had severe sepsis with shock and/or MODS. Risk factors that may be associated with the development of ICUAW in patients with ARDS were specifically examined in this retrospective study by comparing patients diagnosed with ICUAW with those without ICUAW (controls). The occurrence of ICUAW was significantly associated with increased age and with increased blood glucose level; however, the investigators speculated that age may have influenced ICUAW indirectly because of the higher incidence of hyperglycemia in the elderly. The study did not detect a significant difference in duration of sepsis, severity of illness or multiorgan failure, or administration of potentially iatrogenic medications (eg, aminoglycosides, neuromuscular relaxing agents, corticosteroids) between patients with ARDS with and without ICUAW.

The incidence of ICUAW in a general ICU population is difficult to establish given that it depends strongly on the risk factors, diagnostic method, and timing of examination.[6,12] The incidences in 2 general ICU cohorts diagnosed by clinical examination were 25% and 23.8% after 7 days of MV and 10 days of ICU stay, respectively.[11,32] The higher incidence of ICUAW in ARDS versus the general ICU population is not surprising given its connection to sepsis and MODS.

DIAGNOSIS AND PRESENTATION OF INTENSIVE CARE UNIT–ACQUIRED WEAKNESS

At present, no universally accepted diagnostic criteria for ICUAW are available. Diagnosis based on clinical examination of respiratory and peripheral muscle force using handgrip strength and maximal inspiratory pressure has been made.[33,34] It is often difficult to differentiate CIM and CIP on physical examination, and definitive diagnosis requires specific neuromuscular electrophysiology testing and muscle biopsy.

A well-recognized, less frequent clinical presentation of ICUAW is symmetric flaccid paralysis (quadriparesis) with relative sparing of the facial muscles. Respiratory and limb muscles are often affected concurrently in ICUAW.[9] A common presenting feature of ICUAW in the acute setting is failure to wean from MV,[35] but it is often not suspected until the critically ill patient has failed

unsupported breathing and returns to MV. Complications arising from delayed diagnosis of ICUAW highlight the importance of earlier assessments for this condition.[27]

Manual muscle testing using the MRC sum score has been advocated as a primary means of diagnosing ICUAW.[11] This approach provides a global estimate of motor function by combining strength scores obtained from predefined muscle groups in each extremity, yielding a total score ranging from 0 to 60 (full strength). An arbitrarily defined score cutoff of less than 48 has been used to define ICUAW and found to be associated with increased duration of MV and ICU stay, and increased mortality.[9,11,33,35] An inherent limitation of the MRC score is its inability to evaluate patients with impaired cognitive state. A significant proportion of ICU patients were unable to perform MRC testing in one recent study that also found that MRC scores less than 48 had limited clinical predictive value.[36] Diagnostic approaches have been proposed in other reviews of ICUAW.[19,37] A diagnostic algorithm for ICUAW is shown in **Fig. 2**.

Other important factors that may contribute to muscle weakness and poor functional performance in survivors of ARDS include (1) poor prehospital functional status and comorbidity,[2] (2) persistent organ dysfunction,[2] (3) deconditioning and disuse atrophy,[38] and (4) psychological disturbance (mood and cognition).[39] Therefore, it is important to exclude a history of neuromuscular weakness before ICU and assess premorbid function in the ARDS survivor.

The beneficial effects of therapies for ICUAW after hospital discharge can be measured using peripheral muscle strength (eg, MRC score[40]), exercise capacity (eg, 6MW[41]), functional independence measure (FIM score[42]), and health-related quality-of-life scores.[43] At present, minimum clinically important differences (MCIDs) for these outcome measures have not been established in the ICUAW population. Clinical phenotypes of ICUAW that are closely linked to long-term prognosis and therapeutic response will continue to be refined as more studies measuring these outcome variables become available.

PATHOPHYSIOLOGY OF INTENSIVE CARE UNIT–ACQUIRED WEAKNESS

In the context of critical illness, ICUAW has recently gained much attention as a target of organ failure and complication of prolonged ICU care.[1–3] Muscle weakness may result from loss of muscle mass and diminished contractility independently or concurrently caused by a spectrum of nerve dysfunction (CIP) and primary

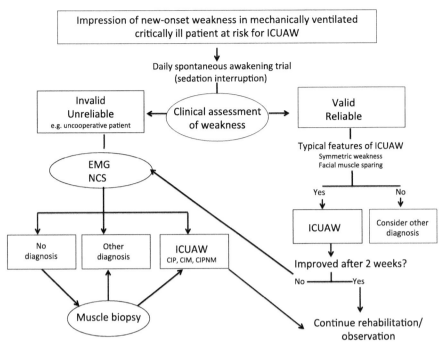

Fig. 2. ICUAW diagnostic algorithm. CIPNM, critical illness polyneuromyopathy; EMG, electromyography; NCS, nerve conduction studies. (*Adapted from* Stevens RD, Marshall SA, Cornblath DR, et al. A framework for diagnosing and classifying intensive care unit-acquired weakness. Crit Care Med 2009;37(10 Suppl):S299–308.)

muscle injury (CIM).[44] Skeletal muscle in ICUAW can display decreased muscle-specific force-generating capacity despite being structurally intact. This functional impairment has been attributed to diminished membrane excitability caused by an acquired sodium channel abnormality,[45] mitochondrial dysfunction,[46] oxidative stress, and potentially impaired excitement-contraction coupling.[14]

Decreased mitochondrial enzyme activity and mitochondrial content in skeletal muscle has been found in animal models of sepsis[47] and in critically ill patients.[48,49] Fredriksson and colleagues[49] found that the pattern of mitochondrial gene expression observed in septic patients with MODS differed from muscle unloading in humans. Mitochondrial dysfunction results in energy loss and depletion leading to muscle atrophy and it is hypothesized that dynamic changes in mitochondrial morphology regulate mitochondrial function and alter signaling pathways linked to atrophy; however, these mechanisms remain unclear.[50]

Muscle atrophy, the net loss of muscle protein and fat-free mass, results when rates of muscle proteolysis exceed those of protein synthesis. Proteolysis is achieved by several cellular signaling networks, but the predominant proteolytic pathway activated in animal models of muscle atrophy is the ubiquitin-proteasome system (UPS)

with the ubiquitin ligases atrogin-1 and muscle-specific RING finger protein-1 (MuRF1) playing key regulatory roles early in the process. Unlike the animal models, analysis of engagement of the UPS in the muscle of critically ill patients has yielded inconsistent results; some studies reported UPS activation and/or upregulation of atrogin-1/MuRF1,[51,52] whereas others found decreased atrogin-1/MuRF1 expression levels,[53,54] implying decreased UPS-mediated proteolysis. These discrepancies are most likely explained by temporal changes in atrogin-1/MuRF1 expression assessed by differing single-time-point studies and by possible discordance between the assessment of the expression level of a limited number of UPS components and proteasome function in studies that do not directly assess muscle proteasome activity.

Autophagy, an intracellular process of bulk degradation of cytoplasmic substrates, is increased in multiple animal models of muscle atrophy.[55,56] Both autophagy and the UPS pathway are activated by the forkhead box O (FoxO) transcription factors, which are induced by immobility, inflammation, nutrient depletion, and cellular stress.[55,57,58] However, the complete depletion of muscle-specific autophagy in mice has also been associated with significant myofiber degeneration and muscle weakness.[59] Thus, the balance of autophagy activation seems essential to skeletal muscle homeostasis. The few studies that have assessed autophagy in ICU patients have showed decreased autophagy in the peripheral muscle but increased autophagy in the diaphragm.[60,61] The contribution of autophagy to ICUAW remains unknown.

Injured muscle grows via hypertrophy of preexisting myofibers and regeneration leading to hyperplasia of muscle tissue. Little is known about the impact of critical illness on regeneration but decreased rates of growth and protein synthesis, resulting from or in conjunction with anabolic resistance, have been suggested to be important components of muscle atrophy in patients with ICUAW.[62] However, several reports have contradicted the theory that anabolic signaling is arrested in ICUAW and instead suggest a possible adaptive anabolic response.[51,53,54] Two major signaling networks control muscle protein synthesis and muscle growth in animal models: the insulinlike growth factor I (IGF-1)/phosphatidylinositol 3 kinase (PI3K)/Akt pathway and the myostatin-Smad2/3 pathway, functioning as positive and negative regulators respectively.[63] The activation of Akt concurrently inhibits the upregulation of proteolysis pathways by preventing nuclear translocation of FoxO transcription factors and subsequently the development of atrophy in an animal model.[64] At present, the significant pathways governing anabolic signaling in patients with critical illness remain to be delineated. Future studies are needed to determine whether pharmacologic upregulation of Akt and inhibition of myostatin restores muscle protein synthesis in ICUAW.[51]

Bed rest reduces mechanical load on skeletal muscles, which has been shown to induce muscle catabolism and decrease muscle contractile strength, even in the absence of critical illness.[38,65] Muscle fiber atrophy begins within hours of immobility in healthy volunteers, resulting in an average of 3% decrease of muscle mass weekly,[66] with more than 50% of muscle atrophy occurring in the initial 2 weeks.[67] Immobility has been shown to increase oxidative stress, leading to accelerated muscle fiber degradation via activation of multiple proteolytic systems in animal models.[58,68] Moderate exercise increases antioxidants to counteract oxidative stress, suggesting potential therapeutic benefits with early rehabilitation in the ICU setting.[46,69–71]

In CIM there is a preferential loss of myosin relative to actin that cannot be explained merely by immobilization.[72] These structural changes are more likely explained by the direct muscle impairment that underlies CIM and indirect muscle impairment caused by axonal degeneration in CIP.[6] Nevertheless, the deleterious effects of critical illness and immobilization may act synergistically to intensify the proinflammatory state and accelerate muscle turnover.[13,31,68,73]

Early identification of ICUAW enables the health care team to limit patient exposure to further risk factors that compound muscle weakness, initiate further investigations, and consider potential interventions and trial enrollment.

NONPHARMACOLOGIC STRATEGIES
Early Rehabilitation Therapy for Disuse Atrophy

Moderate exercise during critical illness has been proposed to counteract the atrophy-inducing effects of the inflammatory state that occurs with inactivity and ICUAW.[69,71] There is increasing evidence showing the benefits of early physical therapy in the ICU. Early rehabilitation is generally defined as physical therapy starting at the period of initial physiologic stabilization, possibly within 24 to 48 hours after initiating MV. Multiple barriers to adopting early mobilization regimens in the ICU have been identified, including safety concerns, patient sedation, and the requirement and cost of a trained multidisciplinary team to minimize the risk of adverse events.[74]

Several observational studies have shown that early rehabilitation is safe and feasible without increased costs.[75–78] Eligibility criteria that have been used to commence early rehabilitation in critically ill patients are (1) the ability to cooperate (neurologic criterion); (2) fraction of inspired oxygen (Fio_2) less than or equal to 0.6 and positive end-expiratory pressure (PEEP) less than or equal to 10 (respiratory criteria); and (3) no requirement for vasopressors or symptomatic orthostasis (cardiovascular criteria). Patients with unstable fractures are excluded from early rehabilitation.[79,80] Patients meeting the neurologic criteria but missing a single cardiac or respiratory criterion can be started cautiously in early rehabilitation trials with close monitoring for physiologic deterioration.[79]

A prospective trial that applied an early activity protocol in a respiratory ICU included 103 patients and found that 41% of activity events occurred in patients on MV. Adverse events were infrequent, occurring in only 1% of all activities, and no event was serious.[75] An observational study of 104 patients with acute respiratory failure requiring MV for more than 4 days who were transferred to an ICU setting with early physical therapy found that the number of patients ambulating had tripled compared with before the intervention.[79] Patients in the study who had not received any sedation were 2-fold more likely to ambulate.

Development and implementation of an early rehabilitation protocol in an ICU setting in which physical therapy was provided infrequently has been shown in one prospective study to increase the proportion of ICU patients receiving physical therapy versus usual care.[76] Patients in the protocol group were far more likely to receive physical therapy (91.5% vs 12.5%; $P \leq .001$) and had earlier mobilization and significantly shorter length of ICU and in-hospital stay. No adverse events were reported and costs of usual care versus mobility protocol were the same.

A 4-phase protocol for progressive mobilization in the ICU has been established with categories at each phase that include education for patient and families, positioning, transfer training, exercises, and a walking program.[81] Patients are classified within 4 phases based on functional status: phase 1, inability to bear weight; phase 2, able to begin transfer training with a walker; phase 3, able to begin walking reeducation; and phase 4, patients transferred out of the ICU. Duration and frequency of training sessions are also specified for patients at each stage in this guideline. The major components of an early rehabilitation protocol necessary for implementing a program in the ICU are summarized in **Table 1**.

One barrier to rehabilitation after ICU discharge in some centers is a lack of physical therapists. To address this issue, a self-help rehabilitation manual

Table 1
Components of an early mobilization implementation protocol

Safety screen (partial checklist to be assessed by team before starting therapy)	Neurologic: ability to cooperate
	Respiratory: $FiO_2 \leq 0.6$ and PEEP ≤ 10, O_2 saturation >88%, and pH >7.25
	Cardiovascular:
	   No requirement for vasopressors
	   Absence of symptomatic orthostasis
	   Absence of cardiac ischemia or arrhythmias
	   Absence of significant bleeding
	Absence of unstable fractures

Staffing and roles within the multidisciplinary team	PT: initial assessment to measure activity and functional impairment. Determine appropriate exercises and advancement of activities Registered nurse: assess sedation, monitor vital signs, assist with care of tubes and arterial and venous catheters RT: alter ventilator settings, discontinue or reestablish MV as needed or ordered by treating physician Treating physician: assess readiness for early mobility and consult PT and multidisciplinary team. Order modifications to sedation, ventilator settings as needed
Equipment	Gait belts, portable telemetry and monitors Walkers and wheelchairs Portable ventilator, oxygen tank, and manual resuscitation bag Cycle ergometers Neuromuscular electrical stimulators
Activities	In-bed exercises (eg, peripheral limb exercises, passive or active) Cycle ergometry Sitting (eg, at the edge of the bed) with or without support Transfer to the chair Pregait standing activities (eg, minisquats) Ambulation
Potential adverse events/complications	Physiologic deterioration/decompensation Extubation Dislodged or nonfunctional line Bleeding
Checklists or guidelines to be established within the protocol	Minimizing/optimizing patient sedation Determining eligibility for early mobilization and consulting early mobilization services Assessing patients for safety early mobilization (starting, stopping, and altering physical activities)

A large number of research articles and documents related to implementing early mobilization of mechanically ventilated ICU patients can be found at www.mobilization-network.org.
Abbreviations: PT, physical therapist; RT, respiratory therapist.

was provided to patients after discharge from ICU with instructions to perform their own physical therapy.[82] A randomized trial compared the self-help manual versus control in a mixed population of 126 post-ICU patients and found that it improved physical function scores at 8 weeks and 6 months after ICU discharge versus usual care.

Cycle Ergometry and Neuromuscular Electrical Stimulation

Novel rehabilitation devices are being studied that may have potential to improve muscle strength in the critically ill, particularly for those unable to move actively because of weakness or sedation. The bedside cycle ergometer may be used to perform active or passive cycling (for sedated patients) at multiple levels of resistance that are individually adjusted. One randomized trial found that patients using the cycle ergometer, in addition to standard mobilization therapies initiated early in ICU rehabilitation, showed no difference in quadriceps force or physical function at ICU discharge.[83] However, it significantly improved quadriceps force, functional scores, and 6MW test (average of 56 m greater in the training group) at hospital discharge. Although this study did not rule out whether extra time spent performing standardized physical therapy was as beneficial as cycling ergometry, it does provide limited evidence associating increased physical activity in the ICU with improved functional outcomes.

There is growing evidence that neuromuscular electrical stimulation (NMES) improves muscular function in the critically ill. NMES applies electrical stimulation using surface electrodes, typically on a target muscle of the lower limbs, to produce visible muscle contractions. It does not require active patient cooperation and has been shown in a small controlled study to increase protein synthesis and quadriceps cross-sectional area in orthopedic patients with knee immobilization.[84] A randomized trial of NMES applied to the lower limb versus sham (52 ICU patients in total) found a significant reduction in ICUAW measured by MRC (27.3% vs 39.3%; $P = .04$).[85]

A systematic review of RCTs that compared NMES versus sham in ICU patients found 5 studies that evaluated strength of different muscle groups and 4 that evaluated muscle mass (thickness or volume).[86] All 5 studies that evaluated muscle strength found an improvement with NMES, whereas only 2 of the 4 studies assessing muscle mass found an improvement. Meta-analysis of these 8 trials was not possible because of high inconsistency in the ICU patient characteristics between studies. However, the data point to moderate treatment effects on muscle strength, but

minimal impact on muscle wasting. Heterogeneity of NMES protocols across studies also limits the ability to generalize of the studies. Compliance and tolerability were generally high, without any adverse events reported in these studies. The only contraindication to use of NMES is the use of NMBAs.[85] The major treatment modalities for early rehabilitation studied in prospective trials are summarized in **Table 2**.

Sedation Interruption

The use of sedation in patients receiving MV has been found to increase the duration of MV and hinder early rehabilitation.[87] A protocol that combined the interruption of sedation with spontaneous breathing trials (SBT) significantly reduced duration of MV versus routine sedation care with SBT in an RCT of 336 ICU patients with respiratory failure.[88] Early rehabilitation performed during periods of interruption of sedation similarly resulted in a significant shortening of duration of MV and improved functional outcomes at hospital discharge and shorter periods of delirium versus interruption of sedation with routine care in one RCT.[89] No differences in duration of ICU stay, hospital stay, or hospital mortality were detected.

Potential Limitations of Early Rehabilitation Therapy

At present the most effective timing, mode, intensity, and frequency of early rehabilitation has not been established in clinical trials.[90] To what extent clinical phenotypes at high risk for limited long-term functional improvement (advanced age, comorbid disease, and poor previous functional status) may benefit from even optimal physical therapies is controversial.[81,91] The significant correlation between the degree of MODS and muscle wasting suggests that physical rehabilitation may only counteract a portion of lost muscle mass in severe critical illness.[54] Although early rehabilitation may be able to attenuate muscle proteolysis and normalize muscle mass in some patients with ICUAW, it may be unable to restore normal muscle strength.[92] Thus therapeutic interventions in addition to early rehabilitation therapy are crucial in order to improve management of ICUAW. Potential pharmacologic adjuncts to early rehabilitation are reviewed briefly later.

VENTILATOR-INDUCED DIAPHRAGM DYSFUNCTION

Controlled MV (CMV) is frequently associated with patient sedation and NMBA, and leads to rapid diaphragmatic atrophy,[7] termed ventilator-induced

Table 2
Specific treatment modalities for early rehabilitation in the ICU studied in positive prospective trials

Treatment Modality/Intervention	Study/Study Design	Patient Population	Primary Outcome/Results
UE/LE exercise	Schweickert et al,[89] 2009 RCT N = 104	Sedated adult ICU patients on MV <72 h	Significantly higher rate of return to independent functional status at hospital discharge (59% in treatment group vs. 35%; P<.02)
Bed exercises and mobilization	Malkoc et al,[120] 2009 N = 510 Prospective intervention group Retrospective case group	Multidisciplinary internal medicine ICU: 51% of patients required MV	Decreased length of MV and ICU stay in intervention group vs controls
Early activity protocol (sitting on chair or edge of bed; ambulation with walker)	Thomsen et al,[79] 2008 Before-after cohort study N = 104	Patients in RICU requiring >4 d of MV	Significant increase in rate of ambulation in patient cohort transferred to an RICU implementing early activity protocol vs pretransfer levels
Cycle ergometry (passive or active) combined with UE/LE exercise	Burtin et al,[83] 2009 RCT N = 67	Single-center surgical and medical ICU patients with expected prolonged stay (at least 12 d after admission to ICU)	Significantly increased 6MWD, quadriceps force, and physical functioning at hospital discharge in treatment group vs controls
IMT with threshold inspiratory device	Martin et al,[97] 2011 RCT N = 69	Single center medical and surgical ICU patients with failure to wean from MV with usual care	IMT significantly improved MIP and weaning outcome compared with sham treatment
NMES	Routsi et al,[85] 2010 RCT N = 52	Patients in the ICU with APACHE score ≥13 capable of assessment with MRC	MRC score was significantly higher in patients with NMES compared with patients who received sham treatment

Abbreviations: 6MWD, 6MW distance; APACHE, acute physiology and chronic health evaluation; IMT, inspiratory muscle training; LE, lower extremity; MIP, maximal inspiratory pressure; RICU, respiratory ICU; UE, upper extremity.

diaphragm dysfunction. Ventilator modes that permit spontaneous breathing, such as airway pressure release ventilation (APRV), have been hypothesized to preserve diaphragm function and reduce the duration of MV. However results from 2 small randomized trials comparing APRV with a controlled mode are conflicting.[93,94] Neurally adjusted ventilator assist (NAVA) facilitates respiratory muscle unloading in proportion to the electrical activity of the diaphragm (a marker of respiratory drive).[95] NAVA has been proposed for use in ICUAW and has been shown to be feasible in a small trial of ICUAW; however, its effect on diaphragm function and weaning remain unknown.[96] At present no recommendation can be made regarding an optimal ventilation mode for the treatment of ARDS. Future trials comparing diaphragm function following CMV versus spontaneous breathing modes are warranted.

Inspiratory Muscle Training

Inspiratory muscle training (IMT) using a threshold device is hypothesized to improve the strength of weakened respiratory muscle and therefore promote earlier liberation from MV. IMT increased the proportion of patients weaned from MV (71% vs 47%; P = .04) in a small single-center RCT involving ICU patients unable to sustain unsupported breathing (mean time on MV was 6 weeks before study intervention).[97] A more recent randomized trial of IMT found that respiratory pressures improved in the intervention group without any significant difference in weaning time.[98] The ability to generalize these studies to the ARDS or ICUAW population is problematic because only a small number of patients with ARDS were enrolled and patients with any type of neuromuscular illness were excluded.

NUTRIENT DEFICIENCY IN CRITICAL ILLNESS

ARDS is characterized by a hypercatabolic state that predisposes to serious nutritional and caloric deficits that may exacerbate muscle weakness and impede recovery.[99,100] Significant gastrointestinal dysfunction contributes to caloric deficiency but whether parenteral nutrition (PN) can improve muscle function is unclear. Optimal timing and routes of feeding have remained controversial and current practice guidelines for nutritional support of critically ill patients differ between North America and Europe.[101,102] A study comparing early and late enteral feeding found increased ventilator-associated pneumonia in the early enteral feeding group and some groups have suggested that underfeeding may reduce muscle wasting and result in shorter duration of MV.[54,103,104] A recent study of ICU patients receiving enteral feeding at day 1 found that net catabolic balance with protein synthesis decreased to rates observed in healthy fasted controls, suggesting a possible adverse effect of higher protein delivery from early feeding in critical illness.[54]

A large multicenter randomized trial compared early initiation of PN (within 48 hours of admission) with initiation after day 8 (late PN), and fewer patients who received late PN remained in the ICU for greater than 3 days and in hospital for greater than 15 days versus early PN.[104] A subanalysis of this trial assessed muscle weakness thrice weekly using the MRC score in 600 patients admitted to the ICU for greater than 1 week.[105] Despite a marked nutritional deficit, fewer patients receiving late PN had weakness on first assessment compared with those receiving early PN (34% vs 43%; P = .03). Furthermore, weakness recovered faster in the late PN group (P = .021). Roughly one-third of the patients in each arm of this study had cardiac surgery, thus the ability to generalize the hypocaloric (late PN) feeding strategy to the ARDS population is uncertain.

To address the conflicting data in previous studies, ARDSnet conducted a large, randomized, multicenter trial that compared full-feeding enteral nutrition (EN) with trophic feeding (25% of estimated caloric needs) for the first 6 days of MV in patients with acute lung injury/ARDS.[106] No difference in the primary end point, ventilator-free days at day 28, was detected. A longitudinal follow-up to assess physical performance at 6 and 12 months after this study in 174 consecutive survivors also did not find any differences between the two groups for any of the physical assessments.[107] A recent RCT compared EN supplemented with PN from days 4 to 8 versus EN in ICU patients receiving less than 60% of their daily energy requirements and found reduction in nosocomial infection.[108] However, there was no difference in time on MV between the two groups. Thus more studies are needed to determine whether the timing and delivery of nutrition in the critically ill can reduce the likelihood of ICUAW while minimizing other adverse effects.

PHARMACOLOGIC STRATEGIES AS ADJUNCTS TO EARLY MOBILITY

At present, no pharmacologic therapies have been approved for the treatment of ICUAW. The anabolic hormone IGF-I increased in-hospital mortality in an RCT of patients with prolonged ICU stay.[109] The increased rate of multiorgan dysfunction and septic shock in the treatment group led the investigators to suspect that IGF-1 exerts an immunomodulatory effect. Grip and hand strength were unaffected by treatment with IGF-I. It has also been postulated that poor delivery of hormones and nutrients to muscle caused by aberrant microvascular perfusion in muscle may explain this anabolic resistance.[62]

Estrogen has been shown to regulate skeletal muscle regeneration and mass recovery in disuse atrophy by activating Akt phosphorylation.[110] The phytoestrogen 8-prenylaringenin prevented loss of muscle mass using a denervation model in mice.[111] Whether this agent can enhance recovery from disuse atrophy or ICUAW in humans by accelerating the blunted Akt pathway should be investigated in future trials.

Clenbuterol, a selective β_2-adrenergic agonist, administered chronically in high doses in multiple animal studies has been shown to increase muscle mass and force-producing capacity. Clenbuterol has been shown to activate the Akt/mammalian target of rapamycin (mTor) pathway and inhibit proteasomal and lysosomal proteolysis independently of Akt, leading to a muscle-sparing effect in animal models of atrophy.[112,113] Concerns have been raised that the beta-agonist–induced shift from oxidative to glycolytic metabolism may result in clinically significant muscle fatigue[114] and that the adverse effects of IGF-1 stimulation may also be applicable to beta-agonist administration.[115]

Bortezomib, a proteasome inhibitor approved for use in multiple myeloma and non-Hodgkin lymphoma, has been shown to prevent atrophy in several animal models,[116,117] but no effect on diaphragm atrophy was found in a rat model, which may be explained by increased calpain activity.[118] There is currently no evidence that bortezomib improves muscle atrophy in humans and the numerous reports of cardiotoxicity linked to bortezomib regimes suggest that long-term administration might adversely affect muscle function.[119] Trials investigating more specific therapies that target the degradation of sarcomeric proteins and impaired muscle contractility are needed.[115]

SUMMARY

Functional impairment caused by weakness and exercise limitation in survivors of ARDS is now recognized as a major complication of this condition that may persist for years after ICU discharge. ICUAW causes increased duration of MV and ICU stay and contributes to persistent weakness after ARDS. Early identification of ICUAW is crucial to tailored patient care; however, therapies for this condition are largely preemptive.

The current ICU culture of excessive sedation and scarcity of physical therapy compounds the burden of ICUAW. Improved outcomes after interruption of sedation combined with spontaneous breathing trials[88] and participation in early rehabilitation[89] has led to the promotion of the ABCDE (awakening and breathing coordination, delirium monitoring, and exercise/early mobility) bundle to reduce the incidence of ICUAW and delirium.[87] This approach highlights the potentially synergistic effects of these therapies on muscle strength, liberation from MV, and long-term functional outcomes in patients with ARDS.

Early exercise therapy, including recent interventions such as ergometry and neuromuscular stimulation, have been found to be safe and cost-effective strategies that may lead to improved functional outcomes, although the details remain to be elucidated. Although early physical therapy may limit muscle atrophy related to immobilization,[80] the wide spectrum of muscle injury among critically ill patients creates a need for specific therapies tailored to the underlying pathophysiologic

processes. Thus, novel therapeutics that target the aberrant pathways that give rise to muscle dysfunction are essential for future management of ICUAW. Drug discovery will likely require a more holistic understanding of these pathways using biological network analysis to integrate multiple sources of experimental data with linkage to functional outcomes.

REFERENCES

1. Herridge MS, Tansey CM, Matte A, et al. Functional disability 5 years after acute respiratory distress syndrome. N Engl J Med 2011;364(14):1293–304. Available at: http://www.ncbi.nlm.nih.gov/pubmed/21470008.
2. Herridge MS, Cheung AM, Tansey CM, et al. One-year outcomes in survivors of the acute respiratory distress syndrome. N Engl J Med 2003;348(8):683–93. Available at: http://www.ncbi.nlm.nih.gov/pubmed/12594312.
3. Bercker S, Weber-Carstens S, Deja M, et al. Critical illness polyneuropathy and myopathy in patients with acute respiratory distress syndrome. Crit Care Med 2005;33(4):711–5. Available at: http://www.ncbi.nlm.nih.gov/pubmed/15818093.
4. Fletcher SN, Kennedy DD, Ghosh IR, et al. Persistent neuromuscular and neurophysiologic abnormalities in long-term survivors of prolonged critical illness. Crit Care Med 2003;31(4):1012–6. Available at: http://www.ncbi.nlm.nih.gov/pubmed/12682405.
5. Deem S, Lee CM, Curtis JR. Acquired neuromuscular disorders in the intensive care unit. Am J Respir Crit Care Med 2003;168(7):735–9. Available at: http://www.ncbi.nlm.nih.gov/pubmed/14522811.
6. Latronico N, Shehu I, Elisa S. Neuromuscular sequelae of critical illness. Curr Opin Crit Care 2005;11(4):381–90.
7. Levine S, Nguyen T, Taylor N, et al. Rapid disuse atrophy of diaphragm fibers in mechanically ventilated humans. N Engl J Med 2008;358(13):1327–35. Available at: http://www.ncbi.nlm.nih.gov/pubmed/18367735.
8. Garnacho-Montero J, Amaya-Villar R, Garcia-Garmendia JL, et al. Effect of critical illness polyneuropathy on the withdrawal from mechanical ventilation and the length of stay in septic patients. Crit Care Med 2005;33(2):349–54.
9. De Jonghe B, Bastuji-Garin S, Durand MC, et al. Respiratory weakness is associated with limb weakness and delayed weaning in critical illness. Crit Care Med 2007;35(9):2007–15.
10. Schefold JC, Bierbrauer J, Weber-Carstens S. Intensive care unit-acquired weakness (ICUAW) and muscle wasting in critically ill patients with severe sepsis and septic shock. J Cachexia

Sarcopenia Muscle 2010;1(2):147–57. Available at: http://www.ncbi.nlm.nih.gov/pubmed/21475702.

11. De Jonghe B, Sharshar T, Lefaucheur JP, et al. Paresis acquired in the intensive care unit: a prospective multicenter study. JAMA 2002;288(22):2859–67. Available at: http://www.ncbi.nlm.nih.gov/pubmed/12472328.

12. Stevens RD, Dowdy DW, Michaels RK, et al. Neuromuscular dysfunction acquired in critical illness: a systematic review. Intensive Care Med 2007;33(11):1876–91. Available at: http://www.ncbi.nlm.nih.gov/pubmed/17639340.

13. Paddon-Jones D, Sheffield-Moore M, Cree MG, et al. Atrophy and impaired muscle protein synthesis during prolonged inactivity and stress. J Clin Endocrinol Metab 2006;91(12):4836–41. Available at: http://www.ncbi.nlm.nih.gov/pubmed/16984982.

14. Batt J, dos Santos CC, Cameron JI, et al. Intensive care unit-acquired weakness: clinical phenotypes and molecular mechanisms. Am J Respir Crit Care Med 2013;187(3):238–46. Available at: http://www.ncbi.nlm.nih.gov/pubmed/23204256.

15. de Jonghe B, Lacherade JC, Sharshar T, et al. Intensive care unit-acquired weakness: risk factors and prevention. Crit Care Med 2009;37(10 Suppl):S309–15. Available at: http://www.ncbi.nlm.nih.gov/pubmed/20046115.

16. Witt NJ, Zochodne DW, Bolton C, et al. Peripheral nerve function in sepsis and multiple organ failure. Chest 1991;99(1):176–84. Available at: http://www.ncbi.nlm.nih.gov/pubmed/1845860.

17. Bednarik J, Vondracek P, Dusek L, et al. Risk factors for critical illness polyneuromyopathy. J Neurol 2005;252(3):343–51. Available at: http://www.ncbi.nlm.nih.gov/pubmed/15791390.

18. de Letter MA, Schmitz PI, Visser LH, et al. Risk factors for the development of polyneuropathy and myopathy in critically ill patients. Crit Care Med 2001;29(12):2281–6. Available at: http://www.ncbi.nlm.nih.gov/pubmed/11801825.

19. Latronico N, Nisoli E, Eikermann M. Muscle weakness and nutrition in critical illness: matching nutrient supply and use. Lancet Respir Med 2013;1(8):589–90.

20. Van den Berghe G, Schoonheydt K, Becx P, et al. Insulin therapy protects the central and peripheral nervous system of intensive care patients. Neurology 2005;64(8):1348–53. Available at: http://www.ncbi.nlm.nih.gov/pubmed/15851721.

21. van den Berghe G, Wouters P, Weekers F, et al. Intensive insulin therapy in critically ill patients. N Engl J Med 2001;345(19):1359–67. Available at: http://www.ncbi.nlm.nih.gov/pubmed/11794168.

22. Van den Berghe G, Wilmer A, Hermans G, et al. Intensive insulin therapy in the medical ICU. N Engl J Med 2006;354(5):449–61. Available at: http://www.ncbi.nlm.nih.gov/pubmed/16452557.

23. Hermans G, De Jonghe B, Bruyninckx F, et al. Interventions for preventing critical illness polyneuropathy and critical illness myopathy. Cochrane Database Syst Rev 2009;(1). CD006832. Available at: http://www.ncbi.nlm.nih.gov/pubmed/19160304.

24. NICE-SUGAR Study Investigators, Finfer S, Chittock DR, et al. Intensive versus conventional glucose control in critically ill patients. N Engl J Med 2009;360(13):1283–97. Available at: http://www.ncbi.nlm.nih.gov/pubmed/19318384.

25. Garnacho-Montero J, Madrazo-Osuna J, Garcia-Garmendia JL, et al. Critical illness polyneuropathy: risk factors and clinical consequences. A cohort study in septic patients. Intensive Care Med 2001;27(8):1288–96. Available at: http://www.ncbi.nlm.nih.gov/pubmed/11511941.

26. Steinberg KP, Hudson LD, Goodman RB, et al. Efficacy and safety of corticosteroids for persistent acute respiratory distress syndrome. N Engl J Med 2006;354(16):1671–84. Available at: http://www.ncbi.nlm.nih.gov/pubmed/16625008.

27. Hough CL, Steinberg KP, Taylor Thompson B, et al. Intensive care unit-acquired neuromyopathy and corticosteroids in survivors of persistent ARDS. Intensive Care Med 2009;35(1):63–8. Available at: http://www.ncbi.nlm.nih.gov/pubmed/18946660.

28. Meduri GU, Golden E, Freire AX, et al. Methylprednisolone infusion in early severe ARDS: results of a randomized controlled trial. Chest 2007;131(4):954–63. Available at: http://www.ncbi.nlm.nih.gov/pubmed/17426195.

29. Leatherman JW, Fluegel WL, David WS, et al. Muscle weakness in mechanically ventilated patients with severe asthma. Am J Respir Crit Care Med 1996;153(5):1686–90.

30. Papazian L, Forel JM, Gacouin A, et al. Neuromuscular blockers in early acute respiratory distress syndrome. N Engl J Med 2010;363(12):1107–16. Available at: http://www.ncbi.nlm.nih.gov/pubmed/20843245.

31. Winkelman C. Inactivity and inflammation in the critically ill patient. Crit Care Clin 2007;23(1):21–34. Available at: http://www.ncbi.nlm.nih.gov/pubmed/17307114.

32. Nanas S, Kritikos K, Angelopoulos E, et al. Predisposing factors for critical illness polyneuromyopathy in a multidisciplinary intensive care unit. Acta Neurol Scand 2008;118(3):175–81. Available at: http://www.ncbi.nlm.nih.gov/pubmed/18355395.

33. Ali NA, O'Brien JM Jr, Hoffmann SP, et al. Acquired weakness, handgrip strength, and mortality in critically ill patients. Am J Respir Crit Care Med 2008;178(3):261–8. Available at: http://www.ncbi.nlm.nih.gov/pubmed/18511703.

34. Tzanis G, Vasileiadis I, Zervakis D, et al. Maximum inspiratory pressure, a surrogate parameter for the assessment of ICU-acquired weakness. BMC

Anesthesiol 2011;11:14. Available at: http://www.ncbi.nlm.nih.gov/pubmed/21703029.

35. De Jonghe B, Bastuji-Garin S, Sharshar T, et al. Does ICU-acquired paresis lengthen weaning from mechanical ventilation? Intensive Care Med 2004;30(6):1117–21. Available at: http://www.ncbi.nlm.nih.gov/pubmed/14767593.

36. Connolly BA, Jones GD, Curtis AA, et al. Clinical predictive value of manual muscle strength testing during critical illness: an observational cohort study. Crit Care 2013;17(5):R229. Available at: http://www.ncbi.nlm.nih.gov/pubmed/24112540.

37. Stevens RD, Marshall SA, Cornblath DR, et al. A framework for diagnosing and classifying intensive care unit-acquired weakness. Crit Care Med 2009;37(10 Suppl):S299–308. Available at: http://www.ncbi.nlm.nih.gov/pubmed/20046114.

38. Ferrando AA, Paddon-Jones D, Wolfe RR. Bed rest and myopathies. Curr Opin Clin Nutr Metab Care 2006;9(4):410–5. Available at: http://www.ncbi.nlm.nih.gov/pubmed/16778570.

39. Wilcox ME, Herridge MS. Long-term outcomes in patients surviving acute respiratory distress syndrome. Semin Respir Crit Care Med 2010;31(1):55–65. Available at: http://www.ncbi.nlm.nih.gov/pubmed/20101548.

40. Kleyweg RP, van der Meche FG, Schmitz PI. Interobserver agreement in the assessment of muscle strength and functional abilities in Guillain-Barre syndrome. Muscle Nerve 1991;14(11):1103–9. Available at: http://www.ncbi.nlm.nih.gov/pubmed/1745205.

41. ATS Committee on Proficiency Standards for Clinical Pulmonary Function Laboratories. ATS statement: guidelines for the six-minute walk test. Am J Respir Crit Care Med 2002;166(1):111–7. Available at: http://www.ncbi.nlm.nih.gov/pubmed/12091180.

42. Linacre JM, Heinemann AW, Wright BD, et al. The structure and stability of the functional independence measure. Arch Phys Med Rehabil 1994; 75(2):127–32.

43. McHorney CA, Ware JEJ, Lu JF, et al. The MOS 36-item Short-Form Health Survey (SF-36): III. Tests of data quality, scaling assumptions, and reliability across diverse patient groups. Med Care 1994; 32(1):40–66.

44. Ruff RL. Why do ICU patients become paralyzed? Ann Neurol 1998;43(2):154–5. Available at: http://www.ncbi.nlm.nih.gov/pubmed/9485055.

45. Allen DC, Arunachalam R, Mills KR. Critical illness myopathy: further evidence from muscle-fiber excitability studies of an acquired channelopathy. Muscle Nerve 2008;37(1):14–22. Available at: http://www.ncbi.nlm.nih.gov/pubmed/17763454.

46. Carre JE, Orban JC, Re L, et al. Survival in critical illness is associated with early activation of mitochondrial biogenesis. Am J Respir Crit Care Med 2010;182(6):745–51. Available at: http://www.ncbi.nlm.nih.gov/pubmed/20538956.

47. Brealey D, Karyampudi S, Jacques TS, et al. Mitochondrial dysfunction in a long-term rodent model of sepsis and organ failure. Am J Physiol Regul Integr Comp Physiol 2004;286(3):R491–7. Available at: http://www.ncbi.nlm.nih.gov/pubmed/14604843.

48. Brealey D, Brand M, Hargreaves I, et al. Association between mitochondrial dysfunction and severity and outcome of septic shock. Lancet 2002;360(9328):219–23.

49. Fredriksson K, Tjader I, Keller P, et al. Dysregulation of mitochondrial dynamics and the muscle transcriptome in ICU patients suffering from sepsis induced multiple organ failure. PLoS One 2008; 3(11):e3686. Available at: http://www.ncbi.nlm.nih.gov/pubmed/18997871.

50. Picard M, Shirihai OS, Gentil BJ, et al. Mitochondrial morphology transitions and functions: implications for retrograde signaling? Am J Physiol Regul Integr Comp Physiol 2013;304(6):R393–406. Available at: http://www.ncbi.nlm.nih.gov/pubmed/23364527.

51. Constantin D, McCullough J, Mahajan RP, et al. Novel events in the molecular regulation of muscle mass in critically ill patients. J Physiol 2011;589(Pt 15):3883–95. Available at: http://www.ncbi.nlm.nih.gov/pubmed/21669975.

52. Tiao G, Hobler S, Wang JJ, et al. Sepsis is associated with increased mRNAs of the ubiquitin-proteasome proteolytic pathway in human skeletal muscle. J Clin Invest 1997;99(2):163–8. Available at: http://www.ncbi.nlm.nih.gov/pubmed/9005983.

53. Jespersen JG, Nedergaard A, Reitelseder S, et al. Activated protein synthesis and suppressed protein breakdown signaling in skeletal muscle of critically ill patients. PLoS One 2011;6(3):e18090. Available at: http://www.ncbi.nlm.nih.gov/pubmed/21483870.

54. Puthucheary ZA, Rawal J, McPhail M, et al. Acute skeletal muscle wasting in critical illness. JAMA 2013;310(15):1591–600.http://www.ncbi.nlm.nih.gov/pubmed/24108501.

55. Zhao J, Brault JJ, Schild A, et al. FoxO3 coordinately activates protein degradation by the autophagic/lysosomal and proteasomal pathways in atrophying muscle cells. Cell Metab 2007;6(6):472–83. Available at: http://www.ncbi.nlm.nih.gov/pubmed/18054316.

56. Wang X, Blagden C, Fan J, et al. Runx1 prevents wasting, myofibrillar disorganization, and autophagy of skeletal muscle. Genes Dev 2005; 19(14):1715–22. Available at: http://www.ncbi.nlm.nih.gov/pubmed/16024660.

57. Sandri M, Sandri C, Gilbert A, et al. Foxo transcription factors induce the atrophy-related ubiquitin

ligase atrogin-1 and cause skeletal muscle atrophy. Cell 2004;117:399–412.

58. Talbert EE, Smuder AJ, Min K, et al. Immobilization-induced activation of key proteolytic systems in skeletal muscles is prevented by a mitochondria-targeted antioxidant. J Appl Physiol (1985) 2013; 115(4):529–38. Available at: http://www.ncbi.nlm. nih.gov/pubmed/23766499.

59. Masiero E, Agatea L, Mammucari C, et al. Auto-phagy is required to maintain muscle mass. Cell Metab 2009;10(6):507–15. Available at: http:// www.ncbi.nlm.nih.gov/pubmed/19945408.

60. Hussain SN, Mofarrahi M, Sigala I, et al. Mechanical ventilation-induced diaphragm disuse in humans triggers autophagy. Am J Respir Crit Care Med 2010;182(11):1377–86. Available at: http:// www.ncbi.nlm.nih.gov/pubmed/20639440.

61. Vanhorebeek I, Gunst J, Derde S, et al. Insufficient activation of autophagy allows cellular damage to accumulate in critically ill patients. J Clin Endocrinol Metab 2011;96(4):E633–45. Available at: http://www.ncbi.nlm.nih.gov/pubmed/21270330.

62. Rennie MJ. Anabolic resistance in critically ill patients. Crit Care Med 2009;37(10 Suppl):S398–9. Available at: http://www.ncbi.nlm.nih.gov/pubmed/ 20046126.

63. Schiaffino S, Dyar KA, Ciciliot S, et al. Mechanisms regulating skeletal muscle growth and atrophy. FEBS J 2013;280(17):4294–314. Available at: http://www.ncbi.nlm.nih.gov/pubmed/23517348.

64. Stitt TN, Drujan D, Clarke BA, et al. The IGF-1/PI3K/Akt pathway prevents expression of muscle atrophy-induced ubiquitin ligases by inhibiting FOXO transcription factors. Mol Cell 2004;14(3):395–403.

65. Chambers MA, Moylan JS, Reid MB. Physical inactivity and muscle weakness in the critically ill. Crit Care Med 2009;37(10 Suppl):S337–46. Available at: http://www.ncbi.nlm.nih.gov/pubmed/20046119.

66. Berg HE, Larsson L, Tesch PA. Lower limb skeletal muscle function after 6 wk of bed rest. J Appl Physiol (1985) 1997;82(1):182–8.

67. Stevens JE, Walter GA, Okereke E, et al. Muscle adaptations with immobilization and rehabilitation after ankle fracture. Med Sci Sports Exerc 2004; 36(10):1695–701.

68. Powers SK, Smuder AJ, Criswell DS. Mechanistic links between oxidative stress and disuse muscle atrophy. Antioxid Redox Signal 2011;15(9):2519–28. Available at: http://www.ncbi.nlm.nih.gov/pubmed/ 21457104.

69. Fan E, Zanni JM, Dennison CR, et al. Critical illness neuromyopathy and muscle weakness in patients in the intensive care unit. AACN Adv Crit Care 2009;20(3):243–53. Available at: http://www.ncbi. nlm.nih.gov/pubmed/19638746.

70. Suhr F, Brenig J, Muller R, et al. Moderate exercise promotes human RBC-NOS activity, NO production

and deformability through Akt kinase pathway. PLoS One 2012;7(9):e45982. Available at: http:// www.ncbi.nlm.nih.gov/pubmed/23049912.

71. Jackson MJ. Control of reactive oxygen species production in contracting skeletal muscle. Antioxid Redox Signal 2011;15(9):2477–86. Available at: http://www.ncbi.nlm.nih.gov/pubmed/21699411.

72. Lacomis D, Petrella JT, Giuliani M. Causes of neuromuscular weakness in the intensive care unit: a study of ninety-two patients. Muscle Nerve 1998;21(5):610–7.

73. Hamburg NM, McMackin CJ, Huang AL, et al. Physical inactivity rapidly induces insulin resistance and microvascular dysfunction in healthy volunteers. Arterioscler Thromb Vasc Biol 2007; 27(12):2650–6. Available at: http://www.ncbi.nlm. nih.gov/pubmed/17932315.

74. Morris PE. Moving our critically ill patients: mobility barriers and benefits. Crit Care Clin 2007;23(1):1–20. Available at: http://www.ncbi.nlm.nih.gov/pubmed/ 17307113.

75. Bailey P, Thomsen GE, Spuhler VJ, et al. Early activity is feasible and safe in respiratory failure patients. Crit Care Med 2007;35(1):139–45. Available at: http://www.ncbi.nlm.nih.gov/pubmed/ 17133183.

76. Morris PE, Goad A, Thompson C, et al. Early intensive care unit mobility therapy in the treatment of acute respiratory failure. Crit Care Med 2008; 36(8):2238–43. Available at: http://www.ncbi.nlm. nih.gov/pubmed/18596631.

77. Needham DM, Korupolu R, Zanni JM, et al. Early physical medicine and rehabilitation for patients with acute respiratory failure: a quality improvement project. Arch Phys Med Rehabil 2010;91(4): 536–42. Available at: http://www.ncbi.nlm.nih.gov/ pubmed/20382284.

78. Zeppos L, Patman S, Berney S, et al. Physiotherapy in intensive care is safe: an observational study. Aust J Physiother 2007;53(4):279–83.

79. Thomsen GE, Snow GL, Rodriguez L, et al. Patients with respiratory failure increase ambulation after transfer to an intensive care unit where early activity is a priority. Crit Care Med 2008;36(4):1119–24. Available at: http://www.ncbi.nlm.nih.gov/pubmed/18379236.

80. Needham DM. Mobilizing patients in the intensive care unit: improving neuromuscular weakness and physical function. JAMA 2008;300(14):1685–90. Available at: http://www.ncbi.nlm.nih.gov/pubmed/ 18840842.

81. Perme C, Chandrashekar R. Early mobility and walking program for patients in intensive care units: creating a standard of care. Am J Crit Care 2009; 18(3):212–21. Available at: http://www.ncbi.nlm. nih.gov/pubmed/19234100.

82. Jones C, Skirrow P, Griffiths RD, et al. Rehabilitation after critical illness: a randomized, controlled

trial. Crit Care Med 2003;31(10):2456–61. Available at: http://www.ncbi.nlm.nih.gov/pubmed/14530751.

83. Burtin C, Clerckx B, Robbeets C, et al. Early exercise in critically ill patients enhances short-term functional recovery. Crit Care Med 2009;37(9):2499–505. Available at: http://www.ncbi.nlm.nih.gov/pubmed/19623052.

84. Gibson JN, Smith K, Rennie MJ. Prevention of disuse muscle atrophy by means of electrical stimulation: maintenance of protein synthesis. Lancet 1988;2(8614):767–70.

85. Routsi C, Gerovasili V, Vasileiadis I, et al. Electrical muscle stimulation prevents critical illness polyneuromyopathy: a randomized parallel intervention trial. Crit Care 2010;14(2):R74. Available at: http://www.ncbi.nlm.nih.gov/pubmed/20426834.

86. Maffiuletti NA, Roig M, Karatzanos E, et al. Neuromuscular electrical stimulation for preventing skeletal-muscle weakness and wasting in critically ill patients: a systematic review. BMC Med 2013;11:137. Available at: http://www.ncbi.nlm.nih.gov/pubmed/23701811.

87. Vasilevskis EE, Ely EW, Speroff T, et al. Reducing iatrogenic risks: ICU-acquired delirium and weakness–crossing the quality chasm. Chest 2010;138(5):1224–33. Available at: http://www.ncbi.nlm.nih.gov/pubmed/21051398.

88. Girard TD, Kress JP, Fuchs BD, et al. Efficacy and safety of a paired sedation and ventilator weaning protocol for mechanically ventilated patients in intensive care (Awakening and Breathing Controlled trial): a randomised controlled trial. Lancet 2008;371(9607):126–34. Available at: http://www.ncbi.nlm.nih.gov/pubmed/18191684.

89. Schweickert WD, Pohlman MC, Pohlman AS, et al. Early physical and occupational therapy in mechanically ventilated, critically ill patients: a randomised controlled trial. Lancet 2009;373(9678):1874–82. Available at: http://www.ncbi.nlm.nih.gov/pubmed/19446324.

90. Denehy L, Berney S. Physiotherapy in the intensive care unit. Phys Ther Rev 2006;11(1):49–56.

91. Morris PE, Herridge MS. Early intensive care unit mobility: future directions. Crit Care Clin 2007;23(1):97–110. Available at: http://www.ncbi.nlm.nih.gov/pubmed/17307119.

92. Batt J, Dos Santos CC, Herridge MS. Muscle injury during critical illness. JAMA 2013;310(15):1569–70. Available at: http://www.ncbi.nlm.nih.gov/pubmed/24108459.

93. Varpula T, Valta P, Niemi R, et al. Airway pressure release ventilation as a primary ventilatory mode in acute respiratory distress syndrome. Acta Anaesthesiol Scand 2004;48(6):722–31.

94. Putensen C, Zech S, Wrigge H, et al. Long-term effects of spontaneous breathing during ventilatory support in patients with acute lung injury. Am J Respir Crit Care Med 2001;164(1):43–9.

95. Cordioli RL, Akoumianaki E, Brochard L. Nonconventional ventilation techniques. Curr Opin Crit Care 2013;19(1):31–7. Available at: http://www.ncbi.nlm.nih.gov/pubmed/23235544.

96. Tuchscherer D, Z'Graggen WJ, Passath C, et al. Neurally adjusted ventilatory assist in patients with critical illness-associated polyneuromyopathy. Intensive Care Med 2011;37(12):1951–61. Available at: http://www.ncbi.nlm.nih.gov/pubmed/22048718.

97. Martin AD, Smith BK, Davenport PD, et al. Inspiratory muscle strength training improves weaning outcome in failure to wean patients: a randomized trial. Crit Care 2011;15(2):R84. Available at: http://www.ncbi.nlm.nih.gov/pubmed/21385346.

98. Condessa RL, Brauner JS, Saul AL, et al. Inspiratory muscle training did not accelerate weaning from mechanical ventilation but did improve tidal volume and maximal respiratory pressures: a randomised trial. J Physiol 2013;59(2):101–7.

99. Krzak A, Pleva M, Napolitano LM. Nutrition therapy for ALI and ARDS. Crit Care Clin 2011;27(3):647–59. Available at: http://www.ncbi.nlm.nih.gov/pubmed/21742221.

100. Villet S, Chiolero RL, Bollmann MD, et al. Negative impact of hypocaloric feeding and energy balance on clinical outcome in ICU patients. Clin Nutr 2005;24(4):502–9. Available at: http://www.ncbi.nlm.nih.gov/pubmed/15899538.

101. Martindale RG, McClave SA, Vanek VW, et al. Guidelines for the provision and assessment of nutrition support therapy in the adult critically ill patient: Society of Critical Care Medicine and American Society for Parenteral and Enteral Nutrition: Executive Summary. Crit Care Med 2009;37(5):1757–61. Available at: http://www.ncbi.nlm.nih.gov/pubmed/19373044.

102. Singer P, Berger MM, Van den Berghe G, et al. ESPEN guidelines on parenteral nutrition: intensive care. Clin Nutr 2009;28(4):387–400. Available at: http://www.ncbi.nlm.nih.gov/pubmed/19505748.

103. Ibrahim EH, Mehringer L, Prentice D, et al. Early versus late enteral feeding of mechanically ventilated patients: results of a clinical trial. JPEN J Parenter Enteral Nutr 2002;26(3):174–81. Available at: http://www.ncbi.nlm.nih.gov/pubmed/12005458.

104. Casaer MP, Mesotten D, Hermans G, et al. Early versus late parenteral nutrition in critically ill adults. N Engl J Med 2011;365(6):506–17. Available at: http://www.ncbi.nlm.nih.gov/pubmed/21714640.

105. Hermans G, Casaer MP, Clerckx B, et al. Effect of tolerating macronutrient deficit on the development of intensive-care unit acquired weakness: a subanalysis of the EPaNIC trial. Lancet Respir Med 2013;1(8):621–9.

106. National Heart, Lung, and Blood Institute Acute Respiratory Distress Syndrome (ARDS) Clinical Trials Network, Rice TW, Wheeler AP, Thompson BT, Steingrub J, et al. Initial trophic vs full enteral feeding in patients with acute lung injury: the EDEN randomized trial. JAMA 2012;307(8):795–803. Available at: http://www.ncbi.nlm.nih.gov/pubmed/22307571.

107. Needham DM, Dinglas VD, Morris PE, et al. Physical and cognitive performance of patients with acute lung injury 1 year after initial trophic versus full enteral feeding. EDEN trial follow-up. Am J Respir Crit Care Med 2013;188(5):567–76. Available at: http://www.ncbi.nlm.nih.gov/pubmed/23805899.

108. Heidegger CP, Berger MM, Graf S, et al. Optimisation of energy provision with supplemental parenteral nutrition in critically ill patients: a randomised controlled clinical trial. Lancet 2013;381(9864): 385–93. Available at: http://www.ncbi.nlm.nih.gov/pubmed/23218813.

109. Takala J, Ruokonen E, Webster NR, et al. Increased mortality associated with growth hormone treatment in critically ill adults. N Engl J Med 1999; 341(11):785–92.

110. McClung JM, Davis JM, Wilson MA, et al. Estrogen status and skeletal muscle recovery from disuse atrophy. J Appl Physiol (1985) 2006;100(6):2012–23. Available at: http://www.ncbi.nlm.nih.gov/pubmed/16497837.

111. Mukai R, Horikawa H, Fujikura Y, et al. Prevention of disuse muscle atrophy by dietary ingestion of 8-prenylnaringenin in denervated mice. PLoS One 2012;7(9):e45048. Available at: http://www.ncbi.nlm.nih.gov/pubmed/23028754.

112. Goncalves DA, Silveira WA, Lira EC, et al. Clenbuterol suppresses proteasomal and lysosomal proteolysis and atrophy-related genes in denervated rat soleus muscles independently of Akt. Am J Physiol Endocrinol Metab 2012;302(1):E123–33. Available at: http://www.ncbi.nlm.nih.gov/pubmed/21952035.

113. Kline WO, Panaro FJ, Yang H, et al. Rapamycin inhibits the growth and muscle-sparing effects of clenbuterol. J Appl Physiol (1985) 2007;102(2): 740–7. Available at: http://www.ncbi.nlm.nih.gov/pubmed/17068216.

114. Ryall JG, Lynch GS. The potential and the pitfalls of beta-adrenoceptor agonists for the management of skeletal muscle wasting. Pharmacol Ther 2008; 120(3):219–32. Available at: http://www.ncbi.nlm.nih.gov/pubmed/18834902.

115. Sandri M. Protein breakdown in muscle wasting: role of autophagy-lysosome and ubiquitin-proteasome. Int J Biochem Cell Biol 2013;45(10):2121–9. Available at: http://www.ncbi.nlm.nih.gov/pubmed/23665154.

116. Supinski GS, Vanags J, Callahan LA. Effect of proteasome inhibitors on endotoxin-induced diaphragm dysfunction. Am J Physiol Lung Cell Mol Physiol 2009;296(6):L994–1001. Available at: http://www.ncbi.nlm.nih.gov/pubmed/19376888.

117. Park JW, Kim KM, Oh KJ, et al. Proteasome inhibition promotes functional recovery after peripheral nerve reperfusion injury. J Trauma 2009;66(3): 743–8. Available at: http://www.ncbi.nlm.nih.gov/pubmed/19276748.

118. Agten A, Maes K, Thomas D, et al. Bortezomib partially protects the rat diaphragm from ventilator-induced diaphragm dysfunction. Crit Care Med 2012;40(8):2449–55. Available at: http://www.ncbi.nlm.nih.gov/pubmed/22809912.

119. Xiao Y, Yin J, Wei J, et al. Incidence and risk of cardiotoxicity associated with bortezomib in the treatment of cancer: a systematic review and meta-analysis. PLoS One 2014;9(1):e87671. Available at: http://www.ncbi.nlm.nih.gov/pubmed/24489948.

120. Malkoc M, Karadibak D, Yildirim Y. The effect of physiotherapy on ventilatory dependency and the length of stay in an intensive care unit. Int J Rehabil Res 2009;32(1):85–8. Available at: http://www.ncbi.nlm.nih.gov/pubmed/19011583.

Index

Note: Page numbers of article titles are in **boldface** type.

A

Abuse
  alcohol
    ARDS related to, 625–629
Acute lung injury (ALI)
  early. *See* Early acute lung injury (EALI)
Acute respiratory distress syndrome (ARDS)
  acute
    steroids for, **781–795**. *See also* Steroid(s), for
      ARDS
  approach to patient with, **685–696**
    diagnosis, 688–691
    identifying patients at risk, 686–688
    introduction, 685–686
    patient evaluation, 691–693
  beyond single-nucleotide polymorphisms in,
    673–684
  consensus criteria on
    limitations of, 609–611
  defined, 729–730
  diagnosis of, 688–691
    EALI, 689–690
  direct *vs.* indirect
    clinical differences, 640–644
      pathologic findings, 640–641
      patient outcomes, 644
      radiographic appearance, 641
      respiratory mechanics, 641–642
      response to treatment, 643–644
      risk factors–related, 643
    experimental models of, 644–645
  disruption of alveolar-capillary barrier in, 797–798
  early
    treatment of
      steroids in
        clinical trials of, 783–785
  early mobilization in, **811–826**
    pharmacologic strategies as adjuncts to,
      820–821
  environmental risk factors for, **625–637**. *See also*
    Environment, in ARDS
  epidemiology of, 611–618
    evolving, **609–624**
    introduction, 609
  evaluation of, 691–693
  evolution of, 609–611
  experimental
    pathogenetic mechanisms of, 644–649
      disruption of alveolar-capillary barrier, 646

histologic injury, 645–646
inflammation, 646–648
markers of epithelial or endothelial
  injury, 645
physiologic dysfunction, 648
therapeutic responses, 648–649
genomics in, **673–684**. *See also* Genomics, in
  ARDS
heterogeneity in
  clinical and biological, **639–653**
  introduction, 639–640
ICU–acquired weakness in, **811–826**. *See also*
  Intensive care unit (ICU)–acquired weakness,
  in ARDS
immunosuppressed patients with
  HIV–infected patients, 703–707. *See also*
    Human immunodeficiency virus (HIV)
    infection, ARDS in
  invasive diagnostic strategies in, **697–712**
    fiber-optic bronchoscopy
      complications of, 706
    HSCT, 701–703. *See also* Hematopoietic
      stem cell transplantation (HSCT),
      ARDS in
    non–HIV, non–organ transplant
      populations, 699–700
    open lung biopsy, 707
  solid-organ transplant recipients, 697–699.
    See also Solid-organ transplant recipients,
    ARDS in
incidence of, 611–615
inflammatory response in
  obesity effects on, 659–660
late
  treatment of
    steroids in
      clinical trials of, 785–789
mimickers of, 692
mortality data, 617–618
muscle wasting in, **811–826**. *See also* Intensive
  care unit (ICU)–acquired weakness, in ARDS
neuromuscular blocking agents in, **753–763**. *See*
  also Neuromuscular blocking agents, in ARDS
nutrient deficiency in, 820
nutrition in, **662–667**. *See also* Nutrition, in ARDS
obesity in, **655–662**. *See also* Obesity, in ARDS
pathogenesis of
  obesity and, 658–659
pathophysiology of

http://dx.doi.org/10.1016/S0272-5231(14)00095-1
0272-5231/14/$ – see front matter © 2014 Elsevier Inc. All rights reserved.

United States Postal Service

Statement of Ownership, Management, and Circulation
(All Periodicals Publications Except Requestor Publications)

1. Publication Title	2. Publication Number	3. Filing Date
Clinics in Chest Medicine	0 0 0 - 7 0 6	9/14/14

4. Issue Frequency	5. Number of Issues Published Annually	6. Annual Subscription Price
Mar, Jun, Sep, Dec	4	$345.00

7. Complete Mailing Address of Known Office of Publication (Not printer) (Street, city, county, state, and ZIP+4®)

Elsevier Inc.
360 Park Avenue South
New York, NY 10010-1710

Contact Person: Stephen R. Bushing
Telephone (Include area code): 215-239-3688

8. Complete Mailing Address of Headquarters or General Business Office of Publisher (Not printer)

Elsevier Inc., 360 Park Avenue South, New York, NY 10010-171■

9. Full Names and Complete Mailing Addresses of Publisher, Editor, and Managing Editor (Do not leave blank)

Publisher (Name and complete mailing address)

Linda Belfus, Elsevier Inc., 1600 John F. Kennedy Blvd., Suite 1800, Philadelphia, PA 19103-2899

Editor (Name and complete mailing address)

Patrick Manley, Elsevier Inc., 1600 John F. Kennedy Blvd., Suite 1800, Philadelphia, PA 19103-2899

Managing Editor (Name and complete mailing address)

Adrianne Brigido, Elsevier Inc., 1600 John F. Kennedy Blvd., Suite 1800, Philadelphia, PA 19103-2899

10. Owner (Do not leave blank. If the publication is owned by a corporation, give the name and address of the corporation immediately followed by the names and addresses of all stockholders owning or holding 1 percent or more of the total amount of stock. If not owned by a corporation, give the names and addresses of the individual owners. If owned by a partnership or other unincorporated firm, give its name and address as well as those of each individual owner. If the publication is published by a nonprofit organization, give its name and address.)

Full Name	Complete Mailing Address
Wholly owned subsidiary of	1600 John F. Kennedy Blvd., Ste. 1800
Reed/Elsevier, US holdings	Philadelphia, PA 19103-2899

11. Known Bondholders, Mortgagees, and Other Security Holders Owning or Holding 1 Percent or More of Total Amount of Bonds, Mortgages, or Other Securities. If none, check box ▶ None

Full Name	Complete Mailing Address
N/A	

12. Tax Status (For completion by nonprofit organizations authorized to mail at nonprofit rates) (Check one)
The purpose, function, and nonprofit status of this organization and the exempt status for federal income tax purposes:
- [ ] Has Not Changed During Preceding 12 Months
- [ ] Has Changed During Preceding 12 Months (Publisher must submit explanation of change with this statement)

PS Form **3526**, August 2012 (Page 1 of 3 (Instructions Page 3)) PSN 7530-01-000-993 **PRIVACY NOTICE:** See our privacy policy in www.usps.com

---

13. Publication Title	14. Issue Date for Circulation Data Below
Clinics in Chest Medicine	June 2014

15. Extent and Nature of Circulation			Average No. Copies Each Issue During Preceding 12 Months	No. Copies of Single Issue Published Nearest to Filing Date
a. Total Number of Copies (Net press run)			729	724
b. Paid Circulation (By Mail and Outside the Mail)	(1)	Mailed Outside-County Paid Subscriptions Stated on PS Form 3541. (Include paid distribution above nominal rate, advertiser's proof copies, and exchange copies)		
	(2)	Mailed In-County Paid Subscriptions Stated on PS Form 3541 (Include paid distribution above nominal rate, advertiser's proof copies, and exchange copies)		
	(3)	Paid Distribution Outside the Mails Including Sales Through Dealers and Carriers, Street Vendors, Counter Sales, and Other Paid Distribution Outside USPS®	218	192
	(4)	Paid Distribution by Other Classes Mailed Through the USPS (e.g. First-Class Mail®)		
c. Total Paid Distribution (Sum of 15b (1), (2), (3), and (4))		▶	947	916
d. Free or Nominal Rate Distribution (By Mail and Outside the Mail)	(1)	Free or Nominal Rate Outside-County Copies Included on PS Form 3541	63	74
	(2)	Free or Nominal Rate In-County Copies Included on PS Form 3541		
	(3)	Free or Nominal Rate Copies Mailed at Other Classes Through the USPS (e.g. First-Class Mail)		
	(4)	Free or Nominal Rate Distribution Outside the Mail (Carriers or other means)		
e. Total Free or Nominal Rate Distribution (Sum of 15d (1), (2), (3) and (4))		▶	63	74
f. Total Distribution (Sum of 15c and 15e)		▶	1,010	990
g. Copies not Distributed (See instructions to publishers #4 (page #3))		▶	207	225
h. Total (Sum of 15f and g)		▶	1,217	1,215
i. Percent Paid (15c divided by 15f times 100)		▶	93.76%	92.53%

16. Total circulation includes electronic copies. Report circulation on PS Form 3526-X worksheet.

17. Publication of Statement of Ownership
If the publication is a general publication, publication of this statement is required. Will be printed in the December 2014 issue of this publication.

18. Signature and Title of Editor, Publisher, Business Manager, or Owner	Date
Stephen R. Bushing Stephen R. Bushing – Inventory Distribution Coordinator	September 14, 2014

I certify that all information furnished on this form is true and complete. I understand that anyone who furnishes false or misleading information on this form or who omits material or information requested on the form may be subject to criminal sanctions (including fines and imprisonment) and/or civil sanctions (including civil penalties).

PS Form **3526**, August 2012 (Page 2 of 3)

Moving?

Make sure your subscription moves with you!

To notify us of your new address, find your **Clinics Account Number** (located on your mailing label above your name), and contact customer service at:

Email: journalscustomerservice-usa@elsevier.com

800-654-2452 (subscribers in the U.S. & Canada)
314-447-8871 (subscribers outside of the U.S. & Canada)

Fax number: 314-447-8029

Elsevier Health Sciences Division
Subscription Customer Service
3251 Riverport Lane
Maryland Heights, MO 63043